PAIN IN CHILDREN AND ADOLESCENTS

Pain Research and Clinical Management

Volume 1

P.D. Wall, *London, U.K.* — Chairman

M.J. Cousins, *Adelaide, Australia*	Anesthesiology
H.L. Fields, *San Francisco, CA, U.S.A.*	Neurology and Neurophysiology
K.M. Foley, *New York, NY, U.S.A.*	Cancer
R.H. Gracely, *Bethesda, MD, U.S.A.*	Psychology
P.J. McGrath, *Ottawa, Ontario, Canada*	Pediatrics
H. Merskey, *London, Ontario, Canada*	Psychiatry
B.A. Meyerson, *Stockholm, Sweden*	Neurosurgery
J. Olesen, *Hellerup, Denmark*	Headache
E. Spangfort, *Huddinge, Sweden*	Orthopedic surgery
T.L. Yaksh, *Rochester, MN, U.S.A.*	Pharmacology

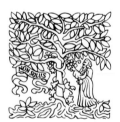

ELSEVIER

AMSTERDAM · NEW YORK · OXFORD

Pain in Children and Adolescents

PATRICK J. McGRATH, Ph.D.

Senior Psychologist (Behavior Program), Career Scientist, Children's Hospital of Eastern Ontario, Adjunct Professor of Psychology and Pediatrics, University of Ottawa, Adjunct Professor of Psychology, Carleton University, Ottawa, Canada

and

ANITA M. UNRUH B.Sc. O.T., M.S.W.

Social Worker, Children's Hospital of Eastern Ontario, and Ottawa Children's Treatment Centre, Ottawa, Canada

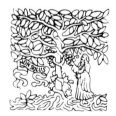

1987

ELSEVIER

AMSTERDAM · NEW YORK · OXFORD

ISBN volume: 0-444-80899-X (hardback)
ISBN volume: 0-444-80921-X (paperback)
ISSN series: 0921-3287

Published by:

Elsevier Science Publishers B.V. (Biomedical Division)
P.O. Box 211
1000 AE Amsterdam
The Netherlands

Sole distributors for the USA and Canada:
Elsevier Science Publishing Company, Inc.
52 Vanderbilt Avenue
New York, NY 10017
USA

Printed in The Netherlands

Contents

Foreword

Anyone who has watched a child suffer severe pain, whether due to minor diseases or major ones such as cancer, feels anguish and a sense of helplessness. Children seem so innocent and vulnerable that it 'hurts' to watch a child suffer. We like to think that the health professionals who look after children are doing everything they can to prevent pain or to relieve it as much as possible. It comes as a terrible shock, then, to find out that our ideas about pain in children are dominated by the myth that children do not feel pain as intensely as adults and therefore require fewer analgesics or none at all. In one study, more than 50% of children who underwent major surgery – including limb amputation, excision of a cancerous neck mass, and heart surgery – were not given any analgesics, and the remainder received woefully inadequate doses. These kinds of outrageous statistics are found in virtually every study that examines the treatment of severe pain in children. Adolescents, who are the butt of another myth – that they will rapidly become drug addicts if they are given narcotic drugs for severe pain – do not fare much better.

Few topics are more worthy of study than pain in children and adolescents, and it is deeply gratifying that Patrick McGrath (a clinical psychologist) and Anita Unruh (trained in both social work and occupational therapy) have written a superb book that does justice to the challenge of the problems they deal with.

Despite the serious, heart-wrenching problems they deal with, McGrath and Unruh have not written a depressing book. Instead, they have presented us with an exciting review of the whole field, full of fascinating information, that will inevitably lead to the better care of children and adolescents in pain. Absurd myths are laid to rest by the force of the excellent data and compelling arguments in favor of more rational, sensible medication and other treatments for the wide variety of pains in young people.

The scholarly introductory chapter, which covers attitudes to pain in children from the earliest records of ancient Egypt and Babylon through the millennia to the present time, inevitably delights the reader. Who can fail to be intrigued and amused by this 3500-year-old Egyptian recipe to placate a crying child: ' ... capsules of the poppy plant; excrement of wasps on the wall; rub together; strain and administer for four days running'? Not all early remedies were so benign; some required near strangulation of the child to produce unconsciousness.

McGrath and Unruh deal with all the major problems of pain encountered in young people. They review the physiological mechanisms of pain as well as the latest techniques that have evolved to measure pain in babies with no language and older children with very little – certainly much less than the adult. Each stage in development is a challenge, and new measurement techniques are evolving for them all. They are described with pros and cons clearly listed and evaluated.

All the different kinds of pain are treated in individual chapters and there is the clear stamp of the authors' wisdom and rich experience on their evaluation of our understanding of the causes of pain and the relative merits of different ways of treating them. The ethical problems inherent in the health care of children and adolescents in pain, and the best way to deliver such care and to pursue research in this rich field round out this outstanding book.

McGrath and Unruh have performed a valuable service by dealing with one of the major problems in the field of pain: how to understand, assess and deal adequately with severe pain in people who are too young to describe their pain and whose complaints are too easily ignored by attributing the cries and screams to other causes. The book covers a broad field and does it so interestingly and competently that readers in all disciplines are certain to benefit. Most important of all, this book will inevitably lead to less suffering in young people – and for this we can all be grateful. It will not happen overnight. It is a goal we must all strive for, and this book will play an important role in the revolution that is in the making.

RONALD MELZACK
McGill University
Montreal, Canada

Preface

'Pain in Children and Adolescents' comprehensively summarizes and integrates the literature in an area that has until very recently been largely neglected. There have been a number of monographs that have examined specific aspects of pediatric pain such as Barlow's (1984) excellent volume on headache, Hilgard and LeBaron's (1984) clinical treatise on hypnosis and pediatric cancer pain, and Apley's (1975) classic on recurrent abdominal pain. Schechter's (1985) outstanding monograph in the Current Problems in Pediatrics series filled a void, but its brevity (67 pages) precluded extensive treatment of any one topic.

Our clinical interest in pain in children has led to a broad-based applied research program which has attempted to elucidate the mechanisms, measurement and alleviation of clinical pain in children. Our patients have taught us to repeatedly reassess each of our hypotheses. The constant interplay between our clinical efforts and our research has not always been comfortable but it has been revealing. The collaboration between us began clinically and has developed into research endeavors.

This volume focusses on pain and pain problems. It does not attempt to extensively review literature on established medical or surgical problems. For example, discussion of the management of the acute abdomen, pathological headache and cancer is very limited. On the other hand, coverage of recurrent abdominal pain, migraine, and pain in pediatric cancer is extensive.

'Pain in Children and Adolescents' is written from the multidisciplinary approach that we have found to be most productive in both our research and in our clinical practice.

We believe that 'Pain in Children and Adolescents' will be of value to all children's health care workers including nurses, physicians and surgeons, social workers, psychologists, occupational therapists and physiotherapists.

Acknowledgements

This book and the research program upon which it is based is the result of the support of many individuals. Dr. J.T. Goodman, Director of Psychology at the Children's Hospital of Eastern Ontario, has freely given encouragement, confidence and wisdom to both of us. Gloria Roseman, Director of Occupational Therapy, and Beth Allan, Director of Social Services, gave enthusiastic support to our research and the writing of this book. Dr. W. Feldman has been a most stimulating collaborator and guide. Dr. Peter Humphreys has been an outstanding co-researcher and supporter in our research. Dr. Ron Barr has always been a most generous and warm friend and colleague. Dr. Toby Gelfand kindly provided critical review and helpful suggestions for the historical chapter. Drs. Mary Ellen Jeans, Judy Beyer, Celeste Johnston, Neil Schechter, Janel Gauthier, Sue Pisterman, Ian Manion, Ray Brunette, Frank Andrasik, Bonnie Stevens, Maria Fitzgerald, Leora Kuttner, Dorthea Ross, Ruth Grunau, Ken Craig and Patricia A. McGrath (who is not related to P.M.) have provided help and encouragement. June Cunningham has been our critic, editor, co-researcher and friend. For 5 years, June ran the day-to-day operation of the psychology research lab. She is responsible for the success of much of our research. Our numerous co-investigators at the Children's Hospital of Eastern Ontario, whom we have not already mentioned, include Drs. Dan Keene and Pierre Jacob, Neurology; Dr. Dick Shipman, Gastro-enterology; Dr. Garry Johnson, Anesthesia; Dr. John Schillinger, Urology; Dr. John Latter, Physiatry; Drs. Jacques D'Astous and Maureen Finnegan, Orthopedy; Drs. Elizabeth Hsu, Brian Luke and Emmanuel Katsanis, Oncology; Dr. Arly Dungy, Dentistry; Carolanne Vair, Jane Goodman and Dr. Denise Alcock, Nursing; and Lorraine Hendry, Physiotherapy. All have been a source of stimulation over the years. We have been blessed with outstanding research secretaries who rescued grants and straightened out our difficulties with patience, competence and enthusiasm. Julie Bishop and Sue Nigra have served their time well. Julie L'Heureux is now our research secretary and was most helpful in the preparation of this volume.

Of course numerous research assistants and graduate students have done most of the work and in the process have become friends and colleagues. We wish to thank: Maureen Lascelles, Mario Cappelli, Helene Martire, Mary-Pat Conklin, Jennifer Dunn-Geier, Maryann Inkster, Libby Bartoli, Michelle Lavoie, Sally Skene, Nadia Kurylyszyn, Iris Richter, Diane Claude, Joanne Chapman, Karen Davies, Muriel O'Hara, Madeleine Guilbert, Robert Schnurr, Lise Erdody, Elvera Unruh, Mary Jean McGrath, Caroline Heick, Barb Nolan, Estelle Couvrier and Amanda George.

The generous financial support of the following agencies have allowed us to pursue our research interests in pediatric pain:
– Ontario Ministry of Health
– Hospital for Sick Children's Foundation
– Ontario Mental Health Foundation
– National Health and Welfare (Canada)
– Children's Hospital of Eastern Ontario Foundation
– Ontario Ministry of Community and Social Services
– Pickering Fund
– Carleton University
– University of Ottawa

The Kiwanis Medical Foundation provided a grant that has made the writing of this book much less onerous. P.M. is supported by a Career Scientist Award of the Ontario Ministry of Health. The Children's Hospital of Eastern Ontario (CHEO) has provided a warm and supportive atmosphere in which to pursue our research and writing. We are exceedingly grateful to have been fortunate enough to work at CHEO, having found that all who work at the Children's share an enthusiasm for their work and a commitment to our children. The library at CHEO epitomizes the spirit of cooperation and collaborative inquiry that is the hallmark of the institution. The library staff (Margaret Taylor, Director) have always been very helpful. We also wish to thank the Media Services Department (Eric Bawden, Director) who have provided graphics support. All royalties from this edition will be donated to the CHEO Foundation.

Dr. Nello Spiteri of Elsevier stimulated, encouraged and prodded in the best tradition of a scientific editor.

We would like to thank our parents and dedicate this book to them: Matt and Jean McGrath and Henry and Mary Unruh who gave us the vision of helping those in pain and pursuing knowledge. Unfortunately, Henry died before this book was finished.

Finally, we would like to thank our patients who have suffered their pain, shown us our mistakes and allowed us to share in their successes.

We remain responsible for any errors or omissions that remain in the volume.

PATRICK MCGRATH
ANITA UNRUH
Ottawa, January 1987

About the authors

Dr. McGrath is a clinical psychologist who graduated from Queen's University in Kingston, Ontario. His major research interests are in pediatric pain, chronic illness in children, and childhood behavior disorders. Dr. McGrath is a Senior Psychologist (Behavior Program) at the Children's Hospital of Eastern Ontario, an Adjunct Professor of Psychology and Pediatrics at the University of Ottawa and Adjunct Professor of Psychology at Carleton University. Dr. McGrath is supported by a Career Scientist Award of the Ontario Ministry of Health.

Ms. Unruh is a social worker and an occupational therapist. She received her O.T. training at the University of Western Ontario in London, Ontario, and her social work degree at Carleton University in Ottawa. Her research interests are in pain in children, social behavior of physically handicapped children and psychological impact of infertility. Ms. Unruh is a social worker at the Ottawa Children's Treatment Centre and at the Children's Hospital of Eastern Ontario.

CHAPTER 1

The history of pain in childhood

With the inborn craving of mankind to know the reason why, the mother sought around for the cause of her child's suffering; sometimes it was obvious in some ill effect of strange food, some bodily wound or injury by man or beast, but more often it was mysterious, some strange effect of the elements, some influence of evil spirits, or spells cast upon him by some enemy or the fascination of an evil eye, and remedies were sought in propitiation of an offended deity, or in charm or incantation; and, as time went on, cause and remedy gathered weight from tradition. Very early also the effects, supposed or real, of herbs had become part of the family lore, and the mother had her simple remedy, gathered from woodland or field for childish ailments *(Still, 1931, p. xvii)*.

1. Introduction

Children experience pain from a number of sources but the two most frequent are pain from injury or disease and pain from childrearing practices. For this reason, historical accounts of pain in childhood encompass two broad historical discussions, that of pediatric medicine and that of childhood itself.

Historians of pediatric medicine (Garrison, 1923; Still, 1931) noted that children in the past were victims of many serious and often fatal illnesses as well as minor complaints, which, poorly treated, became life threatening. Pediatrics developed quite late in the history of medicine, a phenomenon which is often attributed to the indifference felt towards pain and disease in infants and children and the lack of recognition that childhood was a separate state from adulthood (Garrison, 1923; Aries, 1962; DeMause, 1974). Other historians have maintained that the late emergence of pediatrics is in part due to the difficulty in obtaining enough information from children about their pain and discomfort to identify diseases (Garrison, 1923).

Historians of childhood (Payne, 1916; Aries, 1962; Despert, 1965; De-Mause, 1974; Shorter, 1975; Stone, 1977) described a grim picture of childhood. They maintained that children were commonly subjected to harsh and frequently brutal methods of childrearing. Indeed many historians of childhood would agree with DeMause when he wrote:

> The further back in history one goes, the lower the level of child care, and the more likely children are to be killed, abandoned, beaten, terrorized, and sexually abused *(DeMause, 1974, p. 1)*.

However, in our opinion, there is substantial evidence from those who wrote about the medical care of children and provided advice about childrearing, that people in past centuries were also compassionate and caring in their interactions with children. Certainly, historical pediatric writings did recognize that there was a separate state of childhood with unique developmental needs, even though there would seem to have been a constant struggle with the difficulty of measuring and assessing pain and disease in children. Unfortunately, the controversy of what was the reality of childrearing in previous centuries is likely to remain unresolved. Without primary documentation, such as the diaries and autobiographies of parents and children, historical analyses are primarily hypotheses about the experience of pain by children in previous centuries.

Our objective in this chapter is to present an overview of the history of pain in childhood limiting our discussion primarily to medical writings. We will only incidentally be addressing the broader issues of social history. We will begin with the evolution of a concept of pain because prevailing beliefs about pain greatly influence the way in which pain is managed with adults and children. Secondly, we will review historical accounts of pain symptomatology and treatment in childhood. We will see that the common problems of crying, teething and colic have been the concern of parents and physicians for some time. Finally, we will examine the role of pain in childrearing practices.

2. *The evolution of a concept of pain and disease*

> Pain has seized my body. May God tear this pain out (a prayer from a king's daughter in Babylon written on a clay tablet *(quoted in Fulop-Miller, 1938, p. 2)*.

> The wicked man travaileth with pain all his days *(Job 5:17)*.

2.1. *Ancient civilizations*

All ancient civilizations have reflected a global belief in the power of supernatural entities to cause, maintain, and cure pain and disease in accordance with the spiritual goodness or evil of an individual, although these beliefs may have differed in their form. Painful diseases were commonly believed to be caused by personal sin and transgression against the gods for which the individual would be punished by demonic intrusion into the body. Intrusion occurred when objects such as swords, arrows and spears pierced the skin (Procacci and Maresca, 1984). Ancient Egyptians and Assyro-Babylonians believed that vomiting, sneezing, urinating, and sweating were routes for intruding demons to exit from the body (Procacci and Maresca, 1984). In Babylon, it was believed that pain in a specific locality indicated that a demon was eating that part of the body (Garrison, 1923).

Integral to the belief about causation of pain was a hypothesis of where pain was experienced (Sigerist, 1932; Keele, 1962; Procacci and Maresca, 1984). For example, Egyptians believed that the heart was the center of all pain sensation. Two Alexandrians, Herophilus (335–280 B.C.) and Erasistratus (310–250 B.C.) eventually provided evidence that the brain was part of the nervous system with connecting nerves related to movement and sensation (Procacci and Maresca, 1984).

Interference with the authority of the supernatural over pain and disease through the use of human medicine was viewed by many people with varying degrees of suspicion and fear. For example, ancient Judaism sought to suppress animistic concepts or belief in malignant demons by complex regulations and hygienic laws (Castiglioni, 1975). Jewish doctrine maintained that people who called on other gods for healing were severely punished by the one God. Priests were the only people believed to be able to carry out divine will through medical function (Castiglioni, 1975). Such medical function was concerned with physical health only because physical purity was equal to moral purity.

Since most ancient civilizations believed that gods and demons caused pain and disease and that gods had healing powers, treatments relied on convincing the gods through incantations, religious rites, sacrificial offerings, prayer or exorcism of demons (Castiglioni, 1975). In the search to placate deities, religious rituals and herbal remedies were instituted which occasionally had a secondary effect of reducing pain and preventing disease.

2.2. Ancient Greece and Rome

By the 5th and 4th centuries B.C., the ancient Greeks had become increasingly more concerned with the physiology of pain rather than its religious significance (Procacci and Maresca, 1984). There was an enthusiastic debate over whether the heart or the brain was the center of all sensation. Alcmaeon (who was a disciple of Pythagoras, 566–497 B.C.) and Anaxcgoras (500–428 B.C.) argued that the brain was the center of all sensation including pain (Keele, 1962; Procacci and Maresca, 1984).

Plato (about 400 B.C.) adhered to the more ancient beliefs that pain was caused by an external event or intrusion into the body. Both pain and pleasure were the result of an interaction of earth, fire, air and water, with the soul housed in the body. Plato believed that at the beginning of life all these interactions were especially violent so that for an infant all feeling was essentially painful (Keele, 1962).

Aristotle (384–322 B.C.) believed that the heart was the source of all sensation. Pain was not thought to be one of the sensations (sight, smell, hearing, taste and touch). Instead Aristotle believed that pain was produced by interactions between the organ of touch (flesh) and factors in the heart. An increased sensitivity to touch due to the hardness or softness, warmth or coldness of the heart and the contents of the blood resulted in feelings of pain (Keele, 1962). Aristotle also described what would now be considered psychogenic pain. He believed that the idea of a painful experience combined with a minor sensory event could result in an actual physically painful experience (Keele, 1962).

In Rome, there was also a greater concern with the natural or physical causes of pain and with understanding how pain was experienced in the body. Galen (130–200 A.D.), who was a Greek physician working in Rome, referred to the ancient beliefs in which gods were perceived as the source of pain and disease. His comments exemplified the changing beliefs about the causation of pain:

> Just as agriculture promises nourishment to healthy bodies, so does the art of medicine promise health to the sick. Nowhere is this art lacking, for the most uncivilized nations have knowledge of herbs, and other things to hand for the aiding of wounds and diseases... Diseases were (in olden times) ascribed to the anger of the immortal gods, and from them help used to be sought; and it is probable that with no aids against bad health, nonetheless health was generally good because of good habits, which neither indolence nor luxury had vitiated; since it is these two which have afflicted the bodies of men, first in Greece and later among us... *(quoted in Lewis and Reinhold, 1966, p. 311).*

Galen studied extensively the central and peripheral nervous systems. He classified nerves into three groups. There were nerves for sensory function which Galen referred to as soft nerves and nerves for motor function described as hard nerves. A third group of nerves relayed pain messages. Galen believed that the brain was the center of sensibility (Procacci and Maresca, 1984).

Despite the work of Herophilus (335–280 B.C.) and Erasistratus (310–250 B.C.), who identified the brain and nerves of movement and of sensation, and Galen (130–200 A.D.), who expanded their work, Aristotle's argument that pain originated in the heart was the prevailing theory for 23 centuries (Procacci and Maresca, 1984).

2.3. The Middle Ages

After the decline of the Roman empire in the 5th century A.D. (Caton, 1985), Christianity strongly influenced beliefs about pain and disease possibly because it offered new hope for pain relief through the intercession of God at a time of high mortality (Cartwright, 1977). The Christian church was very clear about the causation of pain and disease and about the church's role as healer. As Christian influence became more pronounced, belief in pain and disease occurring from natural sources was increasingly repressed and exchanged for the belief that pain and disease originated with the wrath of God. For example, St. Augustine (5th century A.D.) made the following declaration:

> All diseases of Christians are to be ascribed to demons, chiefly do they torment the fresh baptized, yea even the guiltless newborn infant *(quoted in Haggard, 1929, p. 298)*.

The early Christian church combined its teachings with some ancient Roman beliefs, constructing Roman gods into Christian saints (Cartwright, 1977). For example, the Roman goddess of fever, Febris, was now known as Saint Febronia. The physician had little power since all cures were believed to be miraculous and there were religious proscriptions against some pain-relieving drugs (Todd, 1985). Until the Renaissance, monastic medicine prevailed and the primary medical contribution was the preservation of ancient Greek writings and the expansion of pharmacology (Cartwright, 1977).

2.4. The Arab World

Arabic medicine, which was not influenced by Christianity, flourished during the Middle Ages. In 529 A.D., when the Greek Academy was closed for what were now considered pagan teachings by the Christian world, its scholars fled to Persia. With them they brought priceless medical works from Greece which were translated from the original Greek and Latin into Syriac and Hebrew and later into Arabic (Todd, 1985). The influence of the Greek and Roman physicians is evident in the writings of the Arabic physicians.

A detailed discussion of the nature of pain was elaborated by Avicenna, an Arabic physician from 980 to 1036 A.D. Avicenna based his explanations about pain on his theory of the four temperaments: heat, cold, dryness, and moistness (Gruner, 1930). He believed that Allah had made the human body according to these four temperaments and that each organ or limb had a specific temperament which was most optimal for its function. Avicenna then reasoned that pain was caused by a sudden change in the temperament of the organ or limb. In fact, Avicenna described 15 different types of pain: boring, compressing, corrosive, dull, fatigue pain, heavy pain, incisive, irritant, itching, pricking, relaxing, stabbing, tearing, tension, and throbbing (Gruner, 1930). Avicenna believed that pain could be relieved in three ways. First, the impaired temperament could be reversed. For example, if the area was too hot then cold would be applied to it. Secondly, the material which caused the pain could be dispersed, and thirdly, increased sensitivity to pain could be reduced (Gruner, 1930). Reducing sensitivity was done by using either a remedy that would soothe pain (dill, linseed, chamomile, bitter almond) or one which would stupefy (opium, mandrake, poppy, white and black hyoscyamus, deadly nightshade, lettuce seed, snow or ice-cold water). Avicenna had also experienced the dilemma of providing sufficient relief to ease pain at the risk of causing further harm to the patient:

> Sometimes the method used for alleviating pain acts so slowly that there is a risk of its becoming unbearable before the remedy has come into effect. Thus colic may be cured by purging the small intestine of the material giving rise to it, but this requires time. On the other hand one may give relief speedily, but only at the risk of worse harm in the end. Thus it is possible to apply remedies which will in a case of colic at once make the painful part insensible. The doctor is therefore in a dilemma in such a case, and requires good judgement so as to decide which is more harmful, to preserve the strength or to allow the pain to persist. He has to decide which is worse, the pain, or the danger liable to arise from inducing insensibility of the part. He has to decide which is the more important to avoid, or which is the lesser of two evils. For, should he allow the pain to continue, there is the risk of it increasing so much as to prove fatal; and if he makes the part insensible, this danger is averted and yet some other part is affected adversely. However, one may be able to remedy that, and then if the pain returns in consequence, one may repeat the process *(quoted in Gruner, 1930, pp. 527–528)*.

Finally, Avicenna recognized that pain could be relieved by means other than drugs. For example, the severe pains of flatulence could be alleviated by a hot shower, a warm poultice, dry cupping, walking about, listening to agreeable music or keeping oneself occupied with some very engrossing activity (Gruner, 1930).

2.5. Renaissance to the 20th century

In the Christian world, belief in the power of God, Satan or demons to induce and cure pain and disease eased after the Renaissance but this belief was not entirely lost. In the 16th and 17th centuries, witches were often blamed for causing unexplained pain and disease in their victims including children (Caulfield, 1943). Physicians also, at times, attributed the causation of some illnesses to immorality of the parents or supernatural influences. For example, Metlinger, a German physician of the 15th century believed that convulsions in children were caused either by the mother leaving the room for immoral reasons or by the influence of the stars (Ruhrah, 1925). Thomas Phaer, an English pediatrician of the 16th century, believed that some objects had been given by God a special influence so that if the child wore it strung on its neck, the amulet would ward off epilepsy (Ruhrah, 1925).

However, renewed efforts were made to understand the specific nature of pain. Costaeus, who wrote a book on Annotations to Avicenna in 1595 or 1608 (Gruner, 1930) expanded Avicenna's ideas about pain. He noted that pain was often a symptom of illness but that in some situations it was also the illness itself. He acknowledged that for the patient, pain relief was more important than curing the illness:

> Pain such as a headache may simply be a symptom, that is evidence of an 'intemperamental state', or 'solution of continuity'. But to the patient, it is the thing; it is the malady. Little does it concern the patient that there is an underlying cause to be treated if the practitioner proves unable to relieve his pain *(quoted in Gruner, 1930, p. 159)*.

By the end of the 19th century, there were three conflicting concepts of the nature of pain (Procacci and Maresca, 1984). One was the specificity theory which described pain as one sensation (for example, Blix in 1884 and Goldstein in 1895). Another was the intensive theory in which pain was thought to be the result of intense sensory stimulation such as excessive cold, light or heat (for example, Descartes in the 17th century, Darwin in the 19th century and Erb in 1874). The third was the affective theory originally proposed by Aristotle in which pain was interpreted by the heart (Procacci and Maresca, 1984).

Despite such theories, pain had been associated to such an extent in the minds of people with the will of God, that to seek relief from pain often floundered on the boundary between necessary medical assistance and perceived interference with the will of God. In the last half of the 19th century, anesthesia developed against considerable public and medical resistance (Fulop-Miller, 1938). Although anesthesia was eventually accepted for relief of pain during medical procedures, discussion of the morality of pain relief continued in the 20th century especially in religious institutions. Pope Pius XII himself was required to give his approval for the relief of pain for Catholic parishioners:

> The patient, desirous of avoiding or of relieving pain, may, without any disquietude of conscience, use the means discovered by science which in themselves are not immoral *(quoted in Marshall, 1960, p. 51)*.

The association of pain with religion continued to emphasize that submission to painful suffering by both young and old brought union with Christ who had also suffered for others. For example, in 1947, McFadden wrote the following comments for nurses in Catholic hospitals:

> The nurse must hold it constantly before the eyes of her suffering patient that no one is too small or unimportant to be the concern of God. The outstretched arms of Christ on the crucifix beckon every sufferer to come to Him. Response to this call of Christ will cause pain to be seen in a wholly different light. Suffering will become a medium of union with the Savior of mankind. And the more completely and confidently the suffering soul places itself in the arms of the Crucified, the more certainly will it be using pain as a stepping-stone to its eternal union with God *(McFadden, 1947, p. 121)*.

In the present century, considerable advances were made in understanding the physiological and the psychosocial nature of pain both for adults and children. In chapter 2, these advances will be discussed in depth.

3. Childhood pain symptomatology and treatment

> There can be no Doubt but that a perfect Cure of the Diseases of Children is as much desired by all, as any Thing else whatsoever in the whole Art of Physick. Nor is it of consequence only to the noble, the powerful, and the wealthy, who are desirous of having Heirs, and preserving them, but to all Parents of any Rank whatsoever; for Nature has instilled into all Men an almost invincible Love and Care of their own Offspring *(Walter Harris, 1698, quoted in Ruhrah, 1925, p. 356)*.

Until the 19th century, little systematic study was made of symptoms of pain in children in pediatric writings, but there was general concern with the injuries and diseases of childhood. While these writings do not commonly address the issue of pain, they convey the underlying belief of their writers that all efforts would be made to insure that the infant or child would not suffer needless pain as a result of injury or disease.

3.1. Ancient civilizations

The earliest records of medicine included discussion of the idiosyncratic aches and pains of infancy and childhood even though pediatrics itself was poorly developed.

The Lesser Berlin Papyrus or the Papyrus of Mother and Child (16th century B.C. from Egypt) consisted of tales of wonder and magic charms (Garrison, 1923). The Ebers Papyrus, an Egyptian manuscript written between 1553 and 1550 B.C. but probably belonging to a much older period, identified childhood conditions such as headache, urinary disorders, physical disabilities, and diseases of the eye, scalp, skin, teeth, and ears, as well as worms, fleas, lice, and pruritus, abscesses and tumors (Garrison, 1923). The rest of its small pediatric section relied on prognostications. The papyrus also contained almost 1000 prescriptions to induce evacuation and relieve pain including prescriptions for diarrhea and obstinate vomiting in children (Garrison, 1923; Castiglioni, 1975). For example, the following are prescriptions for the treatment of urinary retention in children:

> What one should do for a child that suffers from urination: xent corn warmed in a pill; if it is an older child let it take this with its nourishment; but if it is an infant, let it be given in the breast milk, the nurse warming it in her mouth and spurting it into the child's mouth *(quoted in Garrison, 1923, p. 14)*.

Among the prescriptions was a drink designed to placate a crying child:

> Capsules of the poppy-plant; excrement of wasps on the wall; rub together; strain and administer for four days running; it will stop immediately *(quoted in Garrison, 1923, p. 14)*.

Variations of this prescription were proposed throughout the centuries especially to reduce crying and sleeplessness in children. It became a controversial prescription after the Renaissance, though it persisted for some time thereafter.

A last resort in treating infant ailments among the Egyptians was the use of dead mice. Skinned mice were found in the alimentary canals of children's mummies as far back as 4000 B.C. (Bettman, 1956).

Similarly, pediatric care in ancient Babylon relied on prognostication about the course of an illness, exorcism, incantations and drugs, most often used in combinations. For example, a cold in the stomach, or gastritis as it would now be known, was treated by giving a mixture of licorice and a number of other drugs diluted in wine. Then the patient was taken out in a boat and incantations were said over him (Garrison, 1923). Another alternative to curing gastritis was administration of a nauseating remedy to drive the demon from the stomach in disgust (Garrison, 1923).

In India, pediatric care also relied on spells and incantations. In the Atharva Veda (from the period 1500–800 B.C.) are two examples of such pediatric charms:

> Headache, head-ailment, earache, anemia, every head disease of thine, do we expel out of thee by incantation.
> Forth from they feet, knees, buttocks, spine, nape, the pains from they head, the disease have I made disappear *(quoted in Garrison, 1923, p. 24)*.

The Suśruta Samhita of India (2nd century B.C.) provided separate dosages of drugs and herbal remedies for children and adults. It recommended administering drugs for children through milk, clarified butter, or in a plaster spread on the breasts of the nurse (Garrison, 1923). The Suśruta Samhita also identified a child's cry and changes in behavior as symptoms of pain and disease. The child was described as constantly touching the affected part or crying if that part of the body was touched. Constant crying indicated general infection. If the illness was in the head, the child would be unable to lift the head, or move about and would keep its eyes closed (Garrison, 1923).

At least two surgical procedures were performed on children in ancient civilizations; trepanation and circumcision. Trepanation consisted of the removal of a piece of skull without damage to underlying blood vessels, the meninges, or the brain (Lisowski, 1967). There is evidence of trepanation in prehistoric times in Europe, Asia, Africa, North, Central and South America, and the procedure persisted throughout subsequent centuries. At one time, it was believed that early surgeons performed trepanation mainly on children and adolescents perhaps because of the frequency of juvenile convulsions (Lisowski, 1967). The reasons for performing trepanation have been therapeutic, magical and ritualistic. For example, during the time of Hippocrates, (about 460–357 B.C.) trepanation was used therapeutically to treat head injuries such as fractures, concussion, or inflammation. At other times, trepanation was performed to free the 'evil spirits' which were causing pain in the head. When this pain was due to headaches, vertigo, neuralgia, coma, delirium, intracranial vascular catastrophes, meningitis, convulsions in epilepsy, intracranial tumors, or mental disease, trepanation sometimes had a therapeutic effect, even though it was performed for magical reasons (Lisowski, 1967). The benefit of trepanation was thought to be in creating an exit so that the evil spirit could leave the head. Trepanation was also used ritualistically as an amulet to ward off evil spirits which might cause pain and disease (Lisowski, 1967).

Circumcision is believed to be one of the oldest surgical procedures (Campbell et al., 1951). It was most often performed from late childhood to adulthood (Wallerstein, 1980) except among Jews where it was performed in infancy. In ancient Egypt and in Israel circumcision was performed for religious and ritualistic reasons (Garrison, 1923).

Strangulation to the point of unconsciousness was used by the Assyrians to allay the pain of circumcision for children. This method of anesthesia was practised in Italy even as late as the 17th century (Collins, 1976).

There is little direct evidence concerning the question of whether physicians worried about pain and disease in children. However, the following letter (about 1800 B.C.) to the king of Mari on the Euphrates conveys the genuine concern of a physician for a child patient:

> To my Lord say this: thus speaks I Aquim-Addu, thy servant. A child who is with me is ill. From beneath his ear, an abscess is discharging. Two physicians of mine are tending him but his disease does not change. Would my Lord, now, dispatch his physician to me ... or an expert physician, that he may examine the disease of the child, and treat him ... *(Maino, 1975, p. 65)*.

3.2. Ancient Greece and Rome

The pediatric writings during the Greco-Roman period continued to differentiate health and disease in children from those of adults and identified more childhood diseases. The Hippocratic writings (5th and 4th centuries B.C.) demonstrate a specific awareness of children's health (Garrison, 1923; Still, 1931). Dosages of herbal remedies and their means of administration considered the constitutional differences of infants and children. The following aphorisms from the Hippocratic writings exemplify the accepted differences in constitution and response to pain between adults and children:

> Old people bear fasting more easily, then adults, much less youths and least of all children. The more active they are, the less they do bear it.
> Fluid diets are beneficial to all who suffer from fevers, but this is especially true in the case of children and the edentulous who are accustomed to such kind of food *(from the 'Aphorisms' quoted in Chadwick and Mann, 1950, p. 150)*.

> Those who are used to bearing an accustomed pain, even if they be weak and old, bear it more easily than the young and strong who are unaccustomed *(from the 'Aphorisms', quoted in Chadwick and Mann, 1950, p. 153)*.

It is intriguing that contrary to popular 20th century thought, the author of the 'Aphorisms' believed infants and children tolerated pain poorly as compared to adults.

The Hippocratic writings also mentioned for the first time the painful gums of children who were teething (Chadwick and Mann, 1950). There was considerable worry that children could die during the time of teething because associated fever could lead to convulsions:

> Not all who are convulsed whilst about teeth, die; many come through it safely *(from 'On Dentition', quoted in Still, 1931, p. 3)*.

Concerns about teething pain were mentioned in virtually all subsequent pediatric texts (Radbill, 1965).

Hippocrates (about 460–357 B.C.), Celsus (25 B.C. – 50 A.D.), Soranus (2nd century A.D.), Galen (130–200 A.D.), Oribasius (325–403 A.D.), Aurelianus (5th century A.D.), Aetius (6th century A.D.) and Aegineta (7th century A.D) all contributed in varying degrees through their writings to the understanding of disease in infancy and childhood. Some attempt was made to examine symptoms of pain in addition to advancing treatment of pain.

Crying was increasingly recognized as a symptom of pain and illness. Galen (130–200 A.D.) wrote no systematic discussion on childhood diseases, but he believed crying was associated with pain and discomfort:

> For as they are devoid of reasoning, their cries and screams and rushing about mean that something is annoying them. So we guess what they want and give it to them before their petulance increases and mind and body become more violently excited. For whether they are teething, or pained in some part from some external cause, or want to pass stool or urine or to eat or to drink, they show constant restless movements as if in distress. It may be that they want warmth when they are cold, or cool when they are hot, or they are in discomfort from their swaddling bands, for even those are a burden especially when they want to turn from side to side or to change the position of any of their limbs: nay, even quiet itself is no small burden to them *(quoted in Still, 1931, p. 34)*.

Aurelianus (5th century A.D.) identified changes in a child's behavior indicating pain and illness due to intestinal worms:

> The child groans in its sleep, rolls about, gnashes its teeth, tends to lie prone, cries out suddenly, or falls silent, is seized with convulsions, sometimes becomes somnolent, the face becomes emaciated and loses its color; the child gets cold and answers questions with difficulty; sometimes throws itself about with outstretched hands, working itself into perspiration *(quoted in Garrison, 1923, p. 47)*.

Celsus (25 B.C.–50 A.D.) emphasized that children should not be treated as if they were adults (Garrison, 1923). Celsus was notable for his discussion of a variety of pediatric surgical procedures such as those for inguinal hernia, repair of harelip and nasal defects, tonsillectomy and treatment of sore eyes by expiration or cauterization of the scalp (Mettler and Mettler, 1947). He also mentioned trepanation for the treatment of hydrocephalus. The following is his discussion of a tonsillectomy:

> The tonsils which are indurated after inflammations ... being covered by a thin capsule that should be scratched round and torn out by the finger: but if they are not got rid of thus, then one might seize them with a hook and cut them out with a knife, then wash the raw place with vinegar and smear the wound with some drug by which bleeding is stopped *(quoted in Still, 1931, p. 20)*.

At times, Celsus used opium and hyoscyamus for pain relief during surgery but it would seem that he used them infrequently:

> Those pills which alleviate pain by causing sleep are called anodynes in Greek. It is bad practice to employ them except in cases of urgent necessity, for they were compounded of powerful drugs and are bad for the stomach. However one may be used, which contains a denarius (about 3 i) each of tears of poppy and galbanum, and two denarii each of myrrh, castoreum and pepper. It is enough to swallow a piece the size of a bean *(quoted in Collins, 1976, p. 4)*.

In Celsus' description of an operation for vesical calculus, he recommended holding the child down by one or, if necessary, two strong men (Still, 1931). More importantly, Celsus was known for his conviction that surgeons needed to be single-minded in order to perform a surgical procedure while the patient was in obvious pain:

> A chirurgien must have a strong, stable and intrepid hand and a mind resolute and merciless; so that to heal him that he taketh in hand, he be not moved to make more haste than the thing requireth, or to cut less than is needful, but which doth all things as if he were nothing affected with their cries, not giving heed to the judgement of the vain common people, who speak ill of chirurgiens because of their ignorance *(quoted in Griffith, 1951, p. 127)*.

Pediatric operations for imperforate anus, urethra, vagina, glans, and ears, removal of fingers in polydactyly, severance of the frenulum of the tongue, circumcision and castration by excision have all been discussed by ancient medical writers including Celsus (Mettler and Mettler, 1947). Although there were various medicines available, such as alcohol, opium and mandragora, to dull pain, it would seem from the comments of Celsus that these drugs were probably inadequate to provide sufficient pain relief.

Soranus (2nd century A.D.) wrote extensively about infantile diseases and the general management of infants and children (Mettler and Mettler, 1947). For pain from teething, Soranus recommended hare's brain, a treatment advocated even as late as the 17th century (Still, 1931). Soranus also suggested:

> Before teething, the gums should be gently rubbed with oil or fats, and the child may be permitted to suck fat bacon without swallowing, but this should cease when the teeth appear. The gums should not be irritated by butter or acid substances, and if there is much inflammation, poulticing and sponging are recommended *(quoted in Garrison, 1923, p. 46)*.

In the 4th century, Oribasius (325–403 A.D.) also prescribed hare's brain for infant teething:

> If they are in pain, smear (the gums) with dog's milk or with hare's brain; this works also if eaten. But if a tooth is coming through with difficulty, smear cyperus with butter and oil-of-lilies over the part where it is erupting *(quoted in Still, 1931, p. 38)*.

Aetius (6th century A.D.) recommended the use of charms to assist the infant through teething:

> He advises the root of colocynth hung on the child in a gold or silver case, or bramble-root, or the tooth of a viper, especially of a male viper, set in gold, or a green jasper suspended on the neck so as to hang down over the stomach *(quoted in Still, 1931, p. 40)*.

These charms would protect the infant from demons who might inflict unnecessary pain.

3.3. The Middle Ages

Little progress was made in understanding pain in childhood during the Middle Ages although there were some incidental references to the diseases of children (Still, 1931). In an old Saxon leech book of 900 A.D., there were prescriptions for the special needs of children including this example of repair of a harelip:

> For harelip pound mastic very small, add the white of an egg, and mingle as thou dost vermilion, cut with a knife (the false edges of the lip), sew fast with silk, then smear without and within with the salve 'ere the silk rot. If it draw together arrange it with the hand: anoint again soon *(quoted in Still, 1931, p. 55)*.

A Practica of about the 12th century also dealt with various childhood ailments. Again it provided a remedy for sleeplessness in children that included an opiate, in this case, mandragora:

> If he suffers from sleeplessness let fomentation be made of cooling herbs such as mallow, solatrum, plantain, lanceola, populeon, and oil of roses or violets, and mix together with the juice of mandragora, purslain and lettuce. Let a rag be soaked in all of these or in one of them and be applied to the forehead and temples; or, let the forehead and temples be smeared with oil of violets mixed with a woman's milk or with oil of roses *(quoted in Garrison, 1923, p. 56)*.

Monastic medicine using drugs, surgery, spells, incantations, prayers, exorcism and the relics of saints prevailed during the Middle Ages (Haggard, 1929; MacKinney, 1937). An intriguing example of monastic medicine is the following description of the Holy Salve, a wound dressing, which was a combination of 60 different herbs with butter and spiritual incantations. It was found in Lacnunga, a physician's handbook in 1000 A.D.:

> And thus shall the butter be made for the holy salve: Let the butter be churned from a cow of all one colour, so that she be all red or all white without markings; and if thou have not butter enough, wash other butter very clean and mix with it. And shred up all the plants together very small; and hallow water with font-hallowing; and put a bowl of it in the butter. Then take a stick and make four prongs to it. Write on the face of the prongs these holy names: Matthew, Luke, Mark, John. Then stir the butter with the stick, the whole vessel. Do thou sing over it these psalms: 'Beati Immaculati', each section thrice over it, and 'Gloria in Excelsis Deo' and 'Credo in Deum Patrem' and recite litanies over it, that is, the names of the saints and 'Deus Meus et Pater' and 'In Principio' and let this charm be sung over it: 'Acre Arcre Arnem Nona Aernem Beoora Aernem: Nidren Arcun Cunao Ele Harassan Fidine'. Sing this nine times, and put thy spittle on the plants and blow on them and lay them by the bowl and afterwards let a mass-priest hallow them. Let him sing these prayers over them: 'Holy Lord, Omnipotent Father, Eternal God: by the laying on of my hands may the enemy, the Devil, depart from the hairs, from the head, from the eyes, from the nose, from the lips, from the tongue, from the undertongue, from the neck, from the breast, from the feet, from the heels, from the whole framework of his members, so that the Devil may have no power over him, neither in his speech nor in his silence, neither in his sleeping nor in his waking, neither by day nor by night, neither in resting nor in running, neither in seeing nor in smiling, neither in writing nor in reading: So be it in the Name of the Lord Jesus Christ, Who redeemed us with His Holy Blood, Who liveth with the Father and reigneth God, world without end. Amen *(quoted in Cartwright, 1977, p. 12)*.

Although in the past, it has been thought that medicine including pediatrics sunk to its lowest level during the Middle Ages (Still, 1931), it is now generally accepted that medicine did not regress. Special interest in the treatment of children's disease continued.

3.4. The Arab World

Rhazes (859–932 A.D.), Avicenna (980–1036 A.D.), Haly Abbas (10th century), and Averros (1126–1191 A.D.) all contributed to the Arabic writings of infant and child care (Still, 1931). However, the latter two authors made only incidental references to the care of children.

Rhazes also wrote about the problem of teething in infants borrowing some of his information from the earlier Roman physician Galen. He believed that if teething was painful it was more likely to produce stronger teeth. Teething in the spring occurred without distress whereas in winter teething was painful. If the gums were swollen and the child in pain, Rhazes prescribed the remedy which was used in ancient Greece and Rome:

> And the treatment of it, when the gum is swollen, is that the gum should be rubbed a little with the finger, and afterwards with oil and hen's fat or hare's brain or dog's milk; and apply to the child's head water in which there have been boiled camomile and dill, and put plasters which have a dispersing effect on his jaws; and if the pain in the part increases after this, take butter and oil of laurels, mix together and apply over the part; or take cow's butter and marrow from the thigh, and apply; and if the points of the teeth have appeared, put over the whole head and neck clean wool, and let some tepid water be sprinkled on the wool each day. If diarrhoea occurs it will be treated along the lines we shall mention *(quoted in Still, 1931, pp. 46–47)*.

Rhazes also prescribed poppy to cure sleeplessness in children:

> For insomnia, oil of violets in vinegar or oleum anetium with lettuce juice are put in the child's nostrils, and, of course, it is allowed to suck syrup of poppies, while the temples and forehead are bathed with oil of opium and crocus *(quoted in Garrison, 1923, p. 54)*.

Avicenna was the most famous of Arabian physicians. Later his work would be frequently referred to by early English pediatricians (Still, 1931). Avicenna wrote extensively about infant and child care as well as their diseases being primarily concerned with treatment.

As had pediatricians before him, Avicenna relied on treating the infant by treating the wet-nurse. For example, infants could not be bled but the wet-nurse could be bled and cupped in its place (Still, 1931). Similarly to his predecessors, Avicenna was also concerned about the pain of teething and recommended:

> For burning pain in the gums apply oil and wax as an epitheme or use salted flesh which is a little 'high' *(quoted in Gruner, 1930, p. 372)*.

His prescription for the treatment of colic was similar:

> Colic. The infant writhes and cries. Hot water applications should be made to the abdomen, using also plenty of warm oil and a little wax *(quoted in Gruner, 1930, p. 377)*.

The prescription of poppy for crying and sleeplessness in infants was also repeated by Avicenna:

> Incessant crying, with loss of sleep. The mouth is constantly whimpering ... For this condition it is necessary to make it sleep if possible, by giving poppy bark and seed, and oil and lettuce and apply poppy oil to the temples and vertex. If this does not suffice prepare the following medicament: Take bugle seed, juniper berry, white poppy, yellow

poppy, linseed, celandine seed, purslane, plantain seed, lettuce seed, fennel seed, aniseed, caraway; some of each is roasted little by little; then all are rubbed together. Add one part of fried fleawort seed which is not powdered. Mix the whole with a like amount of sugar and give two 'drams' as a potion *(quoted in Gruner, 1930, p. 374).*

Avicenna also discussed the use of surgery to relieve water in the skull (now known as hydrocephalus). His discussion was later referred to by Cornelius Roelans (1450–1525) and is of interest to us because it mentions the use of wine and oil to relieve pain in a pediatric operation:

Avicenna says: 'If the water has been scant and retained between the cutis and the cranium, then make one incision widthwise, or if it has been much, make two incisions intersecting each other or three incisions intersecting each other, if there have been very many; and let what is in it be evacuated … Then after the water has been extracted, bind and place wine and oil on the incisions which you have made *(Roelans, quoted in Ruhrah, 1925, pp. 116–117).*

Although Avicenna was not writing specifically about children in this instance, he did discuss the use of wine as an anesthetic:

It is necessary to make a person deeply and profoundly drunk so that pain which has to be inflicted in the treatment of some part of the body may not be felt *(Still, 1931, p. 52).*

He also mentioned that opium, hyoscyamus, or mandragora could be added to the wine to strengthen its sedative effect.

3.5. Renaissance to the 20th century

The Renaissance brought a renewed interest in medicine as a result of the invention of printing in the mid 15th century and the adoption of one language, Latin, as the language of learning (Still, 1931). This renewed interest in medicine also stimulated a greater concern with understanding symptoms and treatment of pain and disease in infants and children. However, many physicians continued to be strongly influenced by the work of the Greeks and the Romans.

In the following centuries, there was more open acknowledgement of the frustration felt by physicians in caring for children who often provided so little evidence of what was ailing them. For example, Harris (1647–1732) wrote:

I know very well in how unbeaten and almost unknown a Path I am treading; for sick Children, and especially Infants, give no other Light into the Knowledge of their Diseases, than what we are able to discover from their uneasy Cries, and the uncertain Tokens of their Crossness; for which Reason, several Physicians of the first Rank have openly declared to me, that they go very unwillingly to take care of the Diseases of Children, especially such as are newly born, as if they were to unravel some strange Mystery, or cure some incurable Disease *(quoted in Ruhrah, 1925, p. 356)*.

This frustration regarding the treatment of children persisted for some time. Hugh Downman (1740–1809), who wrote his pediatric discussion in the form of poetry, also referred to the difficulty in understanding pain symptomatology in children:

Because the child, with reason unendow'd
And power of speech, by words to express his grief
Nature permits not; some believe the source
Of anguish and affections is conceal'd
From every eye, and deem assistance vain
(quoted in Ruhrah, 1925, p. 516).

Nevertheless, Downman believed that a sick child did convey symptoms of pain and illness even if these symptoms were not verbal and he argued that it was necessary to consider such symptoms in treatment rather than to rely on prophecies as cures:

Yet nature, in thy child, tho' not in words,
Speaks plain to those who in her languages vers'd
Justly interpret. Are the different tones
Of woe unfaithful sounds? Can he, whose sight
Hath traced the various muscles in their course,
When irritated in the different limbs,
Retracted, or extended, or supine,
Fix no conclusions on the seat of pain?
Is it of no avail to mark the breath,
How drawn? the face? the motions of the eye?
The salient pulse? the eruptions on the skin?
The skin itself, constructed or relaxed?
The mode of sleep? of waking? heat? or thirst?
From which, and numerous traits beside arranged,
Combined, abstracted and maturely sigh'd,
Judgement its practice forms? Are characters
Like these which ask the nice decypering soul,
Intelligible to beldames old,
Who wrapped in darkness, utter prophecies
And lying oracles, which cheat the ear,
Or followed, to destruction lead the way?
Oh! may good angels, kindling in thy breast
The lamp of reason, guard thee from their snares!
Blind guides assiduous to deceive the blind
(quoted in Ruhrah, 1925, p. 517).

Similarly, Hess in 1849, wrote that pediatrics was the most arduous of the medical specialities because of the difficulty in determining symptoms of pain and disease:

> I have called it the most arduous branch of medical art, and I deem it not less superfluous to dwell upon those circumstances which render it so, arising from the inability or the unwillingness of children to give a proper description of their feelings, or owing to their fretfulness, shyness, and resistance to the proceedings of the physician *(Hess, 1849, p. 341)*.

Even in 1906, Hutchinson wrote:

> With what are called 'subjective symptoms' in children you are not in any way troubled, because there are none. Pediatrics is like veterinary medicine in this, that the patient is unable to give you an account of his sufferings, and you are thrown back entirely on your own observations *(Hutchinson, 1906, p. 5)*.

Despite the difficulty of determining symptoms of pain and disease, physicians began a more systematic search for evidence of pain in children, expanding their observations of children's cries, as well as examining changes in children's facial expressions and sleep habits when they were ill.

3.5.1. Symptoms of pain

3.5.1.1. Cry The cry of infants and children remained the primary tool to measure pain but there was a controversy of opinion about whether crying always indicated discomfort, pain or disease in a child. Some authors maintained that crying was necessary as exercise for the infant. In 1584, Scevole de Sainte-Marthe (treasurer general of one of the provinces of France) wrote a latin poem on infant hygiene after he had extensively studied ancient medical writings to cure an ailment in one of his own children. In the poem he said:

> And moderate cryings come oft not in vain
> They stir a dull and cleanse a watery brain
> *(quoted by Foote, 1919, p. 220)*.

In 1838, Samuel Smiles also believed that crying was an essential exercise:

> Instead of being feared, the practice of crying in children in want of muscular exercise is most beneficial in its effects. Sick and weak children cry a good deal, and but for this, it is almost certain they would not live long. The very first act which an infant performs at birth is to cry, and many of them continue to do so at an average rate of four or five hours a day during the first years of their existence. It cannot for a moment be imagined that all their cries arise from a feeling of pain. It would be an anomaly in the benevolent

working plan of creation and an unmerited infliction of pain on the little innocents, were this the case. Not at all. They cry in default of exercise, or rather for exercise *(quoted in Hardyment, 1983, pp. 55–56)*.

By contrast, Omnibonus Ferrarius (1577), an Italian physician, believed crying always indicated a problem in the infant:

Infants never cry without legitimate cause: having as yet no speech they show their trouble by screaming, anger and restlessness *(quoted in Still, 1931, p. 156)*.

Starr (1895), an American physician from Philadelphia, also believed crying was the chief indicator of pain in children and he regarded crying as unusual in a healthy child:

Crying is the chief, if not the only means that the young infant possesses of indicating his displeasure, discomfort or suffering. Even long after the powers of speech have been developed, the cry continues to be the main channel of complaint. It may be accepted as a rule that a healthy child rarely cries. Of course some acute pain from a fall or accident or blow, will cause crying in the most healthy child, but the storm is quickly over *(Starr, 1895, p. 6)*.

With this increased interest in children's cries, physicians struggled to develop a schema of assessment of pain in children based on different types of cries in an effort to distinguish a pain cry from boredom, frustration or exercise.

Starr (1895), concentrated on associating specific illnesses in children with an individual cry:

Incessant, unappeasable crying is due to one of two causes – namely earache or hunger – and the distinction may be readily made by putting the child to the breast or offering a properly prepared bottle. The hydrencephalic cry, denoting pain in the head, is a sudden, very loud and paroxysmal shriek. Crying during an attack of coughing or for a brief time afterward, and attended with distortion of the features indicates pneumonia. In acute pleuritis the cry also accompanies the cough, but it is produced by movements of the body and by pressure on the affected side. It is louder, indicative of great suffering, and sometimes most difficult to check. Intestinal cry causes crying just before or after evacuation of the bowels, and is associated with wriggling movements of the body and pelvis and with eructation or the passage of flatus. Conditions of general distress or malaise predispose to fits of fretful crying, the paroxysms being excited by any disturbing influence, or even by looking at the little sufferer ... When the cry has a nasal tone, it indicates swelling of the mucous membrane of the nares or other obstructing condition. Thickening and indistinctiveness occur with pharyngeal affections. A loud brazen cry is a precursor of spasmodic croup and in some cases of extreme exhaustion the cry is faint and inaudible. Finally, in severe croupous pneumonia, in extensive pleural effusion, and in rickets ordinary disturbing causes are inoperative for the production of fits of crying, and there is some unwillingness to cry, on account of the action interfering with the respiratory function *(Starr, 1895, p. 6)*.

Holt (1897), who was professor of Diseases of Children at Columbia University from 1901 to 1923, was also concerned with crying and pain in everyday activities. He was emphatic that a child's cry must never be disregarded even if it was the only visible symptom. Holt was particularly concerned that pain in infants less than 2 months of age must not be ignored, that the absence of tears before this time should not be taken as an indication that the young baby did not feel pain. Holt divided children's cries into several functional groups according to whether the cause was due to hunger, indigestion, temper, weakness or exhaustion, discomfort, pain or habit. The characteristics of painful crying depended on the severity of the child's pain. In acute pain, which Holt ascribed to colic and earache, the cry was sharp and piercing with contraction of features, drawing up of the legs, or falling asleep when exhausted and then waking quickly, often with a scream. Crying due to less severe pain was more moaning and less sharp in tone. Interestingly, Holt argued that under the age of 5 months, infants did not cry from temper. He also believed that more delicate children cried more readily. In the fourth edition of his book (1908), Holt continued with the same categorizations of children's cries but he now believed that a newborn needed to cry for about 15–20 min each day to expand the lungs. Similar classifications of pain were also discussed by the physicians Chapin and Pisek (1909) in their pediatric text.

Towards the end of the 19th century, physicians began also to consider altered facial expression and sleep habits as indicative of pain.

3.5.1.2. Facial expression Starr described the following changes in facial expression:

> The picture (of a healthy child) is altered by the onset of any illness, the change being in proportion to the severity of the attack. An expression of anxiety or suffering appears, or the features become pinched and lines are seen about the eyes and mouth. Pain most of all sets its mark upon the countenance, and by noting the features affected it is often possible to fix the seat of serious disease. Thus, contraction of the brow denotes pain in the head; sharpness of the nostrils, pain in the chest; and a drawing up of the upper lip, pain in the abdomen *(Starr, 1895, pp. 3–4)*.

Chapin and Pisek (1909, p. 58) believed that different parts of the child's face revealed pain located in some part of the body. The upper part of the face would indicate pain and disease of the head; altered expression of the middle part of the face was linked to pain in the chest; and the lower part of the face demonstrated pain in the abdominal organs.

3.5.1.3. Sleep Starr also contrasted the changes in sleep which were suggestive of pain:

> The face of a normal sleeping child wears an expression of perfect repose. The eyelids are completely closed, the lips slightly parted, and while a faint sound of regular breathing may be heard, there is no perceptible movement of the nostrils. Incomplete closure of the lids, with more or less exposure of the whites of the eyes, is noted when sleep is rendered unsound by moderate pain and during the course of all acute and chronic diseases, particularly when they assume a grave type *(Starr, 1895, p. 3)*.

Similar descriptions of the changes in facial expression and sleep habits when the child was in pain were also described by Chapin and Pisek (1909).

3.5.2. Treatment of pain

3.5.2.1. Teething Old Greek and Roman remedies for pain continued to be used after the Renaissance. Remedies for teething pain are among the best examples of the lingering influence of the ancient Greek and Roman physicians. Hare's brain, chicken fat or bitches' milk were still applied to children's gums for relief from teething pain. This is exemplified by the following poem written in 1429 by Heinrich von Louffenburg:

> Now when your baby's teeth appear
> You must for these take prudent care
> For teething comes with grievous pain,
> So to my word take heed again.
> When now the teeth are pushing through,
> To rub the gums thou shalt do,
> Take fat from chicken, brain from hare,
> And these full oft on gums shalt smear.
> If ulcers sore thereon should come,
> Then shalt thou rub upon the gum
> Honey and salt and oil thereto.
> But one thing more I counsel you,
> A salve of oil of violet
> For neck and throat and gums to get,
> And also bathe his head awhile
> With water boiled with camomile
> *(quoted in Still, 1931, pp. 91–92)*.

Thomas Phaer (1546), who is known as the father of English pediatricians, also relied on hare's brain for relief from pain during teething:

> About ye seventh moneth, sometime more somtyme lesse, after ye byrth, it is natural for a chyld for to breede teeth, in which time many one is sore vexed with sondry diseases &

peines as swelling of ye gummes & jawes, unquiete cryeing, fever, crampes, palsies, fluxes, reumes and other infirmities, specially whan it is long or ye teeth come forth, for the soner they apere the better and the more ease it is to ye childe. There be divers thinges that are good to procure an easy breeding of teeth, among whom the chiefest is to annoint the gummes with the braynes of an hare myxte with as much capons grece and hony, or any of these thynges alone is exceadynge good to supple the gummes and the synewes. Also it is good to wasshe the chylde two or three tymes in a weeke with warme water of the decoccion of camomyl, hollyhocke and dylle. Fresh butter with a little barly flour or honye, with the fine pouder of frankinsence & liquirice are commended of good authoures for the same entente. And whan the peyne is greatte and intollerable with apostema or inflammacion of the gummes, it is good to make an ointment of oile of roses with the juyce of morelle otherwise called nightshade, and in lack of it annoint the jawes within with a little fresshe butter and honye *(quoted in Still, 1931, p. 121)*.

Sainte-Marthe (1569) wrote about teething pain:

> For teeth the stomach serve, and Life maintain,
> And none can have the Tooth, without the pain.
> The suff'ring Infant tells it by his Cries,
> His drive'ling Mouth he with his fingers plies,
> He strives to help himself, but strives in vain,
> The Nurse's Help must ease him of his Pain
> *(quoted in Ruhrah, 1925, p. 512)*.

He then went on to prescribe the inevitable hare's brains, honey and red coral ring.

Amulets, such as the red coral ring, were often used to ward off teething pain. Omnibonus Ferrarius (1577) wrote:

> A dead man's tooth in the opinion of some, through some particular virtue when hung on the neck of an infant, soothes and disperses the pain of teething *(quoted in Still, 1931, p. 156)*.

James Primerose (1659) advised that the tooth of a dog, wolf or male viper could be hung around the neck to ease teething pain (Still, 1931).

The fear that teething could result in death had continued through the centuries although there was some question now of whether it was teething itself which had resulted in the death. In 1767, George Armstrong wrote:

> I come next to teething, which, in the same manner as was observed on convulsions, is said to carry off a much greater number of children than it actually does; for almost all children that die while they are about teeth, are said to die of teething *(quoted in Seibert, 1940, p. 551)*.

3.5.2.2. Abdominal pain   Abdominal pain, a common childhood complaint, was often discussed by physicians. Vettorio, who was a physician practicing in Bologna, wrote in 1544:

> Pain in the stomach occurs in infants sometimes from flatulence existing in the intestines, sometimes from the coolness of the atmosphere or some other cause chilling the stomach; sometimes it also results from worms biting the intestines *(quoted in Ruhrah, 1925, pp. 139–140)*.

Vettorio recommended that the child's stomach be rubbed with a sponge and hot water, to break up the flatulence or a rag could be soaked in a mixture of common oil with crocus and then applied to the stomach.

Metlinger (1473) prescribed a warm cloth for abdominal pain in children:

> Pain in the abdomen and complaint about the stomach comes at times from gripes or from worms. A warm cloth placed over the little stomach will ease the pain *(quoted in Ruhrah, 1925, p. 21)*.

Bagellardus (1472), in Italy, advised an ancient remedy to reduce abdominal pain from constipation:

> But because up to a month various diseases occur, such as constipation, crying night and day, on this account, while the constipation lasts, the nurse, taking the excrements of a mouse, should infuse it in common edible oil and insert it gently into the child's anus, and if it suffers pains, rub the groin and ribs of the infant with oil of dill *(quoted in Ruhrah, 1925, p. 36)*.

Again there is an example of an amulet which could be used, in this example, from the writings of Sebastian Oestereicher (?–1550) in Alsace, to prevent stomach pain resulting from indigestion:

> Red coral suspended around the suckling's neck, from the mouth to the shoulder, prevents the vomiting of milk and aids in digestion *(quoted in Ruhrah, 1925, p. 138)*.

3.5.2.3. Colic   Colic was not infrequently mentioned by physicians in their discussions of abdominal pain. Thomas Phaer (1546) discussed abdominal pain and colic in the section of his book 'The Boke of Children' (1546) titled 'Of colike and rumblying in the guttes'. He gave similar explanations as to the cause of abdominal pain as had Vettorio (1544) but in addition he provided a discussion of its symptoms:

> Peine in the belly is a common disease of children, it commeth either of worms, or of taking cold, or of evyl mylke, ye signes thereof are to well knowen, for the chylde cannot rest, but cryeth and fretteth it selfe, and manye tymes cannot make theyr uryne, by reason of winde, that oppresseth the neck of the bladder, and is knowen also, by the member in manne chylde, which in thys case, is always stiffe, & pricking, moreover the

noyse and rumblinge in the guttes, hither and thyther, declareth ye chylde to be greved, with winde in the belly, and colike.

Cure

The nourse muste avoyde all maner of meates, that engeder wind, as beanes, peason, butter, harde egges, and suche. Than washe the childes bellye with hote water wherein hathbene sodden comine, dyll and fenel, after that make a playster of oyle and waxe, and clappe it hote upon the belly.

An other good playster for the same entente

Take good stale ale and freshe butter, seeth them with a handfull of comine poudred, and after put it all together into a swines bladder, & bynde the mouth faste, that the licoure yssue not out, then wind it in a cloth, & turne it up and doune upon the belly as hote as the pacient may suffer, this is good for the colike after a sodayne colde, in all ages, but in chyldren ye muste beeware ye applye it not to hote *(quoted in Ruhrah, 1925, p. 180)*.

Colic was also referred to by Sainte-Marthe (1569) in his own poetical style:

> And if with racking Gripes his Belly's rent,
> The Gnawings in his Bowels to prevent,
> Warm Water, and the Parts aggriev'd foment;
> Or else annoint with Oil of Camomile
> His Belly, or with Oil of fragrant Dill,
> Or what old Olives o'er the Fire distil.
> For the kind Heat insinuates by degrees,
> And passes to th' afflicted Place with Ease;
> It drives the Cold out of the Porous Skin,
> And dissipates the Winds that rage within.
> The Causes and Effects of this Disease
> It cures, and gives the patient Infant Ease
> *(quoted in Ruhrah, 1925, p. 513)*.

3.5.2.4. Opium use in treatment Until this time it was not uncommon for opium to be used in medications for children to treat a variety of problems causing pain in childhood with the intention of relieving pain and inducing sleep. However, it was now increasingly recognized that such medication was dangerous for the health of children. Bagellardus (1472) prescribed a medication for sleeplessness but urged that mild remedies be the first strategy:

There happen also to children attacks of wakefulness, through which there come to children sleeplessness and crying which disturb the nurse and everyone in the house. The treatment of this affection, although various remedies have been mentioned by the authorities, should always begin with the milder things, as all things which induce sleep are narcotic and in some degree dulling. So starting with the milder things inunction of the forehead and nose should be done: 1, with oil of violets; 2, with oil of violets and oil of dill, mixed with the milk of the woman who suckles him and with a little wax; 3, with the addition to the above mentioned inunction of little opium or jusquianus or juice of mandragora; 4, do an inunction of ointment of populeon, but with gentle rubbing and in small quantity.

And although according to the view of our authorities it is adviseable to proceed by way of external applications, it does, however, sometimes happen that internal administration has to be used, for instance, let the infant have some food taken in the form of a biscuit soaked in a decoction of white poppy seed, though even Rhazes recommends black poppy or a decoction of it, which I do not at all approve. Our common folk give infants a little of the stuff called 'Quietness', after the prescription of Nicolaus, but this, although he recommends it, should never be given except upon urgent necessity *(quoted in Still, 1931, pp. 61–62)*.

Walter Harris (1647–1732) strongly attacked opiate use for infants:

Further, I may add from repeated experiments, that in Infants the same testaceous Medicines so effectually perform all good Effects of Anodynes, nay of Soporificks (if they are but given in a sufficient Quantity to obtain that End and duly repeated), that they never require the least Assistance of any other Narcoticks, be the pain or Sickness however urgent.

But as Opiates ought never to be exhibited to Infants (except in violent Vomiting, of which more hereafter) I cannot approve of giving heating Medicines, at least in any considerable Quantity, however cordial or wholesome they may commonly be stiled *(quoted in Still, 1931, pp. 298–299)*.

3.5.2.5. Anesthesia in childhood A very significant event in the treatment of pain was the development of anesthesia in the 19th century but it posed considerable difficulties in its application to pediatric surgery. Anesthesia presented a potentially lethal risk to children especially infants. At the same time, assessment and measurement of whether a child was in pain and then the extent of that pain relied on subjective observations of the child. The belief that infants and young children experienced less pain and were easily comforted when they were in pain made it difficult to determine when an anesthetic was necessary for pediatric surgery. For example, Wharton in 1895 maintained that an anesthetic for tracheotomy was not necessary and not worth the risk of obstructed breathing:

Tracheotomy itself is not painful when the dyspnoea is well marked, and after the incision in the skin is made little pain is experienced in the subsequent steps of the operation. In this connection I mention the observation made by Brown-Séquard that an incision of the tissues of the anterior of the neck causes anaesthesia of the surrounding parts, and hence it is only the first incision which gives rise to pain in the tracheotomy *(Wharton, 1895, p. 297)*.

Similarly, W.E. Casselberry (1895) did not feel that an anesthetic was necessary for children during a tonsillectomy:

> The wire snare is an excellent means of abscission when the child is anaesthetized, as when combining this operation with that for 'adenoids'; but otherwise it is slow and painful, and, like the galvano-cautery snare, it requires more time for quietude and adjustment then are available with young children when not anaesthetized. An anaesthetic is not usually necessary when the faucial tonsils alone are to be abscised, although it is decidedly best to administer ether when the combined operation for removal of the faucial tonsils and the naso-pharyngeal 'adenoids' is to be made. Also with unusually exciteable or obstreporous children ether may be administered. The tonsillotome is still the best implement for children who are not anaesthetized, because of the rapidity, precision and comparative ease with this method can be practised. With older children it is best to use a preliminary spraying of 5 percent cocaine solution. Younger children are apt to be terrified of spraying, and it is best to omit it. The pain is not really great *(Casselberry, 1895, p. 439)*.

The problem of anesthesia was especially felt in procedures such as circumcision. The procedure could be swiftly done and when performed on newborns it was difficult to determine if the infant was in pain. As a result, it was often assumed that infants experienced little if any pain during this procedure. Both Bolling in 1930 and Campbell et al. in 1951 did not feel anesthesia was required for this procedure.

In 1938, Thorek wrote that in general, infants did not require an anesthetic:

> Often no anesthesia is required. A sucker consisting of a sponge dipped in some sugar water will often suffice to calm a baby *(Thorek, 1938, p. 2021)*.

Many of the difficulties with anesthesia, postoperative pain relief and pain medication for non-surgical pain problems in infancy and childhood did not receive much attention until the present century. We will discuss these problems in greater detail in the following chapters.

4. Childrearing beliefs and practices

Historians of childhood have commonly argued that childrearing in the past was characterized by brutality and indifference towards children. DeMause (1974) is one of the most vehement proponents of this point of view. We will therefore consider his argument and its limitations prior to reviewing the role of pain in historical childrearing practices.

It is essential to recognize that DeMause biased his investigation by assuming:

> ... the central force for change in history is neither technology nor economics, but the 'psychogenic' changes in personality occurring because of successive generations of parent-child interactions *(1974, p. 3)*.

Integral to this premise, DeMause believed that parents interacted with their children in three different manners. First, the child was an object for the projection of contents from the parent's own unconscious (projective reversal). Second, the parent could use the child as a substitute for a significant person in the parent's life (reversal reaction). Third, the parent could respond empathetically with the child's needs. DeMause argued that parents in previous generations interacted with their children primarily in a projective or reversal reaction creating disastrous parent-child relationships. He argued that parent-child relationships evolved with a general improvement in childrearing practices and he maintained that the further one goes back in history the less likely parents were to have had an empathetic reaction to children. DeMause also maintained that parent-child relationship evolved over six modes from antiquity to the present:

> The series of six modes represents a continuous sequence of closer approaches between parent and child as generation after generation of parents slowly overcame their anxieties and began to develop the capacity to identify and satisfy the needs of their children *(1974, p. 51)*.

The six modes were infanticidal (antiquity to the 4th century A.D.), abandonment (4th – 13th century), ambivalent (14th – 17th century), intrusive (18th century), socialization (19th – mid-20th century) and finally, the helping mode (mid-20th century). DeMause believed that the helping mode resulted in children who were 'gentle, sincere, never depressed, never imitative or group-oriented, strong-willed, and unintimidated by authority' (1974, p. 54).

Analyses such as that of DeMause (1974), which consider only a psychoanalytical perspective in examining historical parent-child relationships to the exclusion of sociological, economic, technological, political, or medical factors of a given time period, rely on an extremely narrow framework. It is unlikely that only one perspective could explain such complex and variable emotion and behavior as that in historical parent-child relationships. More recently, some historians of childhood (Hardyment, 1983; Ozment, 1983; Pollock, 1983; Houlbrooke, 1984) have argued that such historical analyses of childhood as provided by DeMause and others are misrepresentations and distortions of reality. Comprehensive assessment of primary sources, such as pediatric texts and the diaries and autobiographies written by parents do not support an overall conclusion that people in previous centuries were barbaric towards their children.

Of interest in this overview of childrearing practices is whether parents were indifferent to pain in their children, whether children were encouraged to repress pain, whether parents relied on pain as punishment for misbehavior or whether parents and other adults abused children. Finally, the extent to which childrearing advice and practices avoided causing pain and discomfort to children will be explored.

4.1. Ancient civilizations

Infant mortality rates were high as a result of congenital abnormalities, birth trauma, injury and disease. However abandonment, infanticide and child sacrifice were also practiced in many parts of the ancient world. Female infants, illegitimate children, disabled, weak or frail children, twins or triplets, and children who were born to poor families were the most likely to have been poorly cared for (Garrison, 1923). For example in Sparta, infants who did not seem to be healthy and vigorous were exposed in a chasm under Mount Taygetus (Garrison, 1923). A plethora of examples of further abuses of children are discussed by Payne (1916) in his historical review of childhood.

Yet concern for the health and well-being of children is also abundant in the many figurines and reliefs depicting the daily life of children in Egypt, Babylon, and the Orient (Garrison, 1923). The most ancient childcare advice comes from the papyri of Egypt to which we have referred earlier regarding their medical contributions. In his reference to these manuscripts, Castiglioni (1975, p. 59) wrote:

> Worth mentioning is the care that the ancient Egyptians gave to the hygiene of infancy. The newborn was wrapped in large white linen cloths, but not bandaged. After weaning, it was given cow's milk, then vegetables. Up to the age of five, children wore no clothes and played healthy games (ball games, rolling hoops etc.); in the Egyptian museums are found a large number of toys from the ancient tombs for use in games. For older children detailed exercises were prescribed.

In some parts of the world infanticide was severely punished when discovered. For example, Diodorus Siculus in the 1st century A.D. wrote that when ancient Egyptians were found guilty of infanticide they were condemned to continually carry the dead infant in their arms for three days and three nights (Garrison, 1923). Similarly, in Babylon, the value of children is evidenced in the Code of Hammurabi (2250 B.C.). For example, if a woman allowed a suckling to die on her hands and substituted another, her breast was amputated (Garrison, 1923). Infanticide, was uncommon in Egypt, Babylon and Israel (Garrison, 1923).

4.2. Ancient Greece and Rome

In most Greek cities, the father had absolute authority over his children (Lewis and Reinhold, 1966). If the father rejected the child it was abandoned, usually in a public place where it might be possible that the child would be claimed by a passerby. The infant would be carefully wrapped and have trinkets around its neck or in the basket as a way to entice someone to care for it. At Thebes, abandonment was not permitted (Mettler and Mettler, 1947). Instead a father who was unable to provide for his child, brought the infant to the magistrates who would find someone else to look after it. In Rome, a father had absolute authority over his son during the son's entire life:

> ... whether he thought it proper to imprison him, to scourge him, to put him in chains and keep him at work in the fields, or to put him to death ... *(Lewis and Reinhold, 1966, p. 60)*.

This privilege included selling the son as often as three times. For a child, who was less than 3 years old at death, there was no period of mourning (Lewis and Reinhold, 1966). In the Twelve Tables of 449 B.C. it said:

> Quickly kill ... a dreadfully deformed child *(Lewis and Reinhold, 1966, p. 104)*.

The following letter from Hilario to Alis, his wife, in 1 B.C. illustrates the practice of female infanticide although it provides no indication of the feelings of the mother or whether the father's instructions were carried out:

> Know that we are still in Alexandria. Do not worry if they really go home and I remain in Alexandria. I ask you and entreat you to take care of the child, and as soon as we receive our pay I will send it up to you. If you chance to bear a child and it is a boy, let it be; if it is a girl, expose it. You have said to Aphrodisias that I should not forget you. How can I forget you? I ask you, then, not to worry *(Year 29 of Augustus Caesar, Payni 23, quoted in Lewis and Reinhold, 1966, p. 404)*.

In Sparta, which did practise infanticide, childrearing practices concentrated on raising children who had great strength of character and would be able to persevere when in pain or under adversity. Sudhoff (1917) had the following comments about the childrearing practices of Spartan women:

> Upon the same account, the women did not bathe the newborn children with water, as is the custom in all other countries, but with wine, to prove the temper and complexion in their bodies; from a notion they had that epileptic and weakly children waste away upon their being thus bathed, while on the contrary, those of a strong and vigorous habit

acquire firmness and get a temper by it, like steel. There was much care and art, too, used by the nurses: They had no swaddling bands; the children grew up free and unconstrained in limb and form, and not dainty and fanciful about their food; not afraid in the dark, or of being left alone; without any peevishness or ill humor or crying *(quoted in Garrison, 1923, p. 35)*.

Childcare advice in Sparta would have been directed towards rewarding children for control and repression of pain. At one festival, chosen boys were flogged to teach them endurance of pain (Garrison, 1923).

By 18 B.C., in the reign of Augustus in Rome, a program to improve public morality and strengthen marriage and family life was established providing privileges for parents of three or more children and legal disabilities for those without children. Lewis and Reinhold (1966) believed these initial measures were largely ineffective because socio-economic conditions continued to be poor. In 4 A.D., there was a gradual change in Roman law providing tax exemptions to parents who had three or more children and financial rewards for people who raised orphans. In the second century, a protective foundation for female children was established. By 315 A.D., governmental assistance was provided to parents who, due to their poverty, were unable to provide for their children:

> A law shall be written on bronze or waxed tablets or on linen cloth, and posted throughout all the municipalities of Italy, to restrain the hands of parents from infanticide and turn their hopes to the better. Your office shall administer this regulation, so that, if any parent should report that he has offspring which on account of poverty he is unable to rear, there shall be no delay in issuing food and clothing, since the rearing of a newborn infant cannot tolerate delay. For this matter we order that both our fisc and our privy purse shall furnish their services without distinction *(Theodisian Code XI. xxvii. 1; 315 or 329 A.D., Lewis and Reinhold, 1966, p. 483)*.

Such laws reflected a growing concern that the stability of the state relied on stimulation of the birth rate and protection of infants and children (Lewis and Reinhold, 1966). There is also abundant demonstration of affection and concern for children (Garrison, 1923; Drake, 1933; Rosenthal, 1936). The literature of Homer, Herodotus, Euripides and Thucydides all reflected compassion towards the needs of children (Garrison, 1923) and not uncommonly, private Roman citizens made bequests for the support of children (Lewis and Reinhold, 1966).

Most childrearing advice, that was recorded or which we now have, was provided by physicians. The Hippocratic writings do not provide an extensive discussion of childrearing practices but they do give some guidelines concerning the developmental needs of children:

The softest and most moist diets suit young bodies best as at that age the body is dry and has set firm *(from 'A Regime for Health', quoted in Chadwick and Mann, 1950, p. 215)*.

Infants should be bathed for long periods in warm water and given their wine diluted and not at all cold. The wine should be of a kind least likely to cause distention of the stomach and wind *(from 'A Regime for Health', quoted in Chadwick and Mann, 1950, p. 216)*.

Soranus (2nd century A.D.), whose work on labor, delivery and child care was a model for subsequent centuries (Mettler and Mettler, 1947), included the following topics in his discussion of childrearing:

On the care of the baby. How to know what is capable of being reared. How the cord is to be divided. How inunction is to be done. How swaddling should be done. On the baby's lying down. On feeding. On the choice of wet-nurse. What should be done if the milk dries up or becomes unwholesome or too thick or too thin. On the bathing and the rubbing of the baby. How and when to give the breast to the baby. On the separation of the cord. When and how the baby should be freed (from its swaddling bands). How to practise it in sitting and walking. When and how to wean the baby. On teething. On apthae. On rashes and itchings. On wheezing and cough. On flux of the belly *(Still, 1931, pp. 26–27)*.

Although Soranus' work is the earliest known example of such complete and detailed discussion of child management, Soranus himself referred to the work of earlier physicians (Still, 1931).

Galen (130–200 A.D.) was particularly interested in the overall management of children. He firmly believed that good psychological health reduced the likelihood of childhood disease:

...for anger and weeping and grief and excess of sorrow and prolonged wakefulness light up fevers and become causes of various disease... *(quoted in Still, 1931, p. 34)*.

Hence Galen was especially concerned about the crying and fretting of children as is evident in these comments:

If it is not clear what they want and meanwhile the demand is becoming more urgent, let things be put to right by immediately giving whatever is needed and so prevent their becoming exhausted. In the meantime by rocking in the arms and lullabies, such as the more experienced nurses use, one may seek to soothe them. For my own part I have sometimes found as a remedy when the infant was crying and fretting all day and tossing about to an excessive degree, and the nurse at her wit's end and doing no good by putting the child to the breast, that by putting it on its little chair-utensil if it happened to be Nature's need that he was wanting, he has quieted; but he has not quieted so long as she held him still in her arms.

I have also noticed that his cot and his wrappings were too dirty and the infant himself dirty and unwashed, and I have ordered him to be bathed and that she should change his napkins for clean ones, and when these things were done the infant has stopped kicking and has settled off in a long sleep. In this matter there is need not only of forethought but of daily habit *(from 'De Sanitate Tuenda', Lib.i, cap.8, quoted in Still, 1931, pp. 34–35)*.

Galen certainly did not support the infliction of pain as a childrearing practice.

Oribasius (325–403 A.D.) maintained that humane upbringing and education of children was more likely to encourage learning and more optimal physical health than when the parents or teachers were harsh and severe in their methods:

> Now, relaxation and a joyous spirit contribute much to digestion and favorable nutrition; but those who, on the other hand, are insistent in instruction, who resort to sharp reprimands, will make the children servile and timorous and will inspire them with an aversion for the objects of their instruction: it is by beating them that they expect them to learn and recollect things, even at the very moment when they are beaten, when they have lost their courage and presence of mind *(quoted in Ruhrah, 1925, p. 13)*.

John Chrysostom who wrote 'An Address on the Vainglory and the Right Way of Parents to Bring Up Their Children' in 388 also believed that there are more effective approaches to childrearing than physical punishment:

> ... punish him, now with a stern look, now with incisive, now with reproachful, words; at other times win him with gentleness and promises ... Let him at all times fear blows but not receive them ... our human nature has some need for forbearance *(quoted in Lyman, 1974, p. 87)*.

Parents' attitudes about pain and disease in their children are difficult to determine. Inscriptions by parents on the tombstones of their children provide some illustration of parents' feelings. The following is an example of a tombstone inscription for a child who died at the age of 4 years, 5 months, and 20 days in the 2nd or 3rd century B.C. despite the efforts of his father to treat his disease:

> A helpless child am I who have reached this tomb, O traveller; even you who have chanced upon my stony slab will straightway weep at the suffering which I have endured in the brief compass of my life. When the Horae (goddesses of birth) brought me into the light by the travail of my mother, my father joyfully took me up in his hands from the earth, and washed me clean of the impure blood, and he in person placed me in swaddling clothes, and made prayer to the gods which were not to be; for the Fates were the first to make all decisions about me; and my father chose my mother as my nurse and reared me. Forthwith I grew lustily like a young plant and was beloved by all; but in a few seasons the seal of the Fates came upon me, who made me fast with a dread disease about the testicles; but my distressed father healed my dire disease, thus thinking to save my fate by medical treatment. And then, moreover, another disease seized me, most grievous by far, and many times worse than the former; for the metatarsi of my (left)

foot had sepsis in the bones, and so my father's friends performed an operation on me and took out of my bones which were the cause of grief and groans to my parents, and in this way I was healed again as before; not even thus did my ill-boding birth have its full of smiting, but fate again brought upon me another disease of the belly, enlarged my intestines and wasted away other parts, until such time when my mother's hands snatched away life from my eyes; this I suffered in the short space of my life, O stranger, and I, doomed to a sad end, survived by three unwedded sisters (or brothers), have left the hated consumption to those who begat me *(quoted in Meinecke, 1940, pp. 1029–1030)*.

4.3. The Middle Ages

It is very difficult to determine for this period of time the nature of childrearing practices. Although there are stories, poetry, sculptures, and paintings from the Middle Ages, interpreting their significance as evidence of childrearing practices is suspect (Lyman, 1974). Lyman (1974) believed that the legal and religious prohibitions of the first centuries of the Middle Ages had little effect against infanticide, selling of children or abandonment of children but that there was a change in the role of women who became more nurturant as mothers.

In the later centuries of the Middle Ages, it was customary to write biographical or autobiographical accounts of religious people, especially saints. Since these accounts were hagiographies, they were also bound by the conventions and expectations of the clergy (McLaughlin, 1974). It is unknown to what extent these accounts reflected the childrearing practices of ordinary people. McLaughlin (1974) discussed two such documents from the 11th century which provide the most extensive descriptions of infancy and childhood of this period. One is the biography of Peter Damian, who was a spiritual reformer and saint, written after his death by John of Lodi, his disciple, and the other is the autobiography of Guibert of Nogent who became an abbott. Both men suffered beatings in their childhood, the first from a brother and sister-in-law and the other by a tutor. Guibert wrote that his mother was distraught by these beatings:

'... she threw off my inner garments and saw my little arms blackened and the skin of my back everywhere puffed up with the cuts from the twigs', she was 'grieved to the heart' and protested bitterly, 'weeping with sorrow', that he should never become a cleric or 'any more suffer so much to get an education' *(quoted in McLaughlin, 1974, p. 108)*.

Other writers were also distressed by the use of physical punishment. For example, St. Anselm chastized a fellow abbott, who unsuccessfully attempted to control the boys in his care by beating them, saying:

... feeling no love or pity, good-will or tenderness in your attitude towards them, they
have in future no faith in your goodness but believe that all your actions proceed from
hatred and malice against them; they have been brought up in no true charity towards
anyone, so they regard everyone with suspicion and jealousy ... Are they not human?
Are they not flesh and blood like you? Would you like to have been treated as you treat
them, and to have become what they are now *(quoted in McLaughlin, 1974, p. 131)*?

About 1200, Walther von der Vogelweide also objected to physical
punishment:

Children won't do what they ought
If you beat them with a rod.
Children thrive, children grow
When taught by words, and not a blow.
(quoted in McLaughlin, 1974, p. 138).

However, Philip of Novara (about 1265) believed that children should be
punished first by words, then by beating with imprisonment used as a last
resort (McLaughlin, 1974).

McLaughlin (1974), Lyman (1974) and Despert (1965) concluded that the
Middle Ages were characterized by cruelty and indifference towards children
although McLaughlin and Lyman also described a slow evolution towards
more compassionate childrearing practices. Unfortunately, without primary
documentation by parents, it is very difficult to determine the role of pain in
childrearing practices.

4.4. The Arab World

Although there is virtually no information about childrearing in the Arab
world, there is a very intriguing discussion about childrearing by the Arabian
physician Avicenna (980–1036 A.D.). The assumption in all his comments was
that childrearing should avoid causing pain or discomfort to the child. The
following are some examples from Avicenna's 'The Canon of Medicine':

In doing this (referring to swaddling) the limbs must be handled very gently. Every part
should be moulded according to its appropriate form – making wide that which should
be wide, slender that which should be slender, doing all as gently as possible between the
tips of the fingers.
While sleeping the head should be at a higher level than the rest of the body, and
someone should watch lest any part of the body (neck, limbs, back) should get into a
twisted position.
After laving, the palms and soles should be gently raised (up and down). It should be
gently wiped dry with soft cloths. Then turn it down on its belly, then back, rubbing
gently all the while, pressing and moulding (and singing gently to it), then back on its

belly to apply the binder. Afterwards instill sweet oil into the nostrils, and bathe the eyes and the lids *(quoted in Gruner, 1930, pp. 364–365)*.

Rather than encouraging repression of pain and discomfort or advising harsh or restrictive methods of childrearing, Avicenna maintained that such activities as humming, singing or talking to the child would strengthen the child's constitution. He also believed that allowing the infant to nurse solved much of a child's discomfort:

> Experience shows that merely to place the mother's nipple into the infant's mouth is a great help towards removing whatever is hurtful to the infant.
> Besides this there are also two other things to be done to help to strengthen the constitution: gentle rocking movements; humming music or some old song, or prattling to the infant, as is customary while placing the babe into its cradle. How much these two practices are to be employed may be judged (individually); the movement is for the benefit of the body, and the music is for the benefit of the mind *(quoted in Gruner, 1930, p. 365)*.

Similarly, Avicenna was concerned that encouragement of the development of children avoid pain and discomfort by excessive zeal or injury:

> When the child begins to creep about, it must not be allowed to make strenuous efforts, or be encouraged to walk or sit erect before the natural desire to do so appears; otherwise there may be injury done to its legs and back. When it first sits up or creeps over the ground, it is best to place it upon a smooth skin, to prevent injury by roughness in the floor. Bits of stick or any objects able to pierce or cut the skin must be kept out of its way. Care must be taken that it does not fall off some elevated place *(quoted in Gruner, 1930, p. 371)*

Although Avicenna was a physician of the Arab world and his discussion does not reflect childrearing in Western Europe, his comments remain particularly striking for their compassion and sensitivity towards children in a time period which is usually associated with brutality and indifference towards children.

4.5. Renaissance to the 20th century

The childrearing advice given to parents from the Renaissance was clearly divided between those who favored restrictive and punitive methods of childrearing in children and those who advocated a more compassionate approach to childrearing.

Mettlinger (1473), who was from Augsburg, Germany, advocated methods of childrearing which would not cause unnecessary pain and discomfort:

When the child cries or trembles in a bath even though it be warm, it should be taken out ... Furthermore, the child in the first six weeks should be kept in a half-darkened room and care should be taken that neither sun nor moon touch it and also that neither cats or any other animal come near it and it should be protected from fright *(quoted in Ruhrah, 1925, p. 77)*.

Mettlinger was also cautious about the use of harsh punishment for children:

One should gradually but regularly accustom badly mannered children to good habits by kindness and punishment until their natures are formed. It should be known that children should not be too severely punished ... In modesty and goodness should parents bring up their children ... Punishment is to be praised when it is just and not too severe and a small fault in a child may be overlooked to prevent a larger one *(quoted in Ruhrah, 1925, p. 97)*.

Two centuries later, Felix Wurtz (1656), a physician who wrote 'The Children's Book', continued to maintain that a compassionate approach to childrearing was preferable to ignoring pain and discomfort in children:

For it is most certain, that Children will not cry, unless they ail somewhat; because it is more ease for them to when quiet: and they are not able to make their complaints any other way but by crying. Hence we are to note, that as soon as man is born into the world, then he is made subject to endure pains. Therefore good notice must be taken what these crying children aileth, wherein they are grieved or pained, that with one thing or other they may be holp *(quoted in Ruhrah, 1925, p. 201)*.

Wurtz (1656) certainly believed that children experienced pain to the same extent if not more so than adults:

If a new skin in old people be tender, what is it you think in a new born Babe? Doth a small thing pain you so much on a finger, how painful is it then to a Child, which is tormented all the body over, which hath but a tender new grown flesh? If such a perfect Child is tormented so soon, what shall we think of a Child, which stayed not in the wombe its full time? surely it is twice worse with him *(quoted in Ruhrah, 1925, pp. 204–205)*.

In contrast to the argument that parents treated their children with cruelty in the 14th–16th centuries (Stone, 1977), there was considerable criticism from writers of the time that parents were excessively indulgent (Ozment, 1983). For example, Courtin in 1671 made the following criticisms:

These little people are allowed to amuse themselves without anyone troubling to see whether they are behaving well or badly; they are permitted to do as they please; nothing is forbidden them; they laugh when they ought to cry, they cry when they ought to laugh, they talk when they ought to be silent, and they are mute when good manners require them to reply. It is cruelty to allow them to go on living in this way. The parents say that when they are bigger that they will be corrected. Would it not be better to deal with them in such a way that there was nothing to correct *(quoted in Aries, 1962, p. 115)*?

However, there were less compassionate views of childrearing. Hersey (a New England minister), Locke and Rousseau (both philosophers) were examples of such views. Hersey wrote the following:

> Begin the work before they can run, before they can speak plainly or speak at all. Whatever pains it costs, conquer their stubbornness; break their wills if you will not damn the child. Therefore let a child from a year old be taught to fear the rod and cry softly. Make him do as he is bid if you whip him ten times running to do it; let none persuade you that it is cruel to do this *(quoted in Hardyment, 1983, p. 8)*.

Locke (1693) and Rousseau (1762) were influential writers on childrearing. While they both advocated 'hardening' of children, meaning strengthening them against life's adversities, they did not advocate corporal punishment. They encouraged the use of light clothes, uncertain mealtimes, freedom to have accidents, cold baths and even blanket-tossing to strengthen a nervous constitution and firing pistols near the head to stimulate endurance (Hardyment, 1983).

Locke believed that very small children were not susceptible to reason and consequently fear and awe were the most useful childrearing tools for parents. He wrote:

> Parents being wisely ordained by Nature to love their children, are very apt, if Reason not watch their natural Affection very warily, are apt, I say, to let it run into Fondness *(quoted in Hardyment, 1983, p. 16)*.

In a similar vein, Rousseau's comments in a popular childrearing manual of 1762 suggested indifference to the pain and discomforts of childhood:

> Fix your eyes on Nature, follow the path traced by her. She keeps children at work, she hardens them by all sorts of difficulties, she soon teaches them the meaning of pain and grief. They cut their teeth and are feverish, sharp colics bring on convulsions, they are choked by fits of coughing or troubled by worms, evil humours corrupt the blood, germs of various kinds ferment it ... One half of the children who are born die before their eighth year ... This is nature's law; why try to contradict it? ... Experience shows that children delicately nurtured are more likely to die. Accustom them therefore to the hardships they will have to face ... Dip them into the waters of the Styx *(quoted in Hardyment, 1983, p. 18)*.

Bathing children in cold water was a popular method of hardening children even into the 19th century. Cobbett (1829), who wrote a book of advice for fathers, maintained that cold water bathing was an essential practice despite pain and discomfort to the child:

A great deal in providing for the health and strength of children depends on their being duly and daily washed, when well, in cold water from head to foot. Their cries testify to what degree they dislike this. They squall and twist and kick about at a fine rate, and many mothers, too many, neglect this, partly from a reluctance to encounter the squalling, and partly, much too often, from what I will not call idleness, but which I cannot apply a milder term than neglect. Well and duly performed it is an hour's good tight work; for besides the bodily labour, which is not very slight when the child gets to be five or six months old, there is the singing to overpower the voice of the child *(quoted in Hardyment, 1983, pp. 57–58)*.

Throughout the period of the Renaissance to the 20th century, there are examples of childrearing advice which leaned either towards more compassionate and even indulgent views of childrearing and those who took a more aggressive view of childrearing that included 'hardening' and/or severe physical punishment. Parents' diaries, which are available for this period because Puritans encouraged the use of diaries as a means of self-reflection, demonstrate a similar division of childrearing beliefs and practices (Pollock, 1983). The most extensive study of parents' diaries and autobiographies, and diaries by children is that of Pollock (1983). She examined a total of 416 manuscripts from the 16th to the 19th century, 96 of these were written by children. All writers were of course literate but they encompassed a wide range of occupations such as farmer, student, preacher, politician, landowner, teacher, poet, spinner, or king. Pollock (1983) concluded that during each century there were both strict and indulgent parents. Parents used physical punishment, deprivation of privileges, advice, lectures, making the child feel ashamed, and remonstrations to discipline their children but the method used varied according to the parent-child relationship rather than a specific time period (Pollock, 1983, p. 199). However, in the first half of the 19th century, there was a stricter control of children though only a minority of children in the diaries were cruelly treated (Pollock, 1983).

Pollock (1983) criticized historians who made selective use of incidents of physical punishment in parents' diaries as evidence of abuses towards children in the past. For example, Samuel Sewall (1652–1730) wrote that he had whipped his son very smartly. His admission has often been used as an example of the strict discipline characteristic of the 17th century (Pollock, 1983). However, in the whole of Sewall's very lengthy diary, this was the only mention of physical punishment. It occurred on a day when his son had disobeyed several times finally throwing a brass article at his sister which bruised and cut her forehead (Pollock, 1983).

The following are some examples of parents who believed that reasoning was more effective than corporal punishment:

Cotton Mather (1663–1728)
The first Chastisement, which I inflict for an ordinary Fault, is, to lett the Child see and hear me in an Astonishment, and hardly able to beleeve that the Child could do so base a Thing, but beleeving that they will never do it again ... I would never come, to give a child a Blow; except in the Case of Obstinacy or some gross Enormity *(quoted in Pollock, 1983, pp. 152–153)*.

Taylor (1743–1819)
I have thought a deal on 'Train up a child in the way he should go'. I have considered the New Testament precepts on the same subject; and I have endeavoured to practice them ... I recollected my being a child myself; how I behaved to my father and how he behaved to me ... I took notice also of other families in the neighbourhood, and attempted to derive some improvement from them. I laboured to preserve the love, esteem and affection of my children ... I made a practice of talking with my children, to instruct them to impress their minds ... I then understood how unreasonable and cruel it was in parents to scold and beat their children for acting in such and such a manner; when they had taken no pains to instruct them that such actions were wrong *(quoted in Pollock, 1983, pp. 156–157)*.

The following is an example of a mother who was prepared to inflict pain as discipline for misbehavior although in this case she did not use it:

Boscawen (1719–1805)
Billy (4 years) is now perfectly recovered (from inoculation), I thank God. Purging discipline all over, but my discipline to begin, for it has been slackened so long it is unknown, how perverse and saucy we are, and how much we deal in the words won't, can't, shan't, etc. Today he would not eat milk for breakfast, but the rod and I went to breakfast with him, and though we did not come into action, nor anything like it, yet the bottom of the porringer was very fairly revealed *(quoted in Pollock, 1983, p. 157)*.

Parents, who used physical punishment with their children, sometimes did so believing it was necessary but feeling remorseful about the action itself:

Macready (1793–1873)
Before I came down my tenderness was put to a severe trial by my dear child (4 years) repeating the offence for which I had punished her yesterday. I felt there was no alternative, and I punished her with increased severity. It cut my heart to look upon the darling little creature's agony, as she promised to be good. I ordered her to be put to bed, and came downstairs in low spirits. God bless the dear child – my heart dotes on her, and I could weep with her, while I make her suffer; but I love her too well to bring her up with false indulgence *(quoted in Pollock, 1983, p. 164)*.

In other families, the parents differed in their own attitudes about the use of corporal punishment which caused conflict between the parents:

Stedman (1744–1797)
This evening some words happened between Mama and Johnny, about his learning, he being today one year at Tiverton School. She said, 'Well what have you learnt in that

time?' which he being affronted at answered, 'so much in one year as you'd have done in two', when she struck him a black eye which made high words between she and I, and she was exceedingly ill all night. (The next day) Johnny now begged her pardon to no purpose; and he went crying to school. She and I again fell out about this, and neither of us took any dinner till in the evening the boy came home, and all was reconciled *(quoted in Pollock, 1983, p. 158)*.

In Pollock's research of autobiographies by children, only three writers referred to being physically punished. Of these, Grant (1797–?) had a particularly cruel upbringing. She and her siblings were shut up in dark cupboards or whipped for misbehavior. Breakfast was supervised by their father with a whip in his hand until she finished her meal. Grant was also exposed to the practice of bathing children in cold water even in winter:

> ... a large long tub, stood in the kitchen court, the ice on top of which had often to be broken before our horrid plunge into it; we were brought down from the very top of the house, four pairs of stairs, with only a cotton cloak over our night-gowns, just to chill us completely before the dreadful shock. How I screamed, begged, prayed, entreated to be saved ... all no use *(quoted in Pollock, 1983, p. 169)*.

Some authors have claimed that child abuse in the past was largely ignored (Pinchbeck and Hewitt, 1969). Pollock reviewed 385 incidences of child neglect and sexual abuse as reported in The Times newspaper from 1785 to 1860. In only 7% of these was the perpetrator found not guilty and Pollock noted 'the fact that the majority of cases were also found guilty meant that the law and society condemned child abuse long before the specific Prevention of Cruelty to Children Act appeared in 1889' (Pollock, 1983, p. 93). In the newspaper accounts, abusing parents were described as unnatural, horrific and barbaric.

The following is an example of a mother's anger towards a nursemaid who abused and neglected her son. Russell, who had gone on a visit, had left her son with a nurse. The nursemaid had been highly recommended to her:

> *K. Russell (1842–1874)*
> It makes my blood boil for my precious little darling, to think what he has to bear. I am too furious. When he cried she used to shake him – when she washed him she used to stuff the sponge in his little mouth – push her finger (beast!) in his dear little throat – say she hated the child, wished he were dead – used to let him lie on the floor screaming while she sat quietly by & said screams did not annoy her it was good for his lungs ... She sat in her room most of the day reading novels and never nursed the baby or spoke to it ... She always put it on wet diapers though the nurse asked her to let her air them & so it often had stomach ache, then she gave it an empty bottle to suck only wind – No wonder it cried and was so unhappy *(quoted in Pollock, 1983, p. 218)*.

The nursemaid was subsequently dismissed.

Parents also felt considerable sorrow over the pain, illness and death of their children (Pollock, 1983). Shelley (1797–1851) commented in her diary when her baby was teething:

> Baby unwell. We are unhappy and discontented *(quoted in Pollock, 1983, p. 138)*.

Todd (1800–1875) was extremely distressed when his 14-month-old daughter was ill:

> I go to her bedside and gaze, and hear her short groans, as long as I can stay and then go away to weep *(quoted in Pollock, 1983, p. 131)*.

When the 18-month-old daughter of Jones (1755–1821) died, he wrote:

> What a gloom overspreads my soul! ... My Soul seems oppressed with a load, which no length of time will ever lighten. O my dear little infant, lying dead under this roof! whose spirit I watched departing yesterday *(quoted in Pollock, 1983, p. 138)*.

Sainte-Marthe (1594), who was the father that researched medical authorities to seek a cure for one of his children and then compiled his information in poetic form, wrote once that nothing was more distressing to a parent than the death of a child:

> Of all the misfortunes incident to humanity, none is so distressing to a feeling mind as the death of children. It is an affliction which preys upon the mind and increases with time. The longer time the sufferer has to reflect upon his loss, the more he thinks what his son, or daughter, might have been ... It is the only evil for which nature has not provided a remedy *(quoted in Hardyment, 1983, p. 8)*.

Unfortunately, diaries were not commonly available prior to the Renaissance and until this period there is little indication of whether parents used pain as an instrument of discipline or how parents felt about pain and suffering in their children. Without such documentation it is extremely difficult to have an accurate analysis of pain in childrearing practices. However, the documentation which does exist also reveals many parents whose concerns about their children were not unlike those of 20th century parents.

5. Summary

In ancient civilizations, concepts about pain were intertwined with beliefs about gods and demons. Over the centuries, however, there grew another interest in the physiological nature of pain but religious or mystical beliefs about pain have often remained in some form.

The difficulty of measuring and assessing the experience of pain in children has always bewildered those who were concerned about children's health. The cry of infants and children was usually relied on as an indicator of pain and disease though, until the 19th century, we do not have any record of other attempts to classify different types of cries with a specific cause. Teething pain has long been considered a serious problem and was discussed in virtually all pediatric texts, along with abdominal pain and colic.

Contrary to our popular assumption that childrearing practices in past centuries were characterized by indifference and brutality towards children with limited appreciation of the unique state of childhood, compassion and caring towards children are not a phenomenon specific to the 20th century. The ancient Egyptian papyri (Lesser Berlin Papyrus or Papyrus of Mother and Child, 16th century B.C. and the Ebers Papyrus 1553 or 1550 B.C.), the Hippocratic writings (5th and 4th centuries B.C.), the works by Galen (130–200 A.D.), Soranus (2nd century A.D.), Avicenna (980–1036 A.D.), Thomas Phaer (1546) and many others demonstrate concern about the needs of infants and children with an evident assumption that people cared about children and were concerned with the prevention and treatment of pain and disease. Similarly, after the Renaissance, when there is more extensive primary documentation from the diaries of parents, compassion and concern about children become even more evident. Both cruelty towards children with failure to understand and care for children as well as sensitivity, insight, and concern about the unique problems of pain in children are not limited to modern times but can be demonstrated in virtually all historical time periods.

References

Aries, P. (1962) (original in French 1960) Centuries of Childhood: A Social History of Family Life (Vintage Books, New York) pp. 9–128.

Bettmann, O.L. (1956) A Pictoral History of Medicine (Charles C. Thomas, Springfield, IL) pp. 1–13.

Bolling, R.W. (1930) Surgery of Childhood, Vol. XV, Clinical Pediatrics (Appleton, New York).

Brock, A.J. (1972) (reprinted from the original 1929) Greek Medicine (Dent, Toronto) pp. 212–228.

Campbell, M., Goettsch, E. and Lyttle, J.D. (1951) Clinical Pediatric Urology (Saunders, Philadelphia, PA, p. 957).

Cartwright, F. (1977) A Social History of Medicine (Longman, New York) pp. 10–15.

Casselberry, W.E. (1895) Diseases of the pharynx and the nasopharynx. In: L. Starr and T.S. Westcott (Eds.), An American Text-Book of the Diseases of Children (Saunders, Philadelphia, PA) pp. 431–456.

Castiglioni, A. (1975) A History of Medicine (Jason Aronson, New York) pp. 3–64.

Caton, D. (1985) The secularization of pain. Anesthesiology 62, 493–501.

Caulfield, E. (1943) Pediatric aspects of the Salem witchcraft tragedy: a lesson in mental health. Am. J. Dis. Child. 65, 788–802.

Chadwick, J. and Mann, W.N. (1950) The Medical Works of Hippocrates: A New Translation from the Original Greek Made Especially for English Readers (Blackwell Scientific Publications, Oxford) pp. 150–160.

Chapin, H.D. and Pisek, G.R. (1909) Diseases of Infants and Children (William Wood, New York) pp. 57–69, 191–210.

Collins, V.J. (1976) Principles of Anesthesiology (Lea and Fegiger, Philadelphia, PA) pp. 3–30.

DeMause, L. (1974) The evolution of childhood. In: L. DeMause (Ed.), The History of Childhood (The Psychohistory Press, New York) pp. 1–73.

Despert, J.L. (1965) The Emotionally Disturbed Child: Then and Now (Robert Brunner, New York) pp. 45–91.

Drake, T.G.H. (1933) Antiques of pediatric interest. J. Pediatr. 2, 347–348.

Foote, J. (1919) Ancient poems of infant hygiene. Ann. Med. Hist. 2, 213–227.

Friedman, A.P. (1972) The headache in history, literature and legend. Bull. N.Y. Acad. Med. 48, 661–681.

Fulop-Miller, R. (1938) (translated by Eden and Cedar Paul) Triumph over Pain (Literary Guild of America, New York) pp. 1–10.

Garrison, F.H. (1923) A System of Pediatrics, Vol. 1 (Saunders, Philadelphia, PA) pp. 1–61.

Griffith, E.F. (1951) Doctors by Themselves: An Anthology (Cassell, London) p. 127.

Gruner, O.C. (1930) A Treatise on the Canon of Medicine of Avicenna Incorporating a Translation of the First Book (Luzac, London) pp. 68–71, 158–160, 246–257, 279–280, 362–380, 526–530.

Haggard, H.W. (1929) Devils, Drugs and Doctors: The Story of the Science of Healing from Medicine-Man to Doctor (Heinemann, London) pp. 281–397.

Hardyment, C. (1983) Dream Babies: Child Care from Locke to Spock (Jonathan Cape, London) pp. 1–72.

Hess, A. (1849) On the necessity of practical instruction in the treatment of diseases of children. Lancet 10, 341.

Holt, L.E. (1897) The Diseases of Infancy and Childhood: For the Use of Students and Practitioners of Medicine (Appleton, New York) pp. 1–45.

Holt, L.E. (1908) The Care and Feeding of Children: A Catechism for the Use of Mothers and Children's Nurses, 4th edn. (Appleton, London).

Houlbrooke, R.A. (1984) The English Family 1450–1700 (Longman, New York) pp. 7, 132–165.

Hutchinson, R. (1906) Lectures on Diseases of Children (Edward Arnold, London) pp. 1–5.

Keele, K.D. (1962) Some historical concepts of pain. In: C.A. Keele and R. Smith (Eds.), Proc. Int. Symp. held under the auspices of University Federation for Animal Welfare (Middlesex Hospital, London). pp. 12–27.

Lewis, N. and Reinhold, M. (1966) Roman Civilization: Sourcebook II, The Empire (Harper and Row, New York).

Lisowski, F.P. (1967) Prehistoric and early historic trepanation. In: D. Brothwell and A.T. Sandison (Eds.), Diseases of Antiquity: A Survey of the Diseases, Injuries and Surgery of Early Populations (Charles T. Thomas, Springfield, IL) pp. 651–667.

Lyman, R.B. (1974) Barbarism and religion: late Roman and early medieval childhood. In: L. DeMause (Ed.), The History of Childhood (The Psychohistory Press, New York) pp. 75–100.

McFadden, C.J. (1947) Medical Ethics for Nurses (Davis, Philadelphia, PA) p. 121.

MacKinney, L. (1937) Early Medieval Medicine (Johns Hopkins Press, Baltimore, MD) pp. 1–35.

McLaughlin, M.M. (1974) Survivors and surrogates: children and parents from the ninth to the thirteenth centuries. In: L. DeMause (Ed.), The History of Childhood (The Psychohistory Press, New York) pp. 101–181.

Maino (1975) The Healing Hand (Harvard University Press, Cambridge) pp. 29–140.

Marshall, J. (1960) The Ethics of Medical Practice (Darton, Longman and Todd, London) pp. 51–52.

Meinecke, B. (1940) A quasi-autobiographical case history of an ancient Greek child. Bull. Hist. Med. 8, 1022–1031.

Mettler, C.C. and Mettler, F.A. (1947) History of Medicine (The Blakiston Co., Philadelphia, PA) pp. 691–788.

Ozment, S. (1983) When Fathers Ruled: Family Life in Reformation Europe (Harvard University Press, London) pp. 132–172.

Payne, G.H. (1916) The Child in Human Progress (Putnam, New York) pp. 1–50.

Pinchbeck, I. and Hewitt, M. (1969) Children in English Society, 1780–1880 (Routledge and Kegan Paul, London).

Pollock, L.A. (1983) Forgotten Children: Parent-Child Relations from 1500 to 1900 (Cambridge University Press, Cambridge) pp. 28–95, 143–271.

Procacci, P. and Maresca, M. (1984) Pain concept in western civilization: A historical review. In: C. Benedetti and C.R. Chapman (Eds.), Advances in Pain Research and Therapy, Vol. 7 (Raven Press, New York) pp. 1–11.

Radbill, S.X. (1965) Teething as a medical problem: Changing viewpoints through the centuries. Clin. Pediatr. 4, 556–559.

Rosenthal, R. (1936) The ancient Greece: with special reference to the pediatrics of Hippocrates. Minn. Med. 19, 524–534.

Ruhrah, J. (1925) Pediatrics of the Past (Paul B. Hoeber, New York) pp. 28–555.

Seibert, H. (1940) The progress of ideas regarding the causation and control of infant mortality. Bull. Hist. Med. 8, 546–599.

Shorter, E. (1975) The Making of the Modern Family (Basic Books, New York).

Sigerist, H.E. (1970) (originally published in 1932 by W.W. Norton) Man and Medicine: an Introduction to Medical Knowledge (McGrath, Maryland) pp. 76–94.

Starr, L. (1895) The clinical investigation of disease and the general management of children. In: L. Starr and T.S. Westcott (Eds.), An American Text-Book of the Diseases of Children (Saunders, Philadelphia, PA) pp. 3–4.

Still, G.F. (1931) The History of Pediatrics: The Progress of the Study of Diseases of Children up to the End of the XVIIIth Century (Oxford University Press, London) pp. 1–322.

Stone, L. (1977) The Family, Sex and Marriage: In England 1500–1800 (Weidenfeld and Nicolson, London) pp. 75–81, 405–478, 208–215.

Thorek, M. (1938) Modern surgical technique, Vol. III (Lippincott, Montreal) pp. 2021.

Todd, E.M. (1985) Pain: Historical perspectives. In: G.M. Aronoff (Ed.), Evaluation and Treatment of Chronic Pain (Urban and Schwarzenberg, Baltimore, MD) pp. 1–16.

Wallerstein, E. (1980) Circumcision: An American Health Fallacy (Springer, New York) pp. 1–50.

Wharton, H.R. (1895) Tracheotomy. In: L. Starr and T.S. Westcott (Eds.), An American Text-Book of the Diseases of Children (Saunders, Philadelphia, PA) pp. 290–310.

CHAPTER 2

The nature of pain

1. Introduction

This chapter will first review the definition of pain and the implications of this definition for pain research. We shall examine the anatomical and physiological basis of pain and we will then discuss the gate control theory of pain. A brief review of the endogenous opioids will follow. The relationship between the biochemistry of pain and the physiology of pain will end this section on the physical substrate of pain. Of necessity, because of the complexity of the area and the rapidly expanding knowledge base, our discussion will be brief and simplified. We will then focus on developmental and psychosocial influences on pain.

2. Definition of pain

Although pain has always been part of the human experience it was less than 10 years ago that an international group of scientists and practitioners in the area of pain, the International Association for the Study of Pain, agreed on a common definition of pain and pain-related terms. Common definitions are the building blocks of scientific communication and the recent development of such definitions demonstrates the recency of widespread scientific interest in pain. The official IASP definition of pain is:

> Pain is an unpleasant sensory and emotional experience associated with actual or potential tissue damage, or described in terms of such damage.
> *Note*: Pain is always subjective. Each individual learns the application of the word through experiences related to injury in early life *(Merskey, 1986, p. S217)*.

The key issue in this definition is that pain is both a sensory and an emotional experience. It is now unequivocally acknowledged that pain does not bear an invariate relationship to injury and that emotional factors have a dramatic effect on modulating the pain that is experienced.

The fact that pain is always subjective presents difficulty for those who work in the area of childhood pain. The most direct way of tapping subjective experience is through self-report. Pain in the prelingual child cannot be accessed in that way and only second-order, indirect methods such as observing the child's behavior and recording physiological or biochemical changes are available.

The IASP definition also highlights the fact that learning about pain and how to respond to painful situations occurs during childhood. The note accompanying the definition goes on to say that if a person reports pain, even in the absence of any tissue damage or the likelihood of tissue damage, that person's statement should be accepted. This is particularly important with children because adults tend to behave as if children are less credible or less accurate in reporting their pain.

3. Neuroanatomy of pain

The scientific investigation of the nature of pain resulted in increasing our knowledge of the anatomical and physiological basis of pain transmission. The receptors of pain in the skin are primarily, but by no means limited, to high threshold mechanoreceptors (HTMs) and polymodal nociceptors (PMNs) (Lynn, 1984). HTMs accelerate the rate of firing in small myelinated (Aδ) fibers. They are responsive to strong pressure and have a relatively large receptive field. The signal from PMNs are conducted along slower conducting unmyelinated C fibers, responding to pressure, heat, and chemical irritation. They primarily have a small receptive field. Much less is known about nociceptors in viscera, muscles, joints, mucous membranes, cornea and teeth but there appears to be some specialization (Fitzgerald, 1984). For example, from the heart there are fine, mostly unmyelinated fibers, signalling ischemia.

The sensory nerves from the receptors enter the spinal column through the dorsal roots and separate into A and C fiber bundles. Many of the fibers bifurcate and both ascend and descend terminating in the dorsal horn, principally in lamina 1 and 2 (substantia gelatinosa). Cells in each lamina give off dendrites which always extend into neighboring or even into more distant laminae where they may contact axons from the periphery and from other cells (Wall, 1984). From the dorsal horn a number of parallel ascending pathways including the spinothalamic, spinoreticular, spinomesencephalic, spinocervical and second-order dorsal column tracts ascend ipsilaterally and contralaterally to the thalamus, reticular formation, periaqueductal grey, superior colliculus, and the intercollicular nucleus. Projections then occur to the cortex and to the limbic system. Throughout, there are collateral pathways and connections providing a complex, rich, overlapping and redundant information system (Willis, 1984).

Examination of the neural basis of pain has generated a number of theories. The early theories of pain were concerned with intensity and postulated that pain was the result of overstimulation of any one of the senses. Some of these theorists hypothesized the existence of switching mechanisms that channelled strong impulses into one part of the brain or other. Other theorists suggested that highly specialized receptors were responsible for pain. As the scientific evidence expanded, these early theories were replaced by more sophisticated accounts. Melzack and Wall (1965) formulated the gate control theory in an attempt to account for the many conflicting observations about pain. The theory has been one of the most productive theories in medicine and although there have been critics of the gate control theory, none have been able to propose a theory that better accounts for the data.

4. Gate control theory

The gate control theory is based on observation of the response to acute sudden events stimulating the skin. It is clear that, as well, there are slow onset modulating mechanisms that are important in clinical pain and other mechanisms when one considers non-cutaneous, deep tissue pain.

Basically, the theory (Melzack and Wall, 1965, 1982; Wall, 1984) proposes that a neural mechanism, primarily located in the substantia gelatinosa layer in the dorsal horns of the spinal cord, acts as a gate to increase or decrease the flow of nerve impulses from the receptors via peripheral fibers to the central nervous system. As is represented in the diagram (Fig. 1) the substantia gelatinosa receives axons directly and indirectly from both large diameter and small diameter fibers. As well, the dendrites of cells in deeper laminae project into the substantia gelatinosa. Cells in the substantia gelatinosa interconnect and influence each other via the Lissauer's tract on the same side and by means of commisural fibers that cross the cord. The gating is usually thought to be presynaptic but postsynaptic gating also occurs. The spinal gating is influenced by the relative amount of activity in the large diameter and small diameter fibers. Inputs from afferents signalling innocuous events carried by

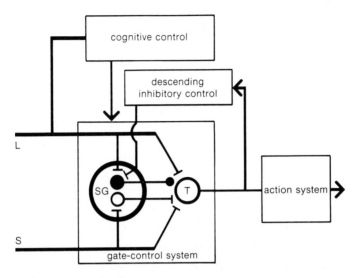

Fig. 1. The gate control theory: Mark II. The new model includes excitatory (white circle) and inhibitory (black circle) links from the substantia gelatinosa (SG) to the transmission (T) cells as well as descending inhibitory control from brainstem systems. The round knob at the end of the inhibitory link implies that its action may be presynaptic, postsynaptic, or both. All connections are excitatory, except the inhibitory link from SG to T cell. (Reprinted with permission of the authors and the publisher from Melzack and Wall, 1982, p. 235).

large myelinated fibers (Aß fibers) activate inhibitory interneurons that block the input from the classic nociceptors to the spinal cord transmission (T) cells.

Descending control of the gate has received particular attention in the past few years. There are multiple systems that may be important in this process. These include central cognitive mechanisms such as attention, anxiety, anticipation and past experience. Such brain inputs, as well as direct brain stimulation, produce descending messages transmitted by large diameter rapidly conducting fibers (the central control trigger) that produce relative analgesia. Their transmission may be, in part, mediated by the endorphin system. Non-opioid systems also are operative. When the output of the spinal cord transmission cells exceeds a threshold, the action system is activated and pain is experienced.

The gate control theory accounts for and was the direct impetus for the development of a number of pain control techniques including transcutaneous electrical nerve stimulation (Wall and Sweet, 1967), dorsal column stimulation (Krainick and Thoden, 1984) and brain stimulation (Turnbull,

1984). The theory also has proved a physiological explanation for the psychological factors that have a major influence on pain.

5. Endogenous opioids

The opioids, beginning with opium, have, for centuries, been used in pain relief. Thus it was not surprising that the isolation of an endogenous opioid peptide from the pig brain (Hughes et al., 1975) triggered a great deal of interest. Although some of the initial hope for new non-addictive opioid analgesics appears now not to be realized, the endogenous opioids have generated a great deal of scientific and popular excitement.

At least 18 active opioid peptides (Woolf and Wall, 1983) in three distinct families have been identified. The enkephalins, the endorphins and the dynorphins each derive from precursor polypeptides and have distinct distribution patterns. The different families of opioid peptides have different affinities for binding with the four major categories of receptors: μ (mu), κ (kappa), δ (delta), and σ (sigma) (Jaffe and Martin, 1985). The general, but oversimplified, view is that analgesia is mediated through μ receptors (Terenius, 1984). The substantia gelatinosa, the periaqueductal grey and the rostral ventromedial medulla are thought to be the major sites of action of the endorphin-mediated analgesia system (Terenius, 1984) but the peripheral nerve endings and the higher centers of the limbic system and cortex have also been implicated (Millan, 1986). It is clear that the endorphin-mediated analgesia system is not the only system and there appear to be several different endorphin-mediated systems (Fields and Basbaum, 1984; Millan, 1986). Systemically administered opioids are thought to act by mimicking the actions of the endorphins at synapses.

The relationship between the endogenous opioids and the neurotransmission of pain impulses is not clear. Areas such as the midline nuclei of the brainstem and the substantia gelatinosa are richly endowed with endogenous opioid receptors and respond to locally administered opioids by producing analgesia. Moreover, naloxone, an opiate receptor antagonist, does block the analgesic action of opioids. Woolf and Wall (1983) have suggested that the endogenous opioids do not function as classical neurotransmitters but in a more subtle and longer lasting manner.

The role of these peptides in pain is not clear and the field is, at this time, rife with contradictory data (Woolf and Wall, 1983). Indeed a recent review of the endogenous opioids concluded:

> ...to formulate the question 'what is the role of opioids in the control of pain' may seem legitimate but is probably so over-simplified as to be dangerously misleading if not actually meaningless *(Millan, 1986, p. 333)*.

No clinically useful results have yet been generated from this research. However, research on the endogenous opioids has led to advances in the understanding of the action of the opioids (Jaffe and Martin, 1985) and in beginning to detail the mechanism of descending control of pain (Fields and Basbaum, 1984). There are hopes for specific new analgesic drugs based on the endogenous opioid peptides (Terenius, 1984).

6. Congenital insensitivity to pain

Since virtually everyone feels pain, the total absence of the ability to feel pain in spite of intact physiology is fascinating. Sternbach (1968) has provided one of the most thoughtful discussions of this syndrome which is most accurately termed congenital universal insensitivity to pain (McMurray, 1955). The syndrome is extraordinarily rare and must be distinguished from indifference to pain that may be secondary to psychosis or retardation and from insensitivity due to known lesions or neuropathy. Sternbach (1968) noted that the disorder might provide insight into three questions: 'Does pain enhance the probability of survival?'; 'Is a pain sense needed for normal personality development?'; and finally 'How does the syndrome enhance our understanding of the mechanism of pain?'. Sternbach (1968) carefully reviewed the documented cases and concluded that serious injury and in some cases, premature death resulted from insensitivity. Sternbach (1968) also noted that although personality problems did occur in some cases, normal development was possible without a sense of pain. The variability of the patients with congenital insensitivity to pain suggests that the defect can occur at several different points and that there is not one pain center whose altered function would eliminate pain.

7. Developmental factors

The sensation of pain is subjective. It is extremely variable between individuals and even within one individual and may be influenced by a variety of factors such as personality characteristics, family responses to pain, cultural attitudes towards pain, past pain experiences, circumstances at the time of tissue damage, amount of tissue damage, absence or presence of chronic intractable pain, reinforcement of pain behavior through treats or excessive sympathy, and personal coping mechanisms (Craig, 1983). In infancy and childhood, additional considerations such as changes in threshold and tolerance, individual differences in responses to pain, memory for pain, perceptions of pain, symptom reporting and the use of coping strategies occur as the child develops.

7.1 Threshold and tolerance

Pain threshold refers to the point at which a stimulus is first experienced as painful whereas pain tolerance is the point at which the painful stimulus can no longer be endured (Wolff, 1983). Experimentally, pain threshold is usually correlated with physiological measures of the sensory components of pain. In contrast, pain tolerance is generally correlated with psychological variables related to the affective aspects of pain (Wolff, 1983). Pain threshold and tolerance are indirect measures of pain as emphasis is on the stimulus rather than on the response. Pain is, of course, not a stimulus but a response. Returning to the IASP definition we note that 'pain is an unpleasant sensory and emotional experience'. Pain tolerance has limited usefulness as a clinical construct as there is usually no option for stopping clinical pain. However, by analogy, vigorous attempts at escape may be seen as pain tolerance.

The concepts of threshold and tolerance are relevant to two assumptions that have been made about children's pain, (1) neonates do not feel pain, and (2) infants and children have high tolerance for pain and tolerate pain well (Swafford and Allen, 1968). We will consider each in turn.

7.1.1. Do neonates feel pain?

Two lines of evidence can be brought to bear on the first assumption that neonates do not feel pain. The first line of evidence is indirect, deriving from physiological data and, by analogy, from arguments about the value of the pain response to survival of the species. Direct evidence is derived from infants' responses to specific noxious stimuli. There is little systematic data on the functional maturity of human neonatal physiology because of ethical constraints. However, it appears that the neonate's spinal cord is intact and the pain receptors are present. Myelinization is not complete in the neonate and this had been used as evidence for the notion that neonates do not feel pain but react in a simply reflexive way (McGraw, 1941). There is some question as to whether or not the intricate interconnections from pain receptors to the 'gate' in the substantia gelatinosa are complete. The neonate's motor ability to respond to pain also appears to be limited. It is clear that, at least in animals, there are significant physiological developments related to pain after birth. For example, although C fibers appear to be anatomically and neurochemically developed in young rat pups, it is not until the second 10 days of life that functional integrity is obtained (Fitzgerald and Gibson, 1984). In a similar vein, Fitzgerald and Kotzenburg (1986) have shown that the descending inhibitory pathways in the rat that are thought to inhibit response to nociception become functional only between the 9th and 22nd day of life. The lack of inhibitory mechanism may mean that immature pups are more sensitive than their more developed brethren.

The evidence from physiology is unclear. The literature does provide evidence that the neonatal pain neuroanatomy is not fully developed and that there is postnatal development of the pain system.

Bondy (1980) has argued that in the first weeks of life a high threshold to painful stimuli would be adaptive in protecting the infant from the pain of the birth process. On the other hand, an ability to perceive pain and to cry would serve as a signalling system to the parent and would likely preserve the helpless infant from harm.

There is now growing evidence that while the physiological and affective responses to pain are subject to developmental changes, infants do experience pain. The relevant studies are discussed in more detail in chapter 3 on the measurement and assessment of pain, but are briefly summarized here.

Until recently it was thought that young infants responded to a painful stimulus such as a pinprick by a whole body motor response and only weeks or months later developed a localized motoric response withdrawing primarily the affected body part (McGraw, 1941; Barr, 1983). At first glance, it appears that newborns do not have the motoric ability to respond other than with generalized movement in response to any stimulus including pain. Recent research has described the pain response of neonates in much more detail. Grunau and Craig (1987) studied response to heel lance in 77 male and 63 female neonates from the well-baby unit of a major metropolitan hospital. The babies were all healthy and uncircumcised and averaged 43.05 h of age. The authors found that the facial response was dependent on the sleep/wake state of the infant and that facial activity was a reliable measure with 'taut tongue' and 'vertical stretch mouth' being particularly sensitive to state differences. There were also significant differences in response to the various technicians administering the heel lance. In a similar study, Franck (1986) used photogrammetric techniques to evaluate the response to heel lance in ten infants at 4 h of age. She found active avoidance of the stimulus by all infants and seven of the infants used the unaffected leg to swipe at the site of the heel lance. Thus, when the appropriate measures are taken, neonates do appear to react to noxious stimuli in a way that is seen by observers as pain.

The research by Grunau and Craig (1987) is important because it demonstrates that, in keeping with the gate control theory of pain, the pain response of neonates at 2 days of age is not simply a total response to insult. It is a complex response that is altered by ongoing events. Moreover, it is evident that the neonates responded to variations in handling. As well, Franck's (1986) study demonstrated that the neonate actively responds and is not simply reactive to the heel lance.

Infants respond to a sudden painful stimulus such as a pinprick with a pain cry as well as with facial and body movements. Although there is some debate whether there is a specific pain cry (see chapter 3), there is no debate that most babies cry. In general, the pain cry is long and loud, has a sudden onset without any preliminary moaning. It is usually followed by breath holding and then a period of rhythmic bouts of crying (Murray, 1979).

There are physiological responses to pain by neonates. Heart rate and pO_2 have been clearly documented to change in response to circumcision and heel prick (e.g., Williamson and Williamson, 1983; Owens and Todt, 1984).

Finally, there are hormonal and metabolic responses to surgery by neonates (Anand and Aynsley-Green, 1985, 1987; Anand et al., 1987a,b) which may, in part, be due to pain. Plasma epinephrine, plasma norepinephrine, plasma insulin, plasma glucagon, and plasma cortisol responses as well as changes in blood glucose, lactate, pyruvate, and alanine were each related to the severity of the surgical stress as measured by a 5 factor stress score (Anand and Aynsley-Green, 1987).

If full-term infants feel pain the next question is: 'Do preterm neonates feel pain?' The clinical impression is that many preterm infants do not respond to pain (D'Apolito, 1984). However, Field and Goldson (1984) found behavioral and physiological reactivity to heel prick in premature neonates in minimal care and in an intensive care unit. As well, Anand and Aynsley-Green (1985) and Anand et al. (1987a) found that premature neonates did mount a stress response to surgery. Finally, we have found that neonatal nurses believe their premature patients feel pain and they suggest that many procedures in the neonatal intensive care unit cause pain (McGrath et al., 1987). Although scant, the evidence does suggest pain perception in preterm neonates.

Children beyond infancy certainly feel pain but little is known about possible developmental changes in pain threshold. Haslam (1969) examined the relationship between age and the perception of pain or pain threshold in 115 children aged 5–18 years. Her results indicated that pain threshold increased with age so that younger children were more sensitive to pain.

In summary, the indirect evidence is equivocal but if one considers the more direct evidence including behavioral, physiological and endocrine response to presumably painful stimuli, there can be little doubt that neonates feel what we call pain. The burden of proof has now shifted so that it is incumbent on anyone who would argue that neonates do not feel pain to prove their assertion (Owens, 1986). The responsivity of premature infants has not been sufficiently studied to make definitive statements but our best guess is that they too feel pain.

7.1.2. Do children tolerate pain well?

The major evidence that children tolerate pain well is based on clinical observations that following surgery children are often out of their beds playing at a time when adults receiving similar surgery are immobilized by pain.

There is little data bearing on the belief that pain following surgery is less in younger children. However, Leikin (1986) in a study of 127 children between 9 and 14 years, who were undergoing tonsillectomy and adenoidectomy, found that younger children reported fewer symptoms and were perceived by their parents to have fewer symptoms than did older children. We believe the observation that children are more active after surgery than adults. Our opinion is that there may be age differences from infancy to late adolescence in the degree of postsurgery activity and perhaps in postsurgical pain.

Age differences in pain following surgery may be due to differences in the physiological response to the trauma of surgery and the greater physical resiliency of younger children. On the other hand, age differences may be due to age-related variations in pain tolerance. Differences in pain tolerance, if they exist, may be due to physiological differences or to differences in learning. Craig's extensive laboratory data with adults (e.g., Craig, 1983) has clearly shown that pain tolerance can be altered by social learning. It is possible that with increasing age children learn to alter their behavior and to complain with pain.

7.2. Individual differences

Even in early infancy, there are individual differences in children's responses to painful stimuli (Johnston and Strada, 1986; Grunau and Craig, 1987). It has been suggested that these differences are based on temperamental variations (Craig, 1980). However, no research has directly examined that question. Nor has research related the response to a painful stimulus at one time to the response at another time (reliability over time). There are no clear sex differences in the neonate's response to pain. Owens and Todt (1984) found no sex difference in response to heel lance, while Grunau and Craig (1987) found that males showed a more rapid facial response and cry to heel lance.

7.3. Memory for pain

Memory of painful experiences is most often conceptualized as the occurrence of anticipatory or apprehensive behavior to an approaching painful stimulus (Barr, 1983). A white lab coat, an approaching needle, or physical restraint may incite anticipatory pain behavior such as fussing, crying or withdrawal. Anticipatory behavior will vary from none, to exploratory activity to defensive or withdrawal behavior (Barr, 1983).

Defensive behavior such as fighting, crying, and temper tantrums in anticipation to a painful stimulus are observed to occur more frequently from the age of 6 months to 2 or 3 years of age and then such behaviors decrease (Kassowitz, 1958). Prior to 6 months of age such behavior is not obvious (Levy, 1960).

The failure to find memory for pain prior to about 6 months of age may be due to the failure to use appropriate methodology. Memory for pain in infants has been investigated using a classical conditioning paradigm in which a heel rub was paired with heel lance (Owens and Todt, 1984). No evidence for conditioning was found. However, in Franck's (1986) study, latency of withdrawal was shorter in those infants undergoing a second heel lance. This could be a learning phenomenon or it could be due to changes in state or physiology due to the first heel lance.

More work in this area needs to be done. Perhaps one trial learning is not sufficient to produce learning; perhaps the measurement of the conditioned response should include a more sensitive indicator such as facial response (Grunau and Craig, 1987) as well as physiological responses.

Questions concerning the development of memory for pain and the contribution of past pain experiences to later learning of pain-coping strategies are especially significant in managing clinical pain problems. The assumption that infants do not learn from past painful experiences, we believe, contributes to the tendency to undermedicate infants. The long-term effect such undermedication has on the learning of coping strategies in response to painful events warrants further investigation. It may be that children who are not given appropriate analgesics have a greater tendency to cope poorly with later pain. The concern is that patterns of feelings of helplessness and hopelessness engendered by early uncontrolled pain may contribute to later feelings of helplessness and poor coping (Seligman, 1975).

7.4. Perceptions of the meaning of pain

Young children's perceptions of the meaning of pain are dependent both on their level of cognitive ability and on their experiences of pain.

A recent investigation of children's pain has found that children's perceptions of pain are consistent with Piagetian stages (Gaffney and Dunne, 1986, 1987).

Piaget and Inhelder (1969) described children from about the age of 2 years to 7 years as being in the preoperational stage of cognitive development.

Children of this age tend to perceive their world concretely in terms of what they are able to see, touch or manipulate and not by verbal and more abstract thinking. Egocentric thinking occurs when children conceptualize the world primarily from their own perspective. The child will have absolute and total belief in his own perception of events and therefore does not check for errors in his logic (Gaffney and Dunne, 1987). Such thinking makes it difficult for the child to perceive that a painful procedure may be of benefit to his or her health because the child is concerned only with the fact that the event caused pain. Children's reasoning is also transductive, meaning that children will put two events together without defining their causal relationship, so that cause and effect may be interchangeable (Gaffney and Dunne, 1987). For example, a child may go to the doctor's office for a vaccination and then believe when she goes to the same office because she is ill that she will get a needle. Gaffney and Dunne (1987) investigated the developmental progression of children's perceptions of pain in 680 children aged 5–14 years. There were over 30 children of each sex for each age. Children were given a ten item sentence completion task which was designed to elicit children's ideas about pain such as definitions, causes, effects, cures, descriptions and location of pain. The resultant responses could be categorized into 12 different groups related to the causation of pain. They were (1) illness, sickness, or disease, (2) malfunction, that is something was wrong, (3) trauma, (4) transgression involving eating, (5) transgression involving other activities, (6) transgression of adult rules or carelessness, (7) health risk behaviors (such as smoking), (8) transgressions with the implication of punishment, (9) psychological factors (such as nervousness), (10) need states (such as hunger), (11) physiological explanations (for example pain as a warning of something else), and (12) contamination (getting pain from germs). The results of this study were that almost half of the children explained the causation of pain by referring to transgressions or some form of self-causality. Secondly, as anticipated from Piagetian concepts, objective and abstract explanations of pain increased with age. Only one sex difference was found. Girls referred more often to psychological factors as causes of pain.

Similarly, Gaffney and Dunne (1986) used Piaget's three stages of cognitive development (preoperational, concrete operational, and formal operational) to examine developmental changes in these same children's definitions of pain. They concluded that the responses of the children could be categorized into three developmental groups (preoperational, concrete operations and formal operations) and that an age difference could be demonstrated.

Children in the preoperational age group were more likely to attend to perceptually dominant features of a painful experience. They were more likely to define pain as something in the tummy or the head, or as something that hurts. They did not perceive a relationship between pain and illness or think of pain as a symptom of something more serious (Gaffney and Dunne, 1986).

Children of the concrete operational stage retained some of the perceptions of pain which characterized the preoperational period but they began to use more generalized and abstract conceptualizations and thus were capable of forming analogies or mentioning the psychological effects of pain. They would discuss pain as inside them or in a part of the body instead of referring to a specific location. They might mention that pain made one feel unhappy, miserable, or feel like crying (Gaffney and Dunne, 1986).

In the formal operational stage, children had developed an ability for introspection with more abstract thinking enabling them to define pain in physical, psychological and/or psychosocial terms.

Gaffney and Dunne (1986) also noted that there was an overlap between the stages of pain definitions consistent with Piaget's theory. There was no sudden change in a child's perception of pain. Instead, the definition of pain had a gradual development of increasingly more complex and abstract ideas of pain while also retaining some definitions more characteristic of a younger age group. This may explain why children regress in their perceptions of pain when they are stressed by pain or illness.

However, an earlier study by Ross and Ross (1984) came to different conclusions from those of Gaffney and Dunne (1986, 1987). Ross and Ross (1984) studied 994 children aged 5–12 years using semi-structured interviews. They found no age or sex differences regarding pain concepts, definitions of pain, causality of pain or the usefulness of pain as warning signal. Contrary to the expectation that younger children would have attributed some pain to punishment for misbehavior there was scarcely any evidence of such a perception. About 70% of the sample were able to give descriptions of pain using single descriptors such as stabbing, or agonizing as well as whole sentences. 99% of the children felt that what helped them most when they had pain was to have a parent present.

Unfortunately, the studies by Gaffney and Dunne (1986, 1987) and Ross and Ross (1984) suffer from the problems inherent in a retrospective survey. Time may alter one's perceptions of events. Responses to a survey may not adequately reflect behavior in actual pain situations.

7.5. Symptom reporting

Symptom reporting refers to the tendency to be aware of and to report internal physiological states. A child who falls and scrapes her knee might be said to be a relative under-reporter if she ignored the scrape and continued playing. Similarly, a child who gently bumps into a protruding table and cries and spends the next half day in distress, searching for a bruise, would be deemed to be an over-reporter. Although pain is only one symptom that can be reported, it is believed that the tendency to report symptoms is a general predisposition rather than highly specific to one symptom or the other. It is obvious that different people perceive the same symptom in different ways, but our understanding of how symptoms are perceived is limited.

Pennebaker (1982) has most comprehensively discussed the extant literature on symptom reporting but only a few studies pertain to children. Children's willingness to report symptoms by interview was examined by Gochman (1971). He found that the children, who saw themselves as vulnerable and had less control over their lives, were more willing to report symptoms and said they would more likely use medical services. Lewis and Lewis (1982) found that 8–12% of children made over 50% of the visits to a school health service that was available at the child's initiative. Highest visitation was by girls, first borns and children of lower socioeconomic class.

The most impressive data in the area is from Mechanic's 16 year longitudinal study of 350 mother-child dyads (Mechanic, 1980, 1983) examining symptom reporting at the fourth grade and at the eighth grade and again 16 years later. The most frequently reported symptoms were headaches, congested or stuffy nose, muscular aches and pains, coughs and indigestion. Mechanic found that the best prospective predictors of young adults' symptom reporting were the number of family problems reported by the mother, her own report of symptoms such as indigestion, nervousness, headaches, allergies and depression, the number of days the child missed from school and the teacher's report of how stoical the child was. Retrospectively reported negative parental behavior, such as not talking to the child when the child had upset the parent, yelling or shouting at the child, making the child feel guilty and insulting the child were related to greater report of symptoms. These variables were retrospectively collected at the same time as the follow-up and thus must be regarded with caution.

Mechanic (1983) suggested that introspectiveness is the major psychological mechanism mediating symptom reporting. He argued that family problems, psychologically abusive parents, and school absences are important in that they create a climate in which the child's attention is focussed on internal states. He noted that across a number of studies the tendency to pay attention to inner states increases the reporting of symptoms, distress and medical utilization. Mechanic (1983) noted that although there are large cultural and individual differences in introspectiveness and attentiveness to bodily sensations, little is known about how such differences develop.

7.6. Coping strategies

Although we have some evidence that teaching coping strategies to children is helpful in assisting children with painful medical procedures (see for example chapter 10 on cancer pain) and coping with painful syndromes (see chapter 8 on headache), we have little information about the nature of coping strategies children use spontaneously when they are confronted by stressful or painful situations.

Brown et al. (1986) studied 487 children aged 8–18 years (52% female, 43% male and 5% unspecified) from ten different schools to determine the kind of spontaneous coping strategies children in stressful or painful situations used. Children were asked to complete the State-Trait Anxiety Inventory (Spielberger 1970), either the children's version (subjects aged 8–13) or the adult form (subjects aged 14–18). The children were then asked to respond in writing to a cognitive questionnaire, about getting an injection at the dentist, giving a class report and a personal stressful event. For our purposes, we are interested in the responses to the dental situation.

Brown et al. (1986) referred to two possible types of responses, those that reflected coping strategies and those that tended to exaggerate the negative characteristics of the situation which the authors referred to as catastrophizing.

The coping strategies used spontaneously by the children were: (1) positive self-talk (I can take this), (2) attention diversion by thinking of something else or listening to music, (3) relaxation, or (4) thought stopping. Thirty-seven percent of the children were judged to be copers in this situation. Positive self-talk was used most often by all age groups but its frequency of use also increased with age. Thought stopping was used infrequently by all ages. The number of strategies children used to cope with dental pain and the number of copers increased with age.

Catastrophizing strategies were: (1) focusing on negative aspects of the dental situation (I'm afraid; This hurts, I hate shots), (2) thoughts of escape or avoidance (I want to run away), (3) concerns about an unlikely consequence (Will I bleed all over the place?), and (4) concern about the dentist (What if he's a meany?) or negative feelings towards the dentist (I hate him). The most common type of catastrophizing for all ages was dwelling on negative aspects of the dental situation. None of the four types increased or decreased with age.

Children were identified as copers or catastrophizers based on their responses on two of the three situations. Copers for all age ranges reported less anxiety than catastrophizers. Although coping increased with age, 79% of children aged 8–9 years and 54% of children aged 16–18 years were judged as catastrophizers.

There are several methodological problems with this study. The method was a written response to the questionnaire which was administered by the classroom teacher. It is unknown whether children would have responded in the way indicated in their responses when faced with the actual situation. For example, in this study, only 37% of children were judged to be copers in the dental situation. Research examining actual behavior of unselected children in routine dental examination and treatment has found a very low rate of disruptive behavior indicating that most children cope quite well in this situation (Zachary et al., 1985). This study also relies on children's recall of past pain experiences as well as projection of how they might respond in the future. The most accurate representation of children's coping strategies would be a study conducted at the time of a stressful or painful procedure. Another difficulty is that an injection at the dentist and giving a class report are infrequent stressful situations for which the child may not have had sufficient opportunity to develop a coping strategy.

However, Ross and Ross (1984) reported results similar to Brown et al. (1986), finding that only 213 of 994 children reported use of self-initiated coping strategies. Distraction and physical activity, such as clenching the fists, were used most frequently with thought stopping, relaxation/imagery and fantasy being used by a small group. This issue of a low rate of self-initiated or spontaneous coping strategies in children found in both studies raises important issues for pain management in clinical situations. Further research on spontaneous coping strategies during painful procedures would be illuminating.

8. Psychosocial factors

8.1. Familial

The role of the family in causing or maintaining pain especially chronic intractable pain has long been of interest to clinicians and researchers but it has been extremely difficult to determine this role. Variables such as the size of the family, patient's position in the sibship, socioeconomic status of the family, relationship with parents, early experiences of abuse, incidence of pain and illness, similarity between the location of pain in more than one family member, and depression have all been of interest to researchers but have provided conflicting results (Payne and Norfleet, 1986).

There have been two significant problems in much of this research. One is the varying definitions of chronic pain which has hindered the comparability of results of different studies. The second problem is the tendency to assume that chronic pain, which does not respond to traditional medical or surgical intervention, is psychogenic pain (for example see review by Payne and Norfleet, 1986) and therefore the family with a chronic pain patient is a psychosomatic family. Unfortunately, there has been limited recognition that chronic pain may be physical, psychological or a combination of both, and that in each case, familial factors may be involved in maintaining pain expression including non-coping pain behavior. We will discuss this problem further in chapter 13 on chronic intractable pain and chapter 14 on psychogenic pain.

Of primary interest to us in examining the role of the family on pain expression in children is the influence of family members on the child's learning of coping or non-coping behavior in response to acute or chronic intractable pain. For our purposes, a social learning model provides some insight of how members of a family, who are highly significant to each other, teach each other how to respond to painful experiences. We are specifically concerned with how children learn about pain from their family.

This process has been discussed by Craig (1983). Attention to observed painful events, memory for painful stimuli, motivation and sufficient motor skills to reproduce observed behavior are all necessary elements of a child's learning about pain from the family. It is impossible for learning to occur without the child being able to attend to the event. Experiences of pain by others, however, readily draw attention and therefore facilitate a child's learning about what causes pain, how others react to pain and what the consequences of the reaction may be. Such observations are integrated with the child's own experiences with painful events. Observing a painful event experienced by others cannot result in learning unless the child has the ability to remember both what he has observed and what he himself has experienced in similar painful experiences.

The child must also be able to repeat the behavior he has seen and remembers seeing other people use when he has pain. If the child observes significant people in his or her life showing frequent displays of verbal or non-verbal expressions of pain, overreacting to minimal pain or having difficulty obtaining pain relief with resultant feelings of anger and depression, then the child is more vulnerable to learning non-coping pain behavior. For example, the child may pay considerable attention to bodily states, interpret various sensations as pain related, complain or use other illness behavior when experiencing minimal distress, succeed in getting others to give substantial attention or release from the usual expectations and responsibilities, or obtain special privileges for incidences of minimal pain and discomfort.

Although such learning is especially significant for children who frequently learn about their world by observation with imitation and rehearsal, there are virtually no studies which have been concerned with the way in which the family teaches the child coping or non-coping behavior.

The research on family influences on pain is primarily anecdotal, retrospective and focussed on adults. We will discuss family influences in different pain disorders in the following chapters.

A number of studies have looked at pain generically. For example, Edwards et al. (1985) had 128 male and 168 female college students report their experience of pain and the presence of other people with pain in the students' families. The number of pain models was significantly correlated ($r = 0.315$) with the frequency of currently experienced pain. Females tended to model specific pain locations whereas males did not.

Sternbach (1986), in his summary of an American epidemiologic study of pain, reported that there were generational effects. Adults who reported that their parents had suffered from severe pain at some time were more likely themselves to have back pain, muscle pain and joint pain.

No studies have yet overcome the problems of retrospective report and the possibility that individuals with pain may remember relatives with pain better than pain-free individuals. Moreover, some pain problems such as migraine have a genetic component which is difficult to separate from learning factors.

8.2. Cultural

The culture of the family also has an impact on how family members will learn to respond to pain and illness. Culture has an important role in determining whether private pain will be expressed by public pain behavior, what the nature of such behavior will be and where it will take place (Helman, 1984).

Unfortunately, there has been little research of the role of culture in determining pain behavior and the majority of the research concerns adults. However, cultural pain differences among adults could be expected to be transmitted to the children of the culture.

Zborowski (1952) compared attitudes towards pain in three cultural groups from New York City by interviewing patients, doctors, nurses, other health professionals as well as some healthy individuals from each of the cultural groups. The cultural groups were Italian-Americans, Jewish-Americans and Old-Americans. Italians were preoccupied with the sensation of pain and complained a great deal while they were in pain with moaning and crying but once the pain was treated they resumed their normal activities. On the other hand, Jewish patients were also very emotional when in pain and also tended to exaggerate pain symptoms. However, they worried more about the effect of the pain on their health and the overall welfare of their families than about the pain itself. At times, they had difficulty resuming their normal activities because of a preoccupation with the underlying cause of their pain. The Old-American patients were more detached in their response to pain and they were more concerned with not bothering anyone. They also had more positive feelings about hospitalization. This study was marred by the fact that the data collection was subjective and open to the biases and prejudices of the author and the people interviewed. Moreover, immigrants may differ in their responses to pain because they are in the unfamiliar environment of a hospital in a foreign culture. Finally, immigrants may systematically differ from persons of the same culture who do not emigrate.

Woodrow et al. (1972) in a study of 41 119 subjects aged from about 20 to 70 years found that Caucasians tolerated more pain than did people of Oriental background with Blacks in the middle. Pain tolerance decreased with age, and men tolerated more pain than did women.

Sternbach (1986) reported that whites were more likely than blacks or Hispanics to experience pain, especially back pain, muscle pain and joint pain. However, white women had less menstrual and premenstrual pain than did black or Hispanic women.

Zborowski (1952) believed that attitudes towards pain are part of any culture's child-rearing practices. He found that both Jewish-American and Italian-American parents in his study were generally over-protective and overly concerned about their child's health and their children were frequently reminded to avoid fights, possible injuries and catching colds. Crying elicited considerable sympathy. However, Old-American parents were less concerned and expected that the child would not run to the parent for a small problem. Children were taught to anticipate some pain when playing and they were expected not to show excessive distress. Once again we emphasize the subjective nature of this study which may reflect the author's biases more than the actual behavior of the different cultural groups.

There are few studies which have been concerned with the influence of culture on pain expression in children. Abu-Saad (1984) conducted semistructured interviews over a 6 month period with 24 children, aged 9–12 years, in each of three cultural groups, Arab-American, Latin-American and Asian-American. Although there was some variability among the three groups on causes of pain, descriptors of pain, color of pain and feelings about pain, the author provided no information concerning whether any of these differences reached statistical significance. The meaning of the variability of the children's responses on these items is also unclear. Interestingly, children in all three groups chose medicine as their most common coping strategy, and females in all groups found being comforted as helpful. Only a very few children believed there was anything useful about pain. An important limitation of this study is its retrospective nature. Thus it is unknown how children of different cultures would respond during an actual pain experience. The effect of culture on children's pain behavior warrants considerable further investigation.

9. Teaching children about pain

> It's really weird. I'm okay when the thing is happening like when I am in hospital, or I'm having stitches, or a shot, but what is really terrible for me is if I know the night before. I have all these terrible scary feelings and I get sick to my stomach. So we have this house rule, you know, like my mom never tells me till right before and that's how I like it best *(boy, aged 7 years, quoted in Ross and Ross, 1984, p. 187)*.

When it's new, and this is real scary, then I like to know a long time before, like 10 days. I talk to my Mom and I think about it a lot and it gets kinda boring and then I know I can take this. Like whatever happens, I can take this *(girl, aged 8 years, quoted in Ross and Ross, 1984, p. 187)*.

In the conclusion to their survey, Ross and Ross (1984) argued for a greater need for children to learn about pain itself and about coping strategies that are effective in pain management. Such teaching can be done in three different settings: home, school and clinic or hospital.

9.1. Home

When I know I'm gonna get a shot I get so scared my hands get all wet, you know, and I feel real sick to my stomach and like shaky, and I cry even before I get it *(child, quoted in Ross and Ross, 1985)*.

No studies have examined parents deliberately teaching their children about pain. Parents are the most important persons to teach children about pain, first by demonstrations of how they themselves cope with pain, which we discussed earlier, and secondly by preparing the child for a painful event. Parents are often advised to inform school-aged children about hospitalization or a painful procedure several days in advance and with information appropriate to the child's developmental level but no adequate guidelines exist for parents.

Ross and Ross (1984) found considerable diversity in children's preference about the timing of information. However, there was indeed a preference to have a longer rather than shorter period between the timing of information and the actual event. Of 994 children, only 107 children preferred less than a day's notice. Parents ought to be aware of their child's preference and to take this into consideration when providing information. However, the temptation to avoid giving any prior information may be detrimental to the child coping effectively when confronted with a stressful or painful situation.

There is no data to suggest how parents can prevent long term pain problems. For example, it is not clear that encouraging stoicism or teaching coping strategies will result in less likelihood of childhood pain problems or pain problems in adulthood.

9.2. School

Pain has rarely been a topic on a school curriculum even though death, coping with stress, and health maintenance are sometimes addressed. There has been very little research in this area. However, a recent study by Ross and Ross (1985) developed a 20-lesson pain program which was presented to 28, third and fourth graders in a school setting. The lessons were about 18 min in length and presented three times a week to groups of five or six children. The program included the following topics: warning function of pain, value of pain for diagnosis and treatment, common locations of childhood pain, pain description, coping strategies, hospitalization, inappropriate pain behavior. Two tests were developed as pre- and postmeasures to evaluate the program. There was a significant improvement in children's knowledge about pain at post-test and no sex differences were apparent. Unfortunately, it was not possible to assess long-term retention. It is also unknown what effect this teaching program had on actual behavior during a painful event or on the response to recurrent pain.

As McGrath and Manion (1987) have noted, the prevention of pain problems by health education may be a very difficult venture because the presumed impact is remote in time from the program and because we do not know what we should teach children about pain. Indeed such attempts may cause more harm than good. Further research of the effect of teaching programs on the child's behavior during painful experiences such as immunization and their response to headaches and abdominal pain would be extremely helpful in determining the usefulness of implementing such programs.

9.3. Clinic or hospital

Many Children's Hospitals have instituted child life programs or nursing programs which prepare children for hospitalization especially surgery. Although the effect on pain itself has not been measured, the best evidence is that such programs do help children cope (see chapter 4, for further discussion). However, children are rarely prepared for outpatient procedures and no evaluation has been undertaken of such preparation.

References

Abu-Saad, H. (1984) Cultural group indicators of pain in children. Children's Health Care 13, 11–14.

Anand, K.J.S. and Aynsley-Green, A. (1985) Metabolic and endocrine effects of surgical ligation of patent ductus arteriosus in the human preterm neonate: Are there implications for further improvement of postoperative outcome? Mod. Probl. Paediatr. 23, 143–157.

Anand, K.J.S. and Aynsley-Green, A. (1987) Measuring the severity of surgical stress in newborn infants. J. Pediatr. Surg., in press.

Anand, K.J.S., Sippell, W.G. and Aynsley-Green, A. (1987a) Randomized trial of fentanyl anaesthesia in preterm babies undergoing surgery: Effects on the stress response, Lancet i, 243–247.

Anand, K.J.S., Sippell, W.G. and Aynsley-Green, A. (1987b) Does the newborn infant require anaesthesia during surgery? Answers from a randomized trial of halothane anaesthesia. V World Congress on Pain, Hamburg. Pain suppl. 4, S451.

Barr, R. (1983) Variations on the theme of pain: 28A Pain tolerance and developmental change in pain perception. In: M.D. Levine, W.B. Carey, A.C. Crocker and R.T. Gross (Eds.), Developmental Behavioral Pediatrics. (Saunders, Philadelphia, PA) pp. 505–512.

Bondy, A.S. (1980) Infancy. In: S. Gabel and M.T. Erickson (Eds.), Child Development and Developmental Disabilities (Little Brown, Boston, MA) pp. 3–19.

Brown, J.M., O'Keeffe, J., Sanders, S.H. and Baker, B. (1986) Developmental changes in children's cognition to stressful and painful situations. J. Pediatr. Psychol. 11, 343–357.

Christensen, M.F. and Mortenson, D. (1975) Long term prognosis in children with recurrent abdominal pain. Arch. Dis. Child. 50, 110–114.

Craig, K.D. (1980) Ontogenetic and cultural influences on the expression of pain in man. In: H.W. Kosterlitz and L.Y. Terenius (Eds.), Pain and Society (Verlag Chemie, Weinheim) pp. 37–52.

Craig, K.D. (1983) Modeling and social learning factors in chronic pain. In: J.J. Bonica, U. Lindblom and A. Iggo (Eds.), Advances in Pain Research and Therapy, Vol. 5 (Raven Press, New York) pp. 813–827.

D'Apolito, K. (1984) The neonate's response to pain, Matern. Child Nurs. 9, 256–257.

Edwards, P.W., Zeichner, A., Kuczmierczyk, A.R. and Bockowski, J. (1985) Family pain models: The relationship between family history of pain and current pain experience. Pain 21, 379–384.

Field, T. and Goldson, E. (1984) Pacifying effects of non-nutritive sucking on term and preterm neonates during heelstick procedures. Pediatrics 74, 1012–1015.

Fields, H.L. and Basbaum, A.I. (1984) Endogenous pain control mechanisms. In: P.D. Wall and R. Melzack (Eds.), Textbook of Pain (Churchill Livingstone, Edinburgh) p. 142.

Fitzgerald, M. (1984) The course and termination of primary afferent fibres. In: P.D. Wall and R. Melzack (Eds.), Textbook of Pain (Churchill Livingstone, Edinburgh) pp. 34–48.

Fitzgerald, M. and Gibson, S. (1984) The postnatal physiological and neurochemical development of peripheral sensory C fibres. Neuroscience 13, 933–944.

Fitzgerald, M. and Kotzenburg, M. (1986) The functional development of descending inhibitory pathways in the dorsolateral funiculus of the newborn rat spinal cord. Development. Brain Res. 24, 261–270.

Franck, L.S. (1986) A new method to quantitatively describe pain behavior in infants. Nurs. Res. 35, 28–31.

Gaffney, A. and Dunne, E.A. (1986) Developmental aspects of children's definition of pain. Pain 26, 105–117.

Gaffney, A. and Dunne, E.A. (1987) Children's understanding of the causality of pain. Pain 29, 91–104.

Gochman, D. (1971) Some correlates of children's health beliefs and potential health behavior. J. Health Soc. Behav. 12, 148–154.

Grunau, R.V.E. and Craig, K.D. (1987) Pain expression in neonates: Facial action and cry. Pain 28, 395–410.

Hartrick, C.T., Dobritt, D.W. and Eckstein, L. (1986) Letter to the editor. Pain 25, 279–280.

Haslam, D.R. (1969) Age and the perception of pain. Psychon. Sci. 15, 86–87.

Helman, C. (1984) Culture, Health and Illness: An Introduction for Health Professionals (Wright, Bristol) pp. 95–105.

Hughes, J., Smith, T.W., Kosterlitz, H.W., Fothergill, L., Morgan, B.A. and Morris, H.R. (1975) Identification of two related pentapeptides from the brain with potent opiate agonist activity. Nature 258, 577–579.

Jaffe, J.H. and Martin, W.R. (1985) Opioid analgesics and antagonists. In: A.G. Gilman, L.S. Goodman, T.W. Rall and F. Murad (Eds.), Goodman and Gilman's: The Pharmacological Basis of Therapeutics, 7th edn. (Macmillan, New York) pp. 491–531.

Johnston, C.C. and Strada, M.E. (1986) Acute pain response in infants: a multidimensional description. Pain 24, 373–382.

Kassowitz, K.E. (1958) Psychodynamic reactions of children to the use of hypodermic needles. Am. Med. Assoc. J. Dis. Child. 95, 253–257.

Krainick, J.U. and Thoden, U. (1984) Dorsal column stimulation. In: P.D. Wall and R. Melzack (Eds.), Textbook of Pain (Churchill Livingstone, Edinburgh) pp. 701–705.

Leikin, L.J. (1986) Children's Physical Symptom Reporting and the Type A Behavior Pattern. Ph.D. dissertation, University of Ottawa, Ottawa, Canada.

Levy, D.M. (1960) The infant's earliest memory of inoculation: a contribution to public health procedures. J. Genet. Psychol. 96, 3–46.

Lewis, C. and Lewis, M. (1982) Determinants of children's health related beliefs and behaviors. Fam. Commun. Health 2, 85–97.

Lynn, B. (1984) The detection of injury and tissue damage. In: P.D. Wall and R. Melzack (Eds.), Textbook of Pain (Churchill Livingstone, Edinburgh).

McGrath, P.J. and Manion, I.G. (1987) Prevention of pain problems. In: K. Craig and S. Weiss (Eds.), Prevention and Early Intervention: Biobehavioral perspectives (Springer, New York) in press.

McGrath, P.J., Lawrence, J., Martire, H., Vair, C. and McMurray, B. (1987) Nurses' perceptions of pain in the neonatal intensive care unit. Manuscript under review.

McGraw, M.D. (1941) Neural mechanisms as exemplified in the changing reaction of the infant to pinprick. Child Dev. 9, 31–41.

McMurray, G.A. (1955) Congenital insensitivity to pain and its implications for motivational theory. Can. J. Psychol. 9, 121–131.

Mechanic, D. (1980) The experience and reporting of common symptoms. J. Health Soc. Behav. 21, 146–155.

Mechanic, D. (1983) The experience and expression of distress: The study of illness behavior and medical utilization. In: D. Mechanic (Ed.), Health, Health Care and the Health Professions (Springer, New York).

Melzack, R. and Wall, P.D. (1965) Pain mechanisms: a new theory. Science 150, 971–979.

Melzack, R. and Wall, P.D. (1982) The Challenge of Pain (Penguin, Harmondsworth) pp. 195–261.

Merskey, H. (Ed.) (1986) Classification of chronic pain: descriptions of chronic pain syndromes and definitions of pain terms. Pain, suppl. 3.

Millan, M.J. (1986) Multiple opioid systems and pain. Pain 27, 303–347.

Murray, A.D. (1979) Infant crying as an elicitor of parental behavior: an examination of two models. Psychol. Bull. 86, 191–215.

Owens, M.E. (1986) Assessment of infant pain in clinical settings. J. Pain Symptom Manage. 1, 29–31.

Owens, M.E. and Todt, E.H. (1984) Pain in infancy: Neonatal response to heel lance. Pain 20, 77–86.

Payne, B. and Norfleet, M.A. (1986) Chronic pain and the family: a review. Pain 26, 1–22.

Pennebaker, J.W. (1982) The Psychology of Physical Symptoms (Springer-Verlag, New York).

Piaget, J. and Inhelder, B. (1969) The Psychology of the Child (Basic Books, New York).

Ross, D.M. and Ross, S.A. (1984) Childhood pain: the school-aged child's viewpoint. Pain 20, 179–191.

Ross, D.M. and Ross, S.A. (1985) Pain instruction with third- and fourth-grade children: a pilot study. J. Pediatr. Psychol. 10, 55–63.

Seligman, M.E.P. (1975) Helplessness: On Depression, Development and Death (Freeman, San Francisco, CA).

Spielberger, C.D. (1970) Manual for the State-Trait Anxiety Inventory for Children (Consulting Psychologists Press, Palo Alto, CA).

Sternbach, R.A. (1968) Pain: A Psychophysiological Analysis (Academic Press, New York) pp. 95–115.

Sternbach, R.A. (1986) Survey of pain in the United States: The Nuprin Pain Report. Clin. J. Pain 2, 49–53.

Swafford, L.I. and Allan, D. (1968) Pain relief in the pediatric patient. Med. Clin. North Am. 52, 131–136.

Terenius, L. (1984) The endogenous opioids and other central peptides. In: P.D. Wall and R. Melzack (Eds.), Textbook of Pain (Churchill Livingstone, Edinburgh) pp. 133–141.

Turnbull, I.M. (1984) Brain stimulation. In: P.D. Wall and R. Melzack (Eds.), Textbook of Pain (Churchill Livingstone, Edinburgh) pp. 706–714.

Wall, P.D. (1984) Introduction. In: P.D. Wall and R. Melzack (Eds.), Textbook of Pain (Churchill Livingstone, Edinburgh) pp. 1–16.

Wall, P.D. and Sweet, W.H. (1967) Temporary abolition of pain in man. Science 155, 108–109.

Williamson, P.S. and Williamson, M.L. (1983) Physiologic stress reduction by a local anesthetic during newborn circumcision. Pediatrics 71, 36–40.

Willis, W.D. (1984) The origin and destination of pathways involved in pain transmission. In: P.D. Wall and R. Melzack (Eds.), Textbook of Pain (Churchill Livingstone, Edinburgh) pp. 88–99.

Wolff, B.B. (1983) Laboratory methods of pain measurement. In: R. Melzack (Ed.), Pain Measurement and Assessment (Raven Press, New York) pp. 7–13.

Woodrow, K.M., Friedman, G.D., Siegelaub, A.B. and Collen, M.F. (1972) Pain tolerance: differences according to age, sex and race. Psychosom. Med. 34, 548–556.

Woolf, C.J. and Wall, P.D. (1983) Endogenous opioid peptides and pain mechanisms: a complex relationship. Nature 306, 739–740.

Zachary, R.A., Friedlander, S., Huang, L.N., Silverstein, S. and Leggott, P. (1985) Effects of stress-relevant and irrelevant filmed modeling on children's responses to dental treatment. J. Pediatr. Psychol. 10, 383–401.

Zborowski, M. (1952) Cultural components in responses to pain. J. Soc. Issues 8, 16–30.

CHAPTER 3

The measurement and assessment of pain

I often say that when you can measure what you are speaking about, and express it in numbers, you know something about it, but when you cannot measure it, when you cannot express it in numbers, your knowledge is of a meager and unsatisfactory kind; it may be the beginning of knowledge, but you have scarcely, in your thoughts, advanced to the stage of science whatever the matter may be *(Lord Kelvin, quoted in Thomas, 1983, pp. 143–144)*.

1. Problems of pain measurement and assessment

The accurate measurement and assessment of pain in children is one of the most difficult and most crucial challenges facing those who would treat children with pain or conduct research in this area. The validity and reliability of pain measurement and assessment in children has, until recently, been a neglected area of investigation. However, it is a prerequisite to the advancement of pediatric pain as a science and is a precursor to the development and evaluation of more effective means of alleviating pain in children. Only in the last few years has there been an attempt to express in numbers the pain experienced by children.

A universally accepted definition of pain has been difficult to achieve. However the International Association for the Study of Pain has attempted to establish a standard definition of pain as: 'An unpleasant sensory and emotional experience associated with actual or potential tissue damage or described in terms of such damage' (Merskey, 1986, p. S217).

From this definition, one might imagine that pain, even in adults, might be difficult to measure. How can unpleasant sensory and emotional experiences be measured in a scientifically rigorous way? Pain in adults is a measurement problem because pain is a subjective private event that can be measured only indirectly by what people report about their experiences (self-report methods); the way they behave in response to pain (behavioral methods); or how their bodies react to the pain (physiological methods).

At least with adults, there is an opportunity for the person in pain to describe, in detail, how he feels. As well, adults generally have fully developed nervous systems and their cognitive and behavioral competencies are relatively stable.

With children, the problems of pain measurement and assessment are confounded: by children's constantly developing but relatively limited cognitive ability to understand what is being asked of them in pain measurement; by children's limited verbal skills; by our lack of understanding of the developing nervous system and its influence on pain perception in children; by the usually limited experience children have had of pain; by the limited behavioral competencies that children (especially very young children) have and, finally, by the lack of research and our subsequent limited understanding of children's pain behavior and the physiology of pain in children (McGrath et al., 1986).

1.1. The distinction between measurement and assessment

The distinction between measurement and assessment in pain research has not always been clearly drawn. For example, Melzack (1983), in his landmark book 'Pain Measurement and Assessment', does not discuss how these two terms should be differentiated. Measurement refers to the application of some metric to a specific element, usually intensity, of pain. Assessment is a much broader endeavour which encompasses the measurement of the interplay of different factors on the experience of pain. These factors might include the affective response to noxious stimuli; the role of family styles on the perception of pain; the impact on families of having a child in pain; and the meaning of pain to the child and to the family. In the form of an analogy, measurement in pain is like using a ruler or a scale to determine the height or weight of something whereas assessment is deciding whether it is height or weight or volume or density or tensile strength that is important to measure.

Whereas the measurement of pain in children is still in its early stages, research on assessment of pediatric pain has not yet really begun. Although every clinician is faced with the problem of assessment each time a patient needs or requests help, there is a dearth of scientific or professional literature attempting to provide pain assessment strategies for children.

This chapter will first focus on the more specific issues in measurement and then will discuss the assessment of pain in the broader context that this requires. Assessment of pain does require the availability of well developed and validated measurement instruments and it is only once measurement instruments are available that assessment strategies can develop.

1.2. Reasons for measuring pain in children

The measurement of children's pain is of vital importance to researchers and health professionals for several reasons. In some situations, measurement of pain will help in the decision to intervene to relieve pain. For example, the well-documented low rate of use of postoperative analgesics with children (see chapter 4 for an extensive discussion of this issue) may be due, in part, to the lack of well-validated, widely used measurement instruments that are appropriate for gauging children's pain (Eland and Anderson, 1977; Beyer et al., 1983).

The measurement of pediatric pain is also crucial for evaluating methods of pain relief. The lack of studies investigating the effectiveness of pharmacological, surgical, behavioral and psychological methods of pediatric pain relief may be, partially, the result of the paucity of reliable and valid measures.

Measuring children's pain can also be part of determining the correlates of a pain episode and the variables that may cause, ameliorate or worsen the child's pain. For example, pain diaries have been used to assist in the diagnosis of recurrent abdominal pain (McGrath, 1983) (see chapter 6). The diary includes a rating scale for intensity of pain as well as a record of associated symptoms and events. Patterns of the occurrence of pain can be discerned by examining such a record over several weeks.

Finally, the accurate measurement of pain in children is required before we can begin to uncover the nature of pain in children and the development of pain and pain problems across the life span. For example, advances in understanding the physiology of pain in neonates and changes that may occur as the nervous system develops require a way of measuring pain in that age group.

2. Components of pain

Pain can be conceptualized as an event that has several components. Each component of pain is only one way of approaching the entire phenomenon. The three most frequently considered components of pain are the cognitive or self-report component, the behavioral component, and the physiological component. Not only are there multiple components of pain, but for each component there may be several different measurement strategies. There are, of course, other ways of conceptualizing pain measurement than in terms of the cognitive, behavioral and physiological components. Melzack (1983) for example, has argued that pain should be divided into pain sensations and reactions to pain. No one way of conceptualizing pain nor any single component of pain will be the most appropriate to measure pain in every clinical or research situation. In fact, the selection of appropriate measures will determine the clinical or research validity of the measurement strategy. The clinical or research question, rather than a predilection to use a specific measurement instrument should dictate the specific instrument used. The measures of pain that have been developed fit nicely into a component analysis and it is for this reason that this format is used in this chapter. In addition to the three components of pain we will also discuss the stress response that occurs with surgery. The stress response is thought to be, in part, due to pain.

2.1. The cognitive or self-report component of pain

The first component, the cognitive component, refers to the individuals' own report of their feelings, images or statements about the pain that they are experiencing. In many ways, this component is the closest to what the layman means when pain is mentioned. Indeed, the latest definition of pain terms by the International Association for the Study of Pain (Merskey, 1986, p. S217) emphasizes 'pain is always subjective'. Measurement of the cognitive component of pain is the attempt to quantify the 'hurt that we feel'. All cognitive component measures of pain in children rely on the expression by children of what they are experiencing and all have focussed on the intensity of pain rather than on other qualities of the pain experience.

Self-report measures have been widely used with adults and an extensive literature has developed which investigates the reliability and validity of these scales (Melzack, 1983). In the past 10 years, there has been an increasing amount of research concerned with the measurement of self-report of pain with children.

A major problem with all self-report measures of children's pain is that this method is open to serious bias because of the demand characteristics of the specific situation. In other words, the way the child perceives the question will influence the answer. Eland and Anderson (1977) found that following an operation, children may deny pain when they are asked because they fear that if they say they have pain they will get a needle.

Ross and Ross (1984) showed that the reason given for asking the question and the person asking the question makes a substantial difference in the children's responses. For example, if children are asked to describe pain to their mothers they will give different answers than if they are asked to describe pain to a doctor so that the doctor can understand children's pain better. In addition, the type of question and the response options (for example, open-ended questions versus a checklist) may also substantially change the children's answers (Ross and Ross, 1984). The solution is not to eliminate demand and other contextual characteristics from the measurement of pain. This cannot be done. We must, however, be aware that a change of context can substantially influence the measurement of pain. It should be emphasized that contextual influences on pain occur with adults and there is no reason to believe that children are more prone to influence than adults.

The second major problem with measures of the cognitive component of pain is that children often lack the cognitive skills to understand the question or to respond in a meaningful way to the question. For example, 18-month-old children are very unlikely to be able to tell where in their abdomen they are hurting and most 2 year olds will be unable to say if something hurts more or less.

The simple question such as 'How is your pain today?' is the most common clinical method used with children to evaluate their level of pain. Although the simple question is clinically relevant and will continue to be an important part of the clinical encounter, the response to the question is rarely of much use to the clinician. Since this simple question is more a social interchange than a request for careful consideration, it may be particularly open to bias from demand characteristics. Moreover, the question 'How is your pain today?' lacks an associated metric, there is no measurement involved. There are no numbers attached to the responses. Even if specific questions are asked about pain frequency, intensity and duration, retrospective questions are likely to be inaccurate. For example, Andrasik et al. (1985) found that children aged 8–16 years overestimated their frequency of headache by 56%, their intensity by 73% and their duration by 107% when global estimates were compared with a month of actual daily diary keeping. Parents also overestimated frequency by 75%, intensity by 82% and duration by 112%. Overestimation of headache was reduced following treatment. Some of the results could be explained by the fact that, in the condition prior to treatment, the children were asked to estimate the month preceding the initial diary collection against which the global estimates were evaluated. The headaches may have declined during the month that the diary was used. Moreover, patients and parents may have been motivated to exaggerate the severity of headache in order to insure that they obtained treatment. The post-treatment estimates were based on the same month as the month in which the diaries were collected. However, the large discrepancy between the global estimates and the diary recordings do cast doubt on the validity of global questions of pain.

Verbal scales such as the McGill-Melzack Scale (Melzack, 1975) are suitable only for older adolescents who are able to understand adjectives, such as 'quivering', 'smarting', 'lacerating' and 'lancinating', and can choose which words best describe their pain. One of the strengths of the Melzack scale is that it is not restricted to the intensity dimension of pain but also considers and measures affective aspects of pain. The McGill-Melzack scale is both a measurement and an assessment instrument.

Attempts to develop simpler verbal scales for children have been reported (Savedra et al., 1981, 1982; Beales, 1982; Jeans, 1983; Tesler et al., 1983) and are discussed in more detail in the assessment section.

Hester (1979) developed a type of numerical scale in which children were presented with four white poker chips. The children were asked to indicate how many pieces of hurt they felt. The concrete nature of the task enabled children aged 4–7 years to readily respond and the results were consistent with their behavior in the pain situation.

In our own lab and in our clinic, children over the age of 9 years routinely complete a numerical-verbal pain scale on which they are asked to rate their headaches on a six point (0–5) scale, four times a day (Table 1). For each number, there is a verbal description of severity of pain. After 5 min of instruction, children are able to use this diary with no difficulty. The inter-rater reliability of this scale, when parents and children independently rated the child's headaches, has been demonstrated. Richardson et al. (1983) compared 16 pairs of adults and their children who rated the child's

TABLE 1
Six point 0–5 numerical-verbal pain scale.

0	No pain
1	Pain – I am only aware of it if I pay attention to it
2	Pain – I can ignore it at times
3	Pain – I can't ignore it but I can do my usual activities
4	Pain – It's difficult for me to concentrate; I can only do easy activities
5	Pain – Such that I can't do anything

headache. Concordance was high for diaries with both a purely behavioral description of the pain and diaries with behavioral and subjective descriptors. Andrasik et al. (1985) found that parents under-reported the frequency of their children's headaches by 40% as measured by the children's diaries in one diary period but they did not underestimate after treatment. There was no under-reporting of the intensity of the children's headaches. We have employed similar scales in measuring recurrent abdominal pain and musculo-skeletal pain in children and have found no difficulties.

The validity and measurement characteristics of happy-sad faces scales on which children report their pain have been investigated by a number of researchers (Jay et al., 1984; Kuttner and LePage, 1984; LeBaron and Zelter, 1984; P.A. McGrath et al., 1985). In faces scales 5–7 faces depicting different degrees of pain are presented to the child and the child chooses the one that most closely approximates his pain. Fig. 1 contains the faces used by Dr. Patricia A. McGrath in her work with a variety of pediatric pain problems.

Faces scales are easily understood by children. They are inexpensive and they have excellent measurement characteristics. For example, P.A. McGrath et al. (1985) used cross-modality matching in which children were asked to match happy-sad faces with the brightness of a light and to rate the faces on a visual analogue scale. The values obtained from the matching procedure were

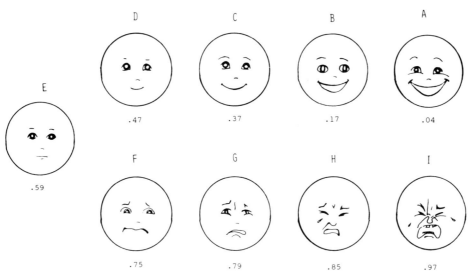

Fig. 1. Faces scale with mean affective magnitude for each face. (Reprinted from P.A. McGrath et al., 1985, with permission of the authors and Raven Press.)

consistent across age, sex and health status of the child as well as being consistent across the two matching procedures. Fig. 1 contains the faces and the associated affective values for each face. The values have been transformed so that the maximum negative value, indicating the most unpleasant feeling, is 1 and the maximum positive value, indicating the most pleasant feeling, is 0. P.A. McGrath et al. (1985) used the faces to measure the affective rather than the sensory aspect of pain. The affective and sensory aspects of pain have been differentially measured in adults (Gracely et al., 1978) but it is not clear that children can make such a discrimination. However, the scale has been properly developed and shows good psychometric properties.

Beyer (1984) has developed an interesting variant of the faces scale. The Oucher is a poster-like device consisting of a vertical numerical scale (0–100) on the left and a vertical six picture photographic scale on the right (Fig. 2). The scale is designed to measure the report of pain intensity in children ages 3–12. Validity data are contained in a series of four articles (Beyer and Aradine, 1986, 1987a,b; Aradine et al., 1987).

Content validity was assessed by having 78 children between the ages of 3 and 7 years rank order the pictures in the Oucher. Forty-one percent sequenced all the photographs while 77% were able to sequence 5 or 6 correctly. Of all the pictures, 85% were placed in the correct sequence (Beyer and Aradine, 1986). Scores on the Oucher correlate highly with visual analogue scores and with Hester's (1979) poker chip measure and correlated poorly with measures of fear, thus showing convergent and discriminant validity (Beyer and Aradine, 1987a,b). Finally, scores on the Oucher were sensitive to analgesia-caused reduction in pain (Aradine et al., 1987). In some of the studies, sub-samples were small but the Oucher appears to have good psychometric properties.

Unfortunately, the recent proliferation of faces-type scales has not led to any agreed upon standard scale. There are major advantages in using faces which have well researched psychometric properties.

The visual analogue scale, which has been extensively used in measurement of adult pain (Huskisson, 1983), can be understood by children over 7 and has evidence of validity. Ratings of pain using the visual analogue scale show expected declines in the postoperative period (Abu-Saad and Holzmer, 1981; Vair, 1981) and were related to behavioral and verbal indicators of pain (Abu-Saad, 1984). The visual analogue scale (Fig. 3) consists of a line (usually 10 cm) either vertical or horizontal with an anchor, such as 'no pain' and 'severe pain' at each end. The child is asked to indicate how much pain he is experiencing.

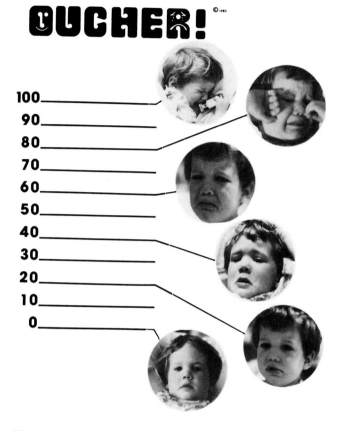

Fig. 2. The Oucher. (Reprinted from Beyer, 1984, with permission of the author and the publisher.)

NO PAIN

**PAIN AS
SEVERE AS
POSSIBLE**

Fig. 3. Visual analogue scale.

It is not clear if a vertical scale is more appropriate than a horizontal scale because children may find it easier to conceptualize the notion of greater or lesser intensity of pain with up and down rather than with left and right. Studies with adults have shown that vertical and horizontal scales correlate but that horizontal scales yield slightly lower scores than vertical scales (Scott and Huskisson, 1979). The visual analogue scale has the advantage of simplicity and, perhaps for this reason, is the most widely used scale. Care must be taken when xeroxing the scale to insure that the process does not alter the length of the line and confound scoring.

Pain thermometers are similar to visual analogue scales but use a graphic representation of a thermometer and a numerical scale (0–10 or 0–100) (Katz et al., 1980; Szyfelbein et al., 1985). Children are asked to rate their pain on the thermometer.

Primarily non-verbal methods have also been used to measure the cognitive component of pain. These include asking children to describe the color of their pain or to draw pictures of their pain. Children are reported to typically describe severe pain as being red (Scott, 1978). Other researchers (Eland, 1974; Jeans, 1983; Unruh et al., 1983; Kurylyszyn et al., 1987) have also found that red and black are the most frequent colors used to describe pain. Unfortunately, no validation of color scales or systematic investigation of their utility in clinical situations has been done. Red and black appear to be preferred colors in all pain drawings even in drawings of low intensities of pain (Kurylyszyn et al., 1987). Drawings can be reliably classified by raters (Unruh et al., 1983) and may show developmental differences (Jeans, 1983).

Only one study has examined whether intensity of children's pain can be determined from drawings. Kurylyszyn et al. (1987) found that drawings of different intensity of headache could not be well discriminated on the basis of overall ratings and by examination of specific features of the drawings. Discrimination occurred only for drawings representing extreme levels of pain and was poor for drawings of moderately intense pain.

As can be seen in Fig. 4, these drawings are often evocative and rich in details that can help the clinician to understand how individual children comprehend their pain and the fantasies children have about their pain. Drawings also provide an excellent clinical tool for communicating with children about their pain. They can be used in developing cognitive pain management strategies such as transforming pain and distraction. These potential uses of drawings have not been systematically investigated.

There is, however, no evidence that pain drawings can provide useful information regarding whether pain is of organic or psychogenic etiology or to give indications of the difficulties that the child may be having in coping with pain.

Projective techniques have not been shown to be effective in measurement of intensity of pain in children. For example, Eland (1974) found no

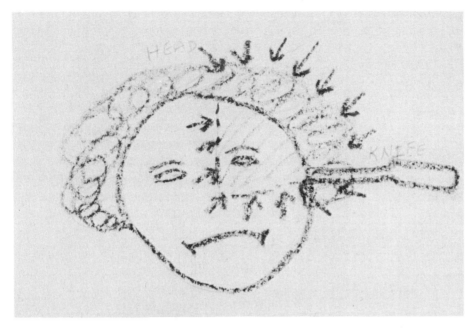

Fig. 4. A 10-year-old child's drawing of her headache. (Printed with permission of the artist.)

relationship between responses to cartoons in which an animal was subjected to a painful experience and the child's own response. However, projective approaches may be of some use in a more broad-based assessment of children's attitudes to painful experiences, perceptions of family response to pain and coping strategies. Lollar et al. (1982) developed a projective pain scale that used 24 pictures to determine how children perceived pain experienced by themselves and their parents. This scale has not been used in clinical pain measurement. It may be useful in determining if children, who are not coping well with pain, project their estimates of pain differently than children who are managing well.

Table 2 summarizes studies on the cognitive component of pain.

More extensive evaluations of the reliability and validity of these instruments for specific situations, different age groups, and varying purposes are now required. The temptation to develop more, new, unvalidated instruments must be resisted. It is unlikely to promote improvements in clinical management or advances in understanding of pain, but will only slow clear communication among clinicians and researchers.

TABLE 2
Cognitive component of pain in children.

Type of strategy	Description	Reference
Simple query	How is your pain?	Ross and Ross, 1984; Andrasik et al., 1985
Verbal scales	McGill-Melzack scale	Melzack, 1975
	Pain words	Savedra et al., 1981, 1982; Jeans, 1983; Tesler et al., 1983; Varni et al., 1987
Numerical scales	Pieces of hurt	Hester, 1979
	Rate your pain from 0 to 5	Richardson et al., 1983; Andrasik et al., 1986
Spatial scales	100 mm line visual analogue	Katz et al., 1980; Abu-Saad and Holzmer, 1981; Vair, 1981; Abu-Saad, 1984; Szyfelbein et al., 1985
Miscellaneous	Color of pain	Eland, 1974; Stewart, 1977; Scott, 1978; Jeans, 1983; Unruh et al., 1983; Kurylyszyn et al., 1987; Varni et al., 1987
	Faces scales	Beyer, 1984; Jay et al., 1984; LeBaron and Zelter, 1984; Kuttner and LePage, 1984; Aradine et al., 1987; Beyer and Aradine, 1987a,b,c
	Drawing of pain	Jeans, 1983; Unruh et al., 1983; Kurylyszyn et al., 1987
	Projectives	Eland, 1974; Scott, 1978; Lollar et al., 1982

2.2. *The behavioral component of pain*

The second component of pain that can be measured is pain behavior. As in all measures of pain assessment, it is not always possible to completely distinguish between pain and other forms of distress. Some researchers have preferred to use the term stress or distress to describe the result of psychological or physical trauma as measured by behavioral or physiological indices (Katz et al., 1980). We choose to use the term pain when the IASP definition of 'an unpleasant sensory and emotional experience associated with actual or potential tissue damage or described in terms of such damage' (Merskey, 1986, p. S217) appears to be met. Even though we cannot directly know the subjective state of infants, the behavior elicited by heel lance and immunization appear to be unpleasant sensory and emotional experience and clearly differ from response to other stimulation. As well, the social validity (Kazdin, 1977) of the response is undoubted. Ordinary adult observers invariably label the response as pain.

2.2.1. *Cry*
Perhaps the most obvious pain behavior in children that can be measured by observation of behavior is crying. The presence or absence of crying is the usual way parents and health professionals determine if a young child is in pain. Since crying is the primary mode of communicating that neonates and young infants have to express their basic needs (Lester, 1985), it is not always known when crying is the result of pain. Crying may be the result of hunger, soiled or wet diapers, excessive heat or cold, boredom, being startled (Ostwald and Murry, 1985) or from anger and fear (Sherman, 1927). In spite of the possibility of factors other than pain causing crying, occurrence and non-occurrence of crying has been used in numerous studies as a measure of pain (Williamson and Williamson, 1983; Field and Goldson, 1984; Owens and Todt, 1984).

The pain cry has been described behaviorally as beginning with an indrawing breath, followed by a long expiratory cry, then another inspiration, then expiratory cries of variable duration (Wolff, 1969).

Wasz-Hockert has described the psychoacoustic properties of the pain cry as researched in a large number of studies over the last 25 years (Wasz-Hockert et al. 1985, pp. 92–93):

> In all our cry studies on the pain cry of healthy full term newborn infants, the mean maximum pitch of the fundamental frequency without shift has been about 650 Hz and the mean minimum pitch about 400 Hz. In 80% of the samples, the pain cry had a falling

or rising/falling melody type with a stable pitch and a duration of approximately 2.5 sec. Shifts with a higher pitch occurred roughly in every third cry. The mean maximum pitch of shift was about 1200 Hz. The mean maximum pitch of the whole cry signal was about 800 Hz when the maximum pitch had been measured from the highest part of either the main fundamental frequency or the shift. The signals were voiced and continuous in about two thirds of the cries. The occurrence of glottal roll was quite common, mainly at the end of the phonations. Vibrato occasionally preceded the glottal roll part. Biphonation, glide, furcation and noise concentration were extremely rare in normal infant crying.

Although Wasz-Hockert et al. (1985) have claimed that the pain cry can be recognized and differentiated by mothers, and is psychoacoustically specific, others have disputed this claim. For example, Muller et al. (1974), in a carefully controlled study, elicited three types of cry (hunger, pain and startle) from four male and four female infants aged 3–5 months. The mothers of these babies and the mothers of a set of like aged babies were asked to identify the first and third 15 s segments of the cries. They misjudged a significant proportion of both the startle and pain cries as hunger cries.

Johnston and Strada (1986) in a study of 14 infants undergoing routine immunization at 2 months or 4 months found such a wide variety in the pain cry responses that they concluded it was not possible to predict whether there was a pain signature to the cry. Indeed, Johnston and Strada noted that the greatest variability of the measured responses across subjects (heart rate, facial expression, body posture and cry) were in the cry. Fig. 5 illustrates the changes in cry over time.

Barr et al. (1987) have also demonstrated that parents' 24 h diary recording of both frequency and duration of infant crying correlate highly and significantly ($r = 0.71$) with a voice-activated recording system. They also found a high and significant relationship between frequency ($r = 0.65$) but not

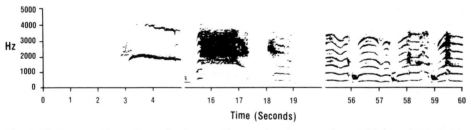

Fig. 5. Electroacoustic tracings of pain cry. Changes in cries over time. Initial cry (at 3–6 s) is high pitched, phonated, flat or slightly falling melody; second cry (at 16–17.5 s) is dysphonated; last cries (at 55–60 s) are phonated, lower pitched, rising-falling melody, and rhythmic. (Reprinted from Johnston and Strada, 1986, with permission of the authors and Elsevier.)

duration of fussing and voice-activated recordings of negative vocalizations (fussing). In other words, mothers can tell us how much their babies cry.

2.2.2. Facial expression

The facial expression of infants receiving injections or having blood taken show a pain pattern consisting of lowering of the brow, broadening of the nasal root, an angular and squarish mouth and tightly closed eyes as specific to pain in this age group (Izard et al., 1980). This system of analysis, known as the maximally discriminative facial movement coding system (MAX), examines patterns of responses and classifies the emotion on the basis of the configuration of the face. This system was used by Johnston and Strada (1986) in the previously mentioned study of immunization pain in infants. They found that the pain expression was the most uniform response to injection. In the period immediately following injection, 11 of the babies had the perfect configuration of pain and the other three had close approximations of the facial expression for pain. With appropriate training, MAX coding has very adequate inter-rater reliability.

Grunau and Craig (1987a) have approached the coding of facial response of infants in pain in a different way by utilizing the strategy developed in Ekman and Friesen's (1978) facial action coding system (FACS). FACS describes facial expression in terms of specific facial muscles underlying skin movements. Whereas MAX codes facial movement in terms of preconceived categories of emotion, FACS codes specific action units without referral to specific global patterns indicative of specific emotions.

Grunau and Craig (1987a) used a revision of the baby FACS originally developed by Ekman and Oster (1979). This coding system scores nine facial movements: brow bulge, eye squeeze, naso-labial furrow, open lips, stretch mouth (vertical), stretch mouth (horizontal), lip purse, taut tongue, and chin quiver. Every 3 s of facial behavior are scored for the presence of each specific movement.

They studied the facial behavior of 140 infants (average age, 43.05 h) who were stimulated by a heel rub (swabbing of the heel) and then by a heel lance. They found that response to the heel rub (presumably a non-painful stimulus) was dependent on the sleep/awake state with quiet/awake babies responding most. Response to heel lance was also state dependent. Although heel lance produced brow action in 96% of the infants, eye squeeze in 96%, naso-labial furrow in 97%, and lip part in 98%, taut tongue and stretch mouth were related to state. Quiet awake infants showed 85% taut tongue and 55% showed stretch mouth. On the other hand, quiet sleep-state infants had 57%

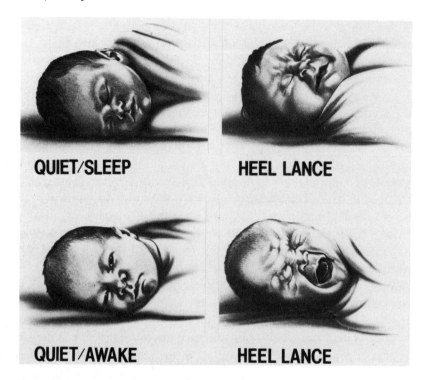

QUIET/SLEEP HEEL LANCE

QUIET/AWAKE HEEL LANCE

Fig. 6. Artist's conception of two babies at rest and in pain. (Reprinted from Grunau and Craig, 1987a, with permission of the authors and Elsevier.)

and 22% respectively. No effects by sex of baby for occurrence of response were found. Males, however reacted quicker. Different technicians showed different effects. Obstetric factors were related to overall facial action. Mothers with greater obstetric medication had children with more vigorous facial action (Grunau and Craig, 1987b). Fig. 6 shows an artist's drawing of two infants exhibiting responses to heel lances.

Although the clinical utility of facial expression as a pain measure has not yet been explored, this research may provide a key to answering questions regarding the beginnings of pain perception in the developing infant. Moreover, facial expression appears to be sensitive enough to test minor variations in handling procedures in order to develop less painful methods.

2.2.3. Other behavior

Other researchers have developed behavioral rating scales for use in assessing pain in young children undergoing discrete painful medical procedures. Katz et al. (1980) compiled a list of behaviors that children exhibit before, during and after bone marrow aspirations (BMA) from their observation of children aged 8 months to 17 years and 9 months. Of the 25 behaviors originally selected, 13 discriminated between children who were rated by nurses as highly anxious and children rated as less anxious. These 13 items comprise the procedure behavior rating scale. Several of the items are peculiar to the BMA procedure and would not be of use in rating pain or distress in other situations. The scale demonstrated inter-rater reliability above 0.85 and good evidence of validity. An extension of this scale has been developed and validated to measure ongoing distress or pain from a discrete event such as bone marrow aspiration but the increased sophistication of the scale has not substantially enhanced its validity (Jay and Elliot, 1984).

In a similar study, Craig et al. (1984) developed a code to measure pain expression in children aged 2–24 months who were undergoing immunization. Items in the scale included: crying, pain vocalization, distortion of face and rigidity of torso. The scale demonstrated inter-rater reliability of most of the items and evidence of validity. This study is discussed in more detail in chapter 5.

Photogrammetric techniques, which have been most widely used in improving athletic performance and in gait analysis, have been used by Franck (1986) to measure response to heel lance. Ten babies aged approximately 4 h were videotaped during heel lance. Videotapes were analysed in 0.01 s increments. Measurements were derived for: time of first cry, time between first movement and cry, duration of cries, number of cries, velocity of first affected leg movement, number of affected first leg movements, time of first unaffected leg movement, number of unaffected leg movements, swiping movements, facial movements and arm movements. Swiping movements refer to movements directed toward the site of stimulation. These measures provide a rich and detailed account of the response to painful stimulation. Although photogrammetry has not been used in clinical measurement, the precision of the technique does yield information about the nature of pain in neonates (see chapter 2).

A group from France (Piquard-Gauvain et al., 1983, 1984) developed a 17 item scale that was completed by nurses and nursing assistants observing children who were hospitalized for cancer treatment. The scale included items on the rest position the child took, protective behavior during movement, somatic complaints and reactions to being medically examined in the painful regions. The scale showed reasonable inter-rater agreement on most items. The clinical utility of the scale has not yet been demonstrated.

One of the few observational studies of postoperative pain in children was conducted by Taylor (1982). She examined 20 children between 18 months and 4 years during the first 3 h after discharge from the recovery room. Taylor recorded occurrence of movements (restlessness, guarding of the operative site, contacting the operative site and grimacing) and of vocalizations (crying, whining, groaning and complaints of pain). Interobserver reliability was high but was based on only 1/60 of the sample. The children exhibited 4373 pain related movements and vocalizations. Taylor (1982) concluded that the children were experiencing pain. Unfortunately data analysis was not very sophisticated and there was no attempt to validate the coding system.

A time sampling method of measuring the behavioral component of pain in the postoperative setting has recently been developed (McGrath et al., 1985). The Children's Hospital of Eastern Ontario pain scale (CHEOPS) presented in Table 3 consists of six behaviors that are observed once every 30 s by a trained observer. Data indicate inter-rater reliability above 0.80 and strong indications of validity as determined by independent ratings by nurses unaware of the CHEOPS score. The scale is also sensitive to clinical intervention as evidenced by changes in the scale in response to intravenous analgesic medication. Using a procedure known as social validation (Kazdin, 1977) it was determined that the behavior measured by the CHEOPS is what most people call pain. Stevens (1986) has recently replicated the findings of reliability and validity of the CHEOPS. The CHEOPS is a valid and reliable behavioral measure of postoperative pain in young children.

Another way of measuring the behavioral aspect of pain is to have experienced adults rate the amount of pain they perceive that a child is suffering. Visual analogue scales, for example, can be used by nurses to rate the amount of pain that children appear to be in.

The visual analogue scale with the anchors of 'no pain' and 'pain as severe as possible' can be completed by independent observers with correlations above 0.80 and excellent correlation with more detailed behavioral methods (McGrath et al., 1985).

Varni and his colleagues (Varni, 1981; Varni et al., 1981; Varni and Gilbert, 1982) have used specific behavioral and self-report measures of pain that were appropriate but idiosyncratic to the individual cases involved. Ratings have been on a 10 point scale and the behaviors used have included drug intake, distance walked, verbal complaints and crying. Inter-rater reliability was consistently obtained but no specific investigations of the more widespread utility of these measures have been presented.

TABLE 3
Behavioral definitions and scoring of CHEOPS. (Reprinted from McGrath et al., 1985, with permission of the authors and Raven Press.)

Item	Behavior	Score	Definition
Cry	No cry	1	Child is not crying
	Moaning	2	Child is moaning or quietly vocalizing; silent cry
	Crying	2	Child is crying, but the cry is gentle or whimpering
	Scream	3	Child is in a full-lunged cry; sobbing: may be scored with complaint or without complaint
Facial	Composed	1	Neutral facial expression
	Grimace	2	Score only if definite negative facial expression
	Smiling	0	Score only if definite positive facial expression
Child verbal	None	1	Child not talking
	Other complaints	1	Child complains, but not about pain, e.g., 'I want to see mommy' or 'I am thirsty'
	Pain complaints	2	Child complains about pain
	Both complaints	2	Child complains about pain and about other things, e.g., 'It hurts; I want mommy'
	Positive	0	Child makes any positive statement or talks about other things without complaint
Torso	Neutral	1	Body (not limbs) is at rest; torso is inactive
	Shifting	2	Body is in motion in a shifting or serpentine fashion
	Tense	2	Body is arched or rigid
	Shivering	2	Body is shuddering or shaking involuntarily
	Upright	2	Child is in a vertical or upright position
	Restrained	2	Body is restrained
Touch	Not touching	1	Child is not touching or grabbing at wound

(continued on next page)

(Table 3 continued)

Item	Behavior	Score	Definition
	Reach	2	Child is reaching for but not touching wound
	Touch	2	Child is gently touching wound or wound area
	Grab	2	Child is grabbing vigorously at wound
	Restrained	2	Child's arms are restrained
Legs	Neutral	1	Legs may be in any position but are relaxed; includes gentle swimming or serpentine-like movements
	Squirming/kicking	2	Definitive uneasy or restless movements in the legs and/or striking out with foot or feet
	Drawn up/tensed	2	Legs tensed and/or pulled up tightly to body and kept there
	Standing	2	Standing, crouching, or kneeling
	Restrained	2	Child's legs are being held down

Field and Goldson (1984) and Dixon et al. (1984) used the neonatal behavioral assessment scale (Brazelton, 1973) to investigate the pacifying effect of non-nutritive sucking in neonates during heelstick procedure. This, of course, should be seen not as a measure of pain but a measure of the outcome of pain.

Table 4 summarizes the studies on the measurement of the behavioral component of pain in children.

Behavioral methods of pain measurement in children offer a great deal to both the researcher and to the clinician. Well-validated measures are available for infants and children undergoing discrete, aversive events and for postoperative pain. These multi-item rating scales require an observer dedicated to the measurement task and thus may not be appropriate in the clinical situation. However, these more sophisticated scales have provided validation for the use of nurses' ratings using a visual analogue scale. Since they do not require dedicated observers, they can be used in the day-to-day world of the clinic or hospital.

2.3. The physiological component of pain

Research studies on the physiological component of pediatric pain have many of the same problems discussed in relation to measurement of the cognitive and behavioral components of pain. For example, physiological

TABLE 4
Behavioral measures of pain in children.

Type of strategy	Description	Reference
Rating of cry	Occurrence of crying	Williamson and Williamson, 1983; Field and Goldson, 1984; Owens and Todt, 1984; Franck, 1986
	Rating by nurses and mothers	Wasz-Hockert et al., 1968, 1985; Muller et al., 1974
Measurement of characteristics of cry	Electroacoustic analysis	Wasz-Hockert et al., 1968, 1985; Lester, 1985; Johnston and Strada, 1986; Barr et al., 1987
Global rating of behavior	Visual analogue scale completed by observer	Martin, 1982; McGrath et al., 1985
Behavior scales	Discrete behaviors coded by observers	Katz et al., 1980; Varni, 1981; Varni et al., 1981; Taylor, 1982; Varni and Gilbert, 1982; Piquard-Gauvain et al., 1983, 1984; Craig et al., 1984; Jay and Elliot, 1984; McGrath et al., 1985; Franck, 1986
Facial	Behaviors coded	Izard et al., 1980; Grunau and Craig, 1987a,b; Johnston and Strada, 1986

responses to pain may not differ from responses to stresses other than pain. Measures of the physiological component of pain have included: heart rate, respiration rate, emotional sweating, transcutaneous pO_2, and endorphins (Table 5).

Williamson and Williamson (1983) found that infants who received penile block for circumcision had lower heart rate than those who did not receive anesthetic blocks. Although this could indicate that changes in heart rate might be an appropriate index of pain in infants, the results are confusing. During parts of the cutting and clamping procedures of the circumcision, the anesthetized group's heart rate was significantly below baseline and indicated a relative bradycardia. As well, in this study, there were significant differences in transcutaneous pO_2 during the circumcision. There were no differences in respiration rate between the two groups. Similarly, Field and Goldson (1984) found that heart rate and respiration correlated with behavioral changes in only one of the two groups of preterm neonates undergoing heelstick procedures. The failure to find congruence was thought to be due to a lack of cardiac-somatic coupling in the neonates in the intensive care unit. Owens and Todt (1984) established a clear pattern of increased heart rate in response to heel lance in 2-day-old infants. Jay et al. (1984) found that pulse rate and blood pressure were sensitive, reliable and valid measures of distress just prior to bone marrow aspiration in children. Similarly, Mischel et al. (1986) found good correlations between heart rate and a behavioral measure of pain/distress (similar to Katz et al. (1980) scale) in children undergoing banding of their teeth by an orthodontist.

TABLE 5
Physiological measures of children's pain.

Physiological measure	Reference
Heart rate	Field and Goldson, 1984; Owens and Todt, 1984; Mischel et al., 1986; Johnston and Strada, 1986
Respiration	Williamson and Williamson, 1983; Field and Goldson, 1984
pO_2	Williamson and Williamson, 1983
Sweating	Harpin and Rutter, 1982
Endorphins	Katz et al., 1982; Szyfelbein et al., 1985
Pulse	Jay et al., 1984
Blood pressure	Jay et al., 1984
Hormonal-metabolic changes	Anand et al., 1985, 1987a,b

Johnston and Strada (1986) demonstrated the complexity of the physiological response to pain by analyzing heart rate in intervals of 3 s following immunization. For nine of the 14 babies, the pain response was an initial bradycardia lasting until approximately 9 s after injection, followed by tachycardia which lasted beyond the 1 min observation period. Two of the babies showed heart rate increases from the initial injection; three babies showed no tachycardia until about 15 s after injection and one baby showed no heart rate response to the injection.

Harpin and Rutter (1982) studied 124 infants undergoing heel lance and detected emotional sweating. In babies of 37 weeks gestation or more, palmar sweating increased significantly in infants during heel prick and reduced to baseline as the infant settled. A subsequent study (Harpin and Rutter, 1983) used this measure to evaluate two methods of obtaining heel prick blood samples. This method is similar to the palmar sweat index in which a plastic impression is made to quantify the number of sweat glands that are active (Johnson and Dabbs, 1967). The palmar sweat index was successfully used by Melamed (Melamed and Siegel, 1980) to measure anxiety related to surgery and dental procedures. However, in the previously mentioned study by Jay, with children undergoing bone marrow aspirations, the palmar sweat index was not found to correlate with other measures of distress (Jay et al., 1984).

As Chapman et al. (1985) have emphasized in their recent review of pain measurement in adults, autonomic measures typically habituate over time and thus are unlikely to be suitable as repeated measures of pain. Variations in the utility of autonomic measures across studies may be due to the habituation phenomenon.

Katz et al. (1982) reported on the endorphin levels (β-EP) in the cerebrospinal fluid of 75 children with leukemia undergoing routine lumbar puncture. Positive but small relationships between the β-EP levels and nurses' ratings of anxiety (partial correlation coefficient = 0.31) were found. There was a positive trend but no significant relationship between the procedures behavior rating scale and endorphin levels. These data suggest that the relationship between pain and endorphins as measured in cerebrospinal fluid in children is not clear. The one study examining serum endorphins in children found an inverse relationship between pain reports and plasma iβ-EP level (Szyfelbein et al., 1985). The reasons for the contrasting findings in these two studies is unclear but may be due to the differences between plasma and CF measures of iβ-EP or the fact that Katz used a single measure and Szyfelbein used repeated measures. The use of endorphin levels in the measurement of pediatric pain is sharply limited by the invasive methods required to assay and the difficulty in interpreting the results.

Simple physiological measures of pain in children (such as respiration rate, blood pressure and pulse), although having the intuitive appeal of being precise and concrete, have not been demonstrated to be of sufficient validity to endorse their widespread use as a specific measure of pain in the clinical setting. More complex methods, such as sweating, have the added disadvantage of requiring equipment that is beyond the usual clinical situation. Clearly, much more research is required to determine what physiological indices can be reliably used in pain measurement in children. Physiological measures may provide the tools for a better understanding of developmental changes in pain and the continued unravelling of the physiology of pain.

2.4. The stress response

It is only in recent years that the response to the trauma of surgery in children has been documented. In a series of studies, Anand et al. (1985, 1987a,b) have documented a series of hormonal changes that trigger a cascade of metabolic adjustments that may precipitate increased morbidity and mortality. The main features of the stress response are hyperglycemia and hyperlactatemia associated with the release of catecholamines and the inhibition of insulin secretion. This response is blunted by the appropriate use of anesthesia (Anand et al., 1987a,b). These studies are discussed in more detail in chapter 4.

3. Pain assessment

The initial quote from Lord Kelvin emphasizes the need to put numbers to pain measurement but the search for numbers can be misleading if we rush into this willy-nilly and end up measuring the wrong thing. As Thomas (1983, p. 144), commenting on Kelvin's famous quote, has emphasized:

> The task of converting observations into numbers is the hardest of all, the last task rather than the first thing to be done, and it can be done only when you have learned, beforehand, a great deal about the observations themselves. You can, to be sure, achieve a very deep understanding of nature by quantitative measurement, but you must know what you are talking about before you can begin applying the numbers for making predictions.

To date, virtually all of our pediatric pain measurement strategies have emphasized either occurrence versus non-occurrence or the intensity dimension of pain. Research with adults has suggested that relying solely on intensity is not sufficient. For example, as Melzack (1983, p. 2) has emphasized:

> Describing pain solely in terms of intensity is like specifying the visual world only in terms of light flux without regard to pattern, color, texture, and the many other dimensions of visual experience.

The pain experience encompasses a wide and complex variety of aspects of sensation as well as elements of evaluation, perception, motivation and affect (Melzack, 1983). These in turn are influenced or may be influenced by a wide variety of social, contextual and developmental factors (Craig, 1980). The difficulty in devising assessment strategies is to decide which of the multitude of possible aspects or factors should be tapped.

Although there can be little doubt that intensity is an important dimension of pain, little research has been done to evaluate which of the multitude of possible other factors should be measured in any specific pediatric pain situation.

Two approaches have been suggested. The first approach is to decide what specific question is being asked and then to address that question by means of a specific test instrument. The second way is to attempt to develop a generic assessment strategy that can be used in a variety of pain situations to answer the most common questions that are likely to be important. A combination of these two strategies is possible in which a basic pain assessment is supplemented by specific measures to answer specific questions.

An example of the first strategy is research in our own lab. If the question is to discern if pain is psychogenic, a set of criteria (McGrath, 1983) based on 'time-locking' events of pain with stressful situations or with specific emotional states can be delineated. Validation of this strategy has not, as yet, been undertaken.

Similarly, Dunn-Geier et al. (1986) focussed on evaluation of the reinforcement of coping behavior and expression of pain. We developed a laboratory task to measure the social support provided by mothers to their children in coping with chronic pain. Adolescents who were coping well with chronic pain were compared to adolescents who were not coping well. During an exercise task supervised by their mothers, the interaction between the parent and child was recorded and analyzed using a variant of the Mash et al. (1973) response class matrix. Coping adolescents complained less and their mothers were much less intrusive in the exercise task.

This type of strategy examines the pain behaviors and the reinforcement patterns of copers and non-copers rather than attempting to measure intensity of pain and may be of use in intervention with the families to normalize the family interaction.

The second strategy, that of developing a generic comprehensive, pediatric pain assessment battery which tries to evaluate a variety of factors implicated in a broad range of pain problems, has been modelled on the very productive McGill pain questionnaire developed by Melzack (1975) for assessment of adult pain. The first attempt was by Savedra et al. (1981, 1982) and Tesler et al. (1983). Their questionnaire (reproduced in Tesler et al., 1983) included eight questions. The child was asked to tell three events that have caused pain; circle those words that describe pain from a list of 24 words; report what color their pain was; select how they felt when they had pain from a list of 13 possibilities; describe their worst pain and how it felt; describe what helps when in pain; report what is good about pain; and finally mark on a silhouette where their pain occurs. The questionnaire was intended for children aged 9–12. This group has published descriptive data on how hospitalized and non-hospitalized children respond. However, no reliability or validity data have been published. Nor has the questionnaire been used to evaluate specific groups of children suffering pain.

Development of clinically oriented instruments has been undertaken by P.A. McGrath et al. (1985) and by Varni and Thompson (1985). They have developed questionnaires that are similar. For example, P.A. McGrath et al. (1985) asked questions about the duration, frequency, and location of pain. The child is asked to describe the temporal pattern and the quality of pain. Visual analogue scales are used to assess the intensity of the pain, the emotions related to the pain, and expectations for relief. Facial scales are used to measure the affective component (how the child feels) of the pain experience. Faces are also used to ask children how they feel in a variety of painful (i.e., toothache, spanking, bee sting) and non-painful (i.e., birthday present, wake up, being teased) experiences.

The Varni/Thompson pediatric pain questionnaire asks the child to rate present pain and worse pain on a visual analogue scale. The child is asked to select colors to represent different severities of pain and to indicate on a body outline the severity of pain by coloring the outline. The child is also asked to select words which describe his pain from a list. Their parents are also asked to report on the intensity, sensory, affective, evaluative aspects of pain and the location of pain.

At present, there is little data evaluating the usefulness of these assessment batteries. Thompson et al. (1987) and Varni et al. (1987) have recently published research on pain in juvenile rheumatoid arthritis using the Varni/ Thompson battery. This work is discussed in chapter 9.

4. Summary

It is evident that the task of measuring children's pain is not impossible and that pediatric pain is increasingly being considered a topic worthy of both clinical consideration and of research. Pain assessment on the other hand has really not yet begun. A great deal of thinking and research is required to insure that appropriate factors of the pain experience are being measured.

Progress in understanding and treatment of pain in children will depend on continuing advances in the measurement and assessment of pain.

5. Clinical implications

(1) Routine measurement of children's pain should be implemented in all health care situations where it is reasonably expected that pain will occur.
(2) Pain measurement should be geared to the state and age of the child. Behavioral and physiological methods are appropriate for preschool or comatose patients. Self-report methods are appropriate for school-age children.

6. Future directions

(1) Research is needed on the utility of measures in evaluating interventions for pain. The sensitivity of different measures to bio-behavioral and analgesic interventions is required.
(2) Measurement of infant pain, particularly in sick infants is needed.
(3) Further validation of existing measures of children's pain is required. New measures should be developed only where appropriate measures do not exist. One area in which new, validated measures are needed is the measurement of pain in severely mentally and physically disabled children (especially postoperative pain). Current measures are not appropriate and these children frequently require surgical intervention.
(4) Validation of assessment measures should be undertaken.

References

Abu-Saad, H. (1984) Assessing children's responses to pain. Pain 19, 163–171.

Abu-Saad, H. and Holzmer, W.L. (1981) Measuring children's self assessment of pain. Issues Compr. Pediatr. Nurs. 5, 337–349.

Anand, K.J.S., Brown, M.J., Causon, R.C., Christofides, N.D., Bloom, S.R. and Aynsley-Green, A. (1985) Can the human neonate mount an endocrine and metabolic response to surgery. J. Pediatr. Surg. 20, 41–48.

Anand, K.J.S., Sippell, W.G. and Aynsley-Green, A. (1987a) Randomized trial of fentanyl anaesthesia in preterm babies undergoing surgery: Effects on the stress response. Lancet i, 243–247.

Anand, K.J.S., Sippell, W.G. and Aynsley-Green, A. (1987b) Does the newborn infant require anaesthesia during surgery? Answers from a randomised trial of halothane anaesthesia. Vth World Congress on Pain, Hamburg. Pain suppl. 4, S451.

Andrasik, F., Burke, E.J., Attanasio, V. and Rosenblum, E.L. (1985) Child, parent and physician reports of a child's headache pain: Relationships prior to and following treatment. Headache 25, 421–425.

Aradine, C.R., Beyer, J.E. and Tompkins, J.M. (1987) Children's pain perception after analgesia: A study of instrument construct validity. J. Pediatr. Nurs., in press.

Barr, R.G., Kramer, M.S., Leduc, D.G., Boisjoly, C., McVey, L. and Pless, I.B. (1987) Validation of a parental diary of infant cry/fuss behavior by a 24-hour voice-activated infant recording (VAR) system. Manuscript under review.

Beales, J.G. (1982) The assessment and management of pain in children. In: P. Karoly, J.J. Steffen and D.J. O'Grady (Eds.), Child Health Psychology: Concepts and Issues (Pergamon, Toronto) pp. 154–179.

Beyer, J.E. (1984) The Oucher: A User's Manual and Technical Report (The Hospital Play Equipment Co., Evanston, IL).

Beyer, J.E. and Aradine, C.R. (1986) Content validity of an instrument to measure young children's perceptions of the intensity of their pain. J. Pediatr. Nurs. 1, 386–395.

Beyer, J.E. and Aradine, C.R. (1987a) Patterns of pediatric pain intensity: A methodological investigation of a self-report scale. Clin. J. Pain, in press.

Beyer, J.E. and Aradine, C.R. (1987b) The convergent and discriminant validity of a self-report measure of pain intensity for children. Child. Health Care, in press.

Beyer, J.E., DeGood, D.E., Ashley, L.C. and Russell, G.A. (1983) Patterns of postoperative analgesic use with adults and children following cardiac surgery. Pain 17, 71–81.

Brazelton, T.B. (1973) Neonatal Behavioral Assessment Scale (Heinemann Medical Books, London).

Chapman, C.R., Casey, K.L., Dubner, R., Foley, K.M., Gracely, R.H. and Reading, A.E. (1985) Pain measurement: An overview. Pain 22, 1–31.

Craig, K.D. (1980) Ontogenetic and cultural influences on the expression of pain in man. In: H.W. Kosterlitz and L.Y. Terenius (Eds.), Pain and Society (Verlag Chemie, Weinheim) pp. 39–52.

Craig, K.D., McMahon, R.J., Morison, J.D. and Zaskow, C. (1984) Developmental changes in infant pain expression during immunization injections. Soc. Sci. Med. 19, 1331–1337.

Dixon, S., Snyder, J., Holve, R. and Bromberger, P. (1984) Behavioral effects of circumcision with and without anesthesia. Dev. Behav. Pediatr. 5, 246–250.

Dunn-Geier, B.J., McGrath, P.J., Rourke, B.P., Latter, J.L. and D'Astous, J. (1986) Adolescent chronic pain: The ability to cope. Pain 26, 23–32.

Ekman, P. and Friesen, W.V. (1978) The Facial Action Coding System (FACS) (Consulting Psychologists Press, Palo Alto, CA).

Ekman, P. and Oster, H. (1979) Facial expression of emotion. Ann. Rev. Psychol. 30, 527–554.

Eland, J.M. (1974) Children's communication of pain. Master's thesis, University of Iowa, IA.

Eland, J.M. and Anderson, J.E. (1977) The experience of pain in children. In: A.K. Jacox (Ed.), Pain: A Sourcebook for Nurses and Other Health Professionals (Little Brown, Boston, MA) pp. 453–473.

Field, T. and Goldson, E. (1984) Pacifying effects of nonnutritive sucking on term and preterm neonates during heelstick procedures. Pediatrics 74, 1012–1015.

Franck, L.S. (1986) A new method to quantitatively describe pain behavior in infants. Nurs. Res. 35, 28–31.

Gracely, R.H., McGrath, P.A. and Dubner, R. (1978) Ratio scales of sensory and affective verbal pain descriptors. Pain 5, 5–18.

Grunau, R.V.E. and Craig, K.D. (1987a) Pain expression in neonates: Facial action and cry. Pain 28, 395–410.

Grunau, R.V.E. and Craig, K.D. (1987b) Neonatal pain behavior and perinatal events. Manuscript under review.

Harpin, V.A. and Rutter, N. (1982) Development of emotional sweating in the newborn infant. Arch. Dis. Child. 57, 691–695.

Harpin, V.A. and Rutter, N. (1983) Making heel pricks less painful. Arch. Dis. Child. 58, 226–227.

Hester, N.K. (1979) The pre-operational child's reaction to immunization. Nurs. Res. 28, 250–255.

Huskisson, E.C. (1983) Visual Analogue Scales. In: R. Melzack (Ed.), Pain Measurement and Assessment (Raven Press, New York) pp. 33–37.

Izard, C.E., Huebner, R.R., Resser, D., McGiness, G.C. and Dougherty, L.M. (1980) The infants ability to produce discrete emotional expressions. Dev. Psychol. 16, 132–140.

Jay, S.M. and Elliot, C. (1984) Behavioral observation scales for measuring children's distress: The effects of increased methodological rigor. J. Consult. Clin. Psychol. 52, 1106–1107.

Jay, S.M., Ozolins, M., Elliot, C. and Caldwell, S. (1983) Assessment of children's distress during painful medical procedures. J. Health Psychol. 2, 133–147.

Jay, S.M., Elliot, C., Katz, E.R. and Siegel, S.C. (1984) Stress reduction in children undergoing painful medical procedures. Paper presented at the Annual Meeting of the American Psychological Association, Toronto, Canada.

Jeans, M.E. (1983) Pain in children: A neglected area. In: P. Firestone, P. McGrath, and W. Feldman (Eds.), Advances in Behavioral Medicine for Children and Adolescents (Erlbaum, Hillsdale, NJ) pp. 23–38.

Johnson, J. and Dabbs, J. (1967) Enumeration of active sweat glands. Nurs. Res. 16, 273–276.

Johnston, C.C. and Strada, M.E. (1986) Acute pain response in infants: a multidimensional description. Pain 24, 373–382.

Katz, E.R., Kellerman, J. and Seigel, S.E. (1980) Distress behavior in children with cancer undergoing medical procedures: Developmental considerations. J. Consult. Clin. Psychol. 48, 356–365.

Katz, E.R., Sharp, B., Kellerman, J., Marston, A.R., Hershman, J.N. and Siegel, S.E. (1982)

Beta-endorphin immunoreactivity and acute behavioral distress in children with leukemia. J. Nerv. Ment. Dis. 170, 72–77.

Kazdin, A.E. (1977) Assessing the clinical or applied importance of behavior change through social validation. Behav. Modif. 1, 427–449.

Kurylyszyn, N., McGrath, P.J., Cappelli, M. and Humphreys, P. (1987) Children's drawings: What can they tell us about intensity of pain? Clin. J. Pain 2, 155–158.

Kuttner, L. and LePage, T. (1984) The development of pictorial self-report scales of pain and anxiety for children. Unpublished manuscript.

LeBaron, S. and Zelter, L. (1984) Assessment of acute pain and anxiety in children and adolescents by self-reports, observer reports, and a behavior checklist. J. Consult. Clin. Psychol. 52, 729–738.

Lester, B.M. (1985) Introduction: There's more to crying than meets the ear. In: B.M. Lester and C.F.Z. Boukydis (Eds.), Infant Crying: Theoretical and Research Perspectives (Plenum, New York) pp. 1–27.

Lollar, D.J., Smits, S.J. and Patterson, D.L. (1982) Assessment of pediatric pain: An empirical perspective. J. Pediatr. Psychol. 7, 267–277.

McGrath, P.A., DeVeber, L.L. and Hearn, M.T. (1985) Multidimensional pain assessment in children. In: H.L. Fields, R. Dubner and F. Cervero (Eds.), Advances in Pain Research and Therapy (Raven Press, New York) pp. 387–393.

McGrath, P.J. (1983) Psychological aspects of recurrent abdominal pain. Can. Fam. Phys. 29, 1655–1659.

McGrath, P.J., Johnson, G., Goodman, J.T., Schillinger, J., Dunn, J. and Chapman, J. (1985) The CHEOPS: A behavioral scale to measure post operative pain in children. In: H.L. Fields, R. Dubner and F. Cervero (Eds.), Advances in Pain Research and Therapy (Raven Press, New York) pp. 395–402.

McGrath, P.J., Cunningham, S.J., Goodman, J.T. and Unruh, A. (1986) The clinical measurement of pain in children: A review. Clin. J. Pain 1, 221–227.

Mash, E., Terdal, L. and Anderson, K. (1973) The response class matrix: A procedure for recording parent-child interactions. J. Consult. Clin. Psychol. 40, 163–164.

Martin, L.V.H. (1982) Postoperative analgesia after circumcision in children. Br. J. Anaesth. 54, 1263–1266.

Melamed, B. and Siegel, L. (1980) Behavioral medicine: Practical applications in health care (Springer, New York).

Melzack, R. (1975) The McGill pain questionnaire: Major properties and scoring methods. Pain 1, 277–299.

Melzack, R. (Ed.) (1983) Pain Measurement and Assessment (Raven Press, New York) pp. 1–6.

Merskey, H. (Ed.) (1986) Classification of chronic pain: descriptions of chronic pain syndromes and definitions of pain terms. Pain suppl. 3, S217.

Mischel, H.N., Fuhr, R. and McDonald, M.A. (1986) Children's dental pain: The effects of cognitive coping training in a clinical setting. Clin. J. Pain 1, 235–242.

Monk, M. (1980) The nature of pain and responses to pain in adolescent hemophiliacs. Master's thesis, McGill University, Montreal.

Muller, E., Hollien, H. and Murry, T. (1974) Perceptual response to infant crying: Identification of cry types. J. Child Lang. 1, 89–95.

Ostwald, P.F. and Murry, T. (1985) The communicative and diagnostic significance of infant sounds. In: B.M. Lester and C.F.Z. Boukydis (Eds.), Infant Crying: Theoretical and Research Perspectives (Plenum, New York) pp. 139–158.

Owens, M.E. and Todt, E.H. (1984) Pain in infancy: Neonatal reaction to a heel lance. Pain 20, 77–86.

Piquard-Gauvain, A., Rodary, C., Rezvani, A. and Lemerle, J. (1983) Establishment of a new rating scale for the evaluation of pain in young children (2 to 6 years) with cancer. Pain suppl. 2, S25.

Piquard-Gauvain, A., Rodary, C., Rezvani, A. and Lemerle, J. (1984) Development of a new rating scale for the evaluation of pain in young children (2–6 yrs) with cancer. In: R. Rizzi and M. Visentin (Eds.), Pain (Piccin/Butterworths, Padua, Italy) pp. 383–390.

Richardson, G.M., McGrath, P.J., Cunningham, S.J. and Humphreys, P. (1983) Validity of the headache diary for children. Headache 23, 184–187.

Ross, D.M. and Ross, S.A. (1984) The importance of type of question, psychological climate, and subject set in interviewing children about pain. Pain 19, 71–79.

Savedra, M., Tesler, M., Ward, J., Wegner, C. and Gibbons, P. (1981) Description of the pain experience: A study of school age children. Issues Compr. Pediatr. Nurs. 5, 373–380.

Savedra, M., Gibbons, P., Tesler, M., Ward, J. and Wegner, C. (1982) How do children describe pain? A tentative assessment. Pain 14, 95–104.

Scott, J. and Huskisson, E.C. (1979) Vertical or horizontal visual analogue scales. Ann. Rheum. Dis. 38, 560.

Scott, R. (1978) It hurts red: A preliminary study of children's perception of pain. Percept. Mot. Skills 47, 787–791.

Sherman, M. (1927) The differentiation of emotional responses in infants. J. Comp. Psychol. 7, 265–284.

Stevens, B. (1986) Reliability and validity of a behavioral measure of pain. Unpublished manuscript, McMaster University Medical School.

Stewart, M.L. (1977) Measurement of clinical pain. In: A.K. Jacox (Ed.), Pain: A Sourcebook for Nurses and Other Health Professionals (Little Brown, Boston, MA) pp. 107–137.

Szyfelbein, S.K., Osgood, P.F. and Carr, D.B. (1985) The assessment of pain and plasma β-endorphin immunoactivity in burned children. Pain 22, 173–182.

Taylor, P.L. (1982) Post-operative pain in toddler and pre-school age children. Matern. Child Nurs. J. 12, 35–50.

Tesler, M., Ward, J., Savedra, M., Wegner, C.B. and Gibbons, P. (1983) Developing an instrument for eliciting children's descriptions of pain. Percept. Mot. Skills 56, 315–321.

Thomas, L. (1983) Late Night Thoughts on Listening to Mahler's Ninth Symphony (Viking, New York) pp. 143–155.

Thompson, K.L. and Varni, J.W. (1986) A developmental cognitive-behavioral approach to pediatric pain assessment. Pain 25, 283–296.

Thompson, K.L., Varni, J.W. and Hanson, V. (1987) Comprehensive assessment of pain in juvenile rheumatoid arthritis: An empirical model. J. Pediatr. Psychol., in press.

Unruh, A., McGrath, P.J., Cunningham, S.J. and Humphreys, P. (1983) Children's drawings of their pain. Pain 17, 385–392.

Vair, C.A. (1981) The perceptions and coping strategies of seven to twelve year old hospitalized children in response to acute pain. Unpublished Master's thesis, University of Toronto.

Varni, J.W. (1981) Self regulation techniques in the management of chronic arthritic pain in hemophilia. Behav. Ther. 12, 185–194.

Varni, J.W. and Gilbert, A. (1982) Self-regulation of chronic arthritic pain and long-term analgesic dependence in a hemophiliac. Rheum.Rehabil. 22, 171–174.

Varni, J.W. and Thompson, K.L. (1985) Biobehavioral assessment and management of pediatric pain. In: N.A. Krasnegor, J.D. Austen and M.F. Cataldo (Eds.), Child Health Behavior (Wiley, New York).

Varni, J.W., Gilbert, A. and Deitrich, S.L. (1981) Behavioral medicine in pain and analgesia management for the hemophilic child with factor VIII inhibitor. Pain 11, 121–126.

Varni, J.W., Thompson, K.L. and Hanson, V. (1987) The Varni/Thompson pediatric pain questionnaire: 1. Chronic musculo-skeletal pain in juvenile rheumatoid arthritis. Pain 28, 27–38.

Wasz-Hockert, O., Lind, J., Vuorenkoski, V., Partanen, T. and Valanne, E. (1968) The infant cry: A spectrographic and auditory analysis. Clin. Dev. Med. 29, 9–42.

Wasz-Hockert, O., Michelson, K. and Lind, J. (1985) Twenty-five years of Scandinavian cry research. In: B.M. Lester and C.F. Zachariah Boukydis (Eds.), Infant Crying: Theoretical and Research Perspectives (Plenum Press, New York) pp. 83–104.

Williamson, P.S. and Williamson, M.L. (1983) Physiologic stress reduction by a local anesthetic during newborn circumcision. Pediatrics 71, 36–40.

Wolff, P.H. (1969) The natural history of crying and other vocalizations in early infancy. In: B.M. Foss (Ed.), Determinants of infant behavior, Vol. 4 (Methuen, London).

CHAPTER 4

Perioperative and postoperative pain

Pain is soul destroying. No patient should have to endure intense pain unnecessarily. The quality of mercy is essential to the practice of medicine. Here, of all places, it should not be strained (*Angell, 1982, p. 99*).

1. Introduction

Modern surgery has brought major advances in the health care of children. However, a side effect of surgery is the occurrence of perioperative pain and resulting stress and postoperative pain. Perioperative pain, or pain occurring during surgery, has been controlled in children and adults by anesthetic agents. However, in neonates there has been little effort to control perioperative pain. This chapter will first discuss perioperative pain and will then focus on postoperative pain. Different aspects of postoperative pain and the major controversies in the area will be discussed. Clinical guidelines for management of perioperative and postoperative pain will be discussed. Suggestions for future directions in research and policies will be given.

2. Perioperative pain

Anand and Aynsley-Green (1985) have reported that in the 40 published papers that they reviewed, 76% of preterm neonates undergoing thoracotomy for patent ductus arteriosus (the most common surgical procedure in the preterm neonate) received no or only very minimal anesthesia. The practice of not using anesthesia with preterm neonates has been the result of the traditional beliefs that preterm neonates cannot feel pain and that they may develop adverse reactions to any anesthetic. Until recently, virtually no research has examined the effects of the failure to use anesthesia in the neonate. A series of studies by Anand, Aynsley-Green and others have detailed the metabolic and endocrine response to surgery. Anand and

Aynsley-Green (1985) in a study of ten preterm neonates found highly significant hyperglycemia during surgery that persisted for more than 24 h after surgery. They also showed hyperlactacidemia, hyperketonemia and increases in blood glycerol, blood pyruvate and an inhibition of insulin secretion during surgery. They suggested that the preterm neonate does mount a substantial stress response to thoracotomy under minimal anesthesia. In subsequent studies of term and preterm neonates, they (Anand et al., 1985a,b) confirmed the universal hyperglycemia; demonstrated a high correlation (0.95) between adrenaline and glucose; and detailed differences between term and preterm neonates. They also noted differences between neonates subjected to different anesthetic techniques.

In a randomized controlled trial, Anand et al. (1987a) studied 16 preterm neonates who were randomized to two anesthesia groups. Both were given nitrous oxide and curare. In addition, intravenous fentanyl was used in the experimental group. Major differences were found between the two groups in their hormonal response. The non-fentanyl group had the strong adrenaline response and the massive hyperglycemic response documented in their previous research. As well, they experienced high levels of endogenous protein breakdown. The stress response and the protein breakdown were substantially blunted in the fentanyl group. The authors discussed the clinical implications of the massive stress response with the typical minimal anesthetic and concluded it may contribute to morbidity and mortality.

A similar study of 36 term neonates compared response to surgery with muscle relaxants and nitrous oxide with halothane anesthesia to the response without halothane anesthesia (Anand et al., 1987b). They found that the group with halothane did not have as strong a stress response as the group without the benefit of halothane.

Anand et al. (1987a) suggested that although neonates undergoing surgery with reduced anesthesia do not appear to be in pain (perhaps because they are paralyzed and ventilated) the stress response is mediated by nociception from the surgery.

3. Are children undermedicated postoperatively?

A pervasive debate in the literature on pain in children has been whether or not children are undermedicated when compared with adults for postoperative pain. This debate must take into consideration evidence that, in general, pain in children has been neglected in both research and clinical practice

(Jeans, 1983), that most postoperative pain in adults is poorly managed, and that aggressive use of analgesics can virtually eliminate severe pain (Angell, 1982). On one side of the debate is the oft quoted position of Merskey in regards to postoperative pain that 'at birth the response to trauma is minimal' (Merskey, 1970, p. 118) and that before age 5 there are significantly decreased pain thresholds (Merskey, 1970). Perhaps most illustrative is the opinion of Swafford and Allan (1968) who acknowledged that children may be able to experience pain but insisted that:

> Pediatric patients seldom need medication for the relief of pain. They tolerate discomfort well. The child will say he does not feel well, or that he is uncomfortable or that he wants his parents but often he will not relate this unhappiness to pain *(Swafford and Allan, 1968, p. 133)*.

According to this argument, the need for postoperative pain control in infants and young children is minimal or non-existent. On the other side of the debate about the adequacy of postoperative analgesia for children are three studies that have compared analgesics prescribed and given to children and adults.

Eland and Anderson (1977) reported on the management of 25 children aged 4–8 years who were hospitalized for surgery. Although 21 of the children had been ordered analgesics p.r.n., only 12 of the 25 children were given any analgesics. The authors matched 18 of these children with 18 adults with similar diagnoses and found that the children received a total of 24 doses of analgesic while the adults received 372 opioid analgesic doses and 299 non-opioid doses of analgesics.

Similarly, Beyer et al. (1983) compared the postoperative prescription and administration of analgesics following cardiac surgery in 50 children and 50 adults. Children received 30% of the analgesic doses and adults received 70% of doses. Six children were not prescribed any analgesics in the first 3 days postoperatively. Adults were more likely to receive more potent drugs. Dosages for children were more likely to be below recommended levels and by the 5th day postoperatively, children had received ten doses whereas adults had received 136 doses.

Schechter et al. (1986) examined a random sample of 90 adults and 90 children matched for sex with similar diagnoses (appendectomies, hernias, fractured femurs, and burns) and found that depending on diagnostic category, adults received between one-and-a-half to three times the number of doses of opioids than did the children.

In a related study, Mather and Mackie (1983) reviewed the charts of 170 pediatric patients postoperatively. They found that approximately 40% of patients reported pain as moderate or severe on the operative day. For 16% of the children, no analgesic medication was ordered at all. In nearly 50% of the cases where opioids were ordered, the dose was inadequate. In 46% of the cases, the analgesic ordered was substituted with a less potent drug.

However, as Jeans (1984) has emphasized, none of these studies directly measured the amount of pain experienced by the patient. She reported a preliminary study, which indicated that on the basis of self-report, there were no major differences in pain experienced by children and adults undergoing similar surgery. She also found that, at the Montreal Children's Hospital, in which she did the study, children were given similar levels of analgesics as adults in other settings.

4. Are children subjected to unnecessary surgery?

There is good evidence that some surgeries which cause pain to children are unnecessary. Among the two most common surgeries are tonsillectomy and circumcision. Tonsillectomy is usually suggested for children who have seven episodes of tonsillitis within a 1 year period, five or more episodes in each of the 2 preceding years, or three or more episodes in each of the preceding 3 years. A randomized trial to test the benefit of tonsillectomy in children who had met these criteria yielded suggestive evidence that there was no significant benefit for children who underwent tonsillectomy compared with the control children who did not undergo the procedure (Paradise et al., 1984). During the first 2 years after tonsillectomy, there were fewer throat infections, but by the third year after the operation, the frequency of throat infections was the same in both groups. No major side effects were detected in either group.

Similarly, the justification for circumcision (other than for religious reasons) is very tenuous. The lack of justification for circumcision has led the American Academy of Pediatrics (1975) to declare that circumcision had no medical indication. Minor complications occur in one in 15–20 boys and major complications can occur and include amputation of the penis or death (King, 1982). North American parents seem to be the major proponents of circumcision and the rate of circumcision remains at about 80% in the United States (Slotkowski and King, 1982).

The reduction in unnecessary tonsillectomies and circumcisions would substantially reduce postoperative pain in children.

5. Pharmacological methods in postoperative pain

Acetylsalicylic acid and acetaminophen are the major non-opioid analgesics while morphine, codeine, methadone, meperidine, and hydromorphine are the opioid analgesics most commonly used for postoperative pain relief in children.

5.1 Non-opioid analgesics

Acetylsalicylic acid (ASA), whose most common trade name is Aspirin, was introduced in clinical practice in 1899 and herbal remedies that contained salicylates have been in use for centuries (Peterson, 1985). Although ASA is most commonly used in young children for its potent antipyretic and anti-inflammatory effect, it also has an important analgesic effect. Acetylsalicylic acid acts by inhibiting the conversion of arachidonic acid to endoperoxide prostaglandin G_2 which would subsequently be converted to various prostaglandins (Peterson, 1985). Prostaglandins are often released at the site of trauma and they appear to sensitize nociceptors to histamine and bradykinin. Thus ASA appears to desensitize the nerve to chemical environmental factors that might ordinarily produce pain (Schechter, 1985). Current recommended dosages for ASA are 10 mg/kg every 4 h or 60 mg/kg every 24 h. Side effects of ASA include: blood loss from the gastrointestinal tract and interference with platelet functioning. There is a danger of fatal poisoning from ASA. It is important to note that, in children under the age of 3 years, a large proportion of the poisonings and deaths result from therapeutic misuse in an aggressive attempt to control fever rather than accidental poisoning (Peterson, 1985). There are no adequate liquid or suppository preparations but chewable forms are available (Schecter, 1985). There is no tolerance, physical dependence or addiction with ASA.

Acetaminophen also acts by means of prostaglandin antagonism. However, the spectrum of action of acetaminophen is much narrower than acetylsalicylic acid. In particular, acetaminophen has much less anti-inflammatory action. Acetaminophen is the principal metabolite of phenacetin. Phenacetin has long been used in analgesic preparations but possesses serious toxic potential in the form of methemoglobinemia and interstitial nephritis. This toxicity has led to a reduced use of phenacetin in North America. In the therapeutic dosage of 10–15 mg/kg/dose at 4 h intervals up to 65 mg/kg/24 h, acetaminophen has no significant side effects. The pharmacokinetics of acetaminophen have been described by Peterson and Rumack (1978) who noted that for adults the half-life is 1.5–3 h; for children the half-life is 1.0–3.5 h and for neonates half-life is 2.2–5.0 h. Unlike ASA, chronic aggressive therapy with acetaminophen is not likely to lead to poisoning although one therapeutic fatality at a higher dose has been reported (Peterson, 1985). Overdoses of acetaminophen can result in potentially fatal hepatic necrosis. Liquid forms both in the form of an elixir (160 mg/5 ml) and drops (80 mg/0.8 ml) are available and care must be taken not to confuse dosages with each. Suppositories are now available. There is no tolerance, physical dependence or addiction with acetaminophen.

Reye syndrome is a serious and sometimes fatal disorder of non-inflammatory encephalopathy associated with microvesicular fatty degeneration of the liver. The etiology is unknown. Although it is clear that ASA does not cause Reye syndrome, ASA has been implicated in precipitating the syndrome in vulnerable children with varicella or influenza.

At the urging of pediatric associations (e.g., Fulginiti et al., 1982), Canada and the U.S.A. have required warning labels on all ASA products. The U.K. has gone further by announcing that all children's ASA products will be withdrawn from the market.

Subsequent to publicizing the link between ASA and Reye syndrome the consumption of ASA and the incidence of Reye syndrome declined dramatically in the U.S.A. (Barrett et al., 1986).

Recently, benzydamine, a non-steroidal anti-inflammatory agent has been evaluated as a postoperative oral spray or rinse to reduce the pain and swelling following tonsillectomy or tracheal intubation. Benzydamine is reported to have analgesic, anesthetic, anti-inflammatory and antimicrobial effects. Its action is believed to be mediated by inhibition of prostaglandin and thromboxane biosynthesis, inhibiting platelet aggregation and stabilizing cell membranes (Segre and Hammarstrom, 1985).

A number of randomized trials demonstrating efficacy of benzydamine have appeared in the adult literature (Mahon and DeGregorio, 1985) and some of these adult trials have included adolescents in their sample. Only one properly controlled pediatric trial could be found. Giacomelli et al. (1984) reported on a randomized placebo controlled trial with benzydamine nebulized spray administered six times daily for 5 days following tonsillectomy. The subjects were 57 children aged 4–17 years (mean age = 7.5 years). They found statistically significant and meaningful differences between the two groups on pain, difficulty swallowing and measures of inflammation. Young children may not be able to follow instructions sufficiently well to use the oral rinse formulation.

Other non-steroidal anti-inflammatory drugs have been suggested for analgesic use with children. These are discussed in chapter 9 on musculo-skeletal pain.

5.2 Opioid analgesics

The most widely accepted term for the drugs developed from opium and their many natural and synthetic derivatives is now opioids. The term narcotic, although widely used, is considered obsolete for medical purposes (Jaffe and Martin, 1985).

5.2.1. Mode of action

The mode of action of all opioid analgesics is thought to be primarily central and is presumed to be due to their binding to receptor sites located principally in the limbic system, hypothalamus, thalamus, striatum and spinal cord. There is reasonable evidence for the existence of four major groups of receptors that act on the central nervous system: μ (mu), κ (kappa), δ (delta), and σ (sigma) receptors. Analgesia has been linked to both the μ and κ receptors while dysphoria has been associated with the σ receptors which are thought to be related to changes in affective behavior (Jaffe and Martin, 1985).

Morphine and the other opioids produce their analgesic effects in a relatively selective way so that there is no interference with sensory inputs other than pain. The opioids act to reduce pain not only by a direct analgesic effect but also by reducing the reactive component of the pain. In many cases, adult patients report that the pain is still there but it hurts less; there is less suffering.

5.2.2. Side effects of opioids

An issue that has been repeatedly mentioned as a major factor in limiting the use of opioids with children is the fear of addiction. Four terms related to addiction should be defined: tolerance, physical dependence, psychological dependence and abuse. Tolerance (the requirement for increasing dosage for the same effect) and physical dependence (the occurrence of withdrawal symptoms when the drug is discontinued) are characteristic of continued usage of all opioid drugs. Tolerance can interfere with analgesic effectiveness and increasing dosages may be required for analgesia. In some cases, side effects from increasing dosages may be problematic. Dependence is easily controlled by the tapering of opioids to withdraw the drug.

Psychological dependence, which is the precursor of abuse, is not well understood but consists of craving for the drug, the belief that one cannot do without the drug and a drive to seek the drug. Abuse occurs when the individual's normal responsibilities or health are endangered by drug-seeking or drug-taking. Psychological dependence and abuse are more likely to occur with drugs that cause physical dependence but there are a host of other factors that play a major role. Tolerance and physical dependence are common with opioid drug use but this is not a major problem. Psychological dependence and subsequent abuse of opioids prescribed for postoperative pain is extraordinarily rare in adults (less than one tenth of 1%) (Miller and Jick, 1978; Porter and Jick, 1980) and has not been documented in the pediatric age group. As Newburger and Sallan (1981) emphasized, a child undertreated for pain who is desperately and single-mindedly anticipating his next dose exhibits more addictive-like behavior than a properly medicated child who is able to enjoy other activities. A miserly approach, in which analgesia is withheld until the patient proves that they need the analgesic to a skeptical caregiver, is more likely to contribute to exaggerated pain behavior on the part of the patient and would theoretically be more likely to lead to dependence.

Respiratory depression is a very frequent side effect of the opioids. The depression is dose related and the action is primarily the result of the reduction of the responsiveness of the brainstem respiratory centers to increases in carbon dioxide tension. Respiratory depression is of concern because of the resulting danger of respiratory arrest or postoperative atelectasis. As a result, respiration should be monitored on patients taking opioids. Respiratory depression due to the analgesic opioids used with children (which are all agonists) is reversible by use of naloxone, which antagonizes the action of the common analgesic opioids. Respiratory depression from therapeutic doses of opioids must be weighed against the often more troublesome side effects of reduced movement because of postoperative pain and the humanitarian issue of suffering.

Nausea and vomiting occur with opioids because of direct stimulation of the chemoreceptor trigger zone for emesis in the area postrema of the medulla (Jaffe and Martin, 1985). Nausea and vomiting are relatively rare with recumbent patients but quite common (40% and 15% respectively) with ambulatory patients, suggesting a vestibular interaction. Motion sickness medications such as dimenhydrinate are of use in combatting these side effects in affected patients.

Constipation is a frequent side effect of opioid use. The mechanism of action is both central and a direct action on the bowel. Some tolerance develops to the constipating action. Constipation can be treated with stool softeners, laxatives and a high fiber diet.

Flushing of the skin of the face, neck and upper body and sweating due to dilation of the blood vessels are frequent side effects of opioids which occur most often after the first dose. Cooling with a wet facecloth may help reduce this side effect.

5.2.3. *Opioid kinetics in children*

The kinetics of opioids in the pediatric age range have not been thoroughly investigated. In fact, morphine is the only opioid for which much information is available. Dahlstrom et al. (1979) examined the kinetics of morphine and found only minor differences in the kinetic patterns of morphine at ages 0–15 years. The kinetic values obtained for children did not differ from published values for adults with elimination half-life of approximately 2 h. The minimum morphine concentration in plasma needed to suppress the clinical signs of pain during surgery was 65 ng/ml and was uniform across the age range. Recently, Lynn et al. (1984) reported the minimal analgesic level of morphine as 12 ng/ml in a sample of 12 children (mean age 11.3 years) reporting on their pain using a numerical pain scale. Koren et al. (1985), in their study of 12 neonates given morphine intravenously for postoperative analgesia, found a much slower elimination half-life (13.9, plus or minus 6.4 h) than had been previously described by Dahlstrom et al. (1979). They also noted an increased sensitivity to morphine as evidenced by morphine-induced seizures in two babies who had received 32 and 40 μg/kg/h respectively. Consequently, they recommended that the infused dose in newborns should not exceed 15 μg/kg/h.

5.2.4 *Morphine*

Morphine is the standard opioid against which all others are measured. Morphine is dispensed as water-soluble morphine sulfate and is administered orally, subcutaneously, intramuscularly and occasionally intravenously or rectally. The textbook belief is that oral morphine is only about 1/6 as potent as parenteral administration (Jaffe and Martin, 1985). As a result, oral morphine is of limited usefulness (Schecter, 1985). Recently, McQuay et al. (1985) have contested this view and suggested that at low plasma morphine concentrations, the availability of oral morphine was virtually the same as intravenously administered morphine. Morphine used in cancer pain is discussed in chapter 10 while morphine and meperidine in sickle cell crisis are discussed in chapter 11.

Dosages for the opioid analgesics are outlined in Table 1. Suggested

TABLE 1
Pediatric dosages of opioid analgesics.

Drug	Route	Dosage
Codeine phosphate	Oral, i.m., i.v. or s.c.	0.5–1.0 mg/kg dose, every 4–6 h to a maximum of 30 mg/day for 2–6 year olds and 60 mg/day for 6–12 year olds
Morphine sulfate	Oral	0.2–0.3 mg/kg/dose, every 2–4 h to a maximum of 0.8 mg/kg/day
	i.v., i.m. or s.c.	0.1–0.2 mg/kg/dose, every 2–4 h to a maximum of 1.2 mg/kg/day
Meperidine (pethidine) hydrochloride	Oral, i.v., i.m. or s.c.	1–1.5 mg/kg/dose, every 3–4 h to a maximum of 7.5 mg/kg/day
Hydromorphone hydrochloride	Oral, i.m. or s.c.	1–4 mg/dose, every 4–6 h to a maximum of 24 mg daily (For older children only)
	Rectal suppository	3 mg h.s.
Methadone hydrochloride	Oral, i.m. or s.c.	0.1–0.2 mg/kg/dose every 4–6 h to a maximum of 0.7 mg/kg/day

Note: See text for specific cautions. Table prepared in conjunction with S. Brooker, Director of Pharmacy, Children's Hospital of Eastern Ontario.

dosages are estimates and should be carefully titrated against pain and side effects.

5.2.5. Codeine

Codeine is the mildest of the opioid analgesics and is frequently used to control mild to moderate postoperative pain. Since the mode of action is quite different, combinations of codeine and ASA or acetaminophen are more potent than either alone. Codeine also has a strong antitussive effect and is widely used to control coughing in dosages about half that used for analgesia.

5.2.6. Methadone

Methadone is not only an effective analgesic but also widely used as a therapeutic substitute for heroin among addicts because it blocks the withdrawal symptoms and does not produce euphoria. Methadone is well absorbed orally and has a longer duration of action (approximately 12 h) than morphine. Methadone used in cancer pain is discussed in chapter 10.

5.2.7. Pethidine or meperidine
Pethidine or meperidine, although chemically dissimilar, is similar in effect to morphine, except it has less antitussive effect, better oral absorption, and less spasmodic effect on the biliary tract (Jaffe and Martin, 1985). Concern has been raised about the central nervous system excitatory effects of meperidine and the increased risk of seizures with meperidine (Tang et al., 1980; Kaiko et al., 1983). Levels of normeperidine, the only active metabolite, have been correlated with the appearance of adverse neurological signs (Kaiko et al., 1983). A recent trial using both meperidine and morphine infusions found similar low levels of neuromuscular excitability with each drug (Cole et al., 1986). The issue is unclear but patients on meperidine should be carefully monitored for neurological excitation. Patients with low epileptic threshold should probably receive alternate analgesics.

5.2.8. Hydromorphone
Hydromorphone is similar to morphine in effect but more potent.

5.2.9. Fentanyl
Fentanyl is a synthetic opioid which is short acting, showing duration of analgesic action of between 30 and 60 min. Fentanyl is used intravenously for perioperative pain relief and for analgesia in the immediate postoperative time period. Other characteristics are similar to morphine.

5.3. Routes and schedules of administration

Analgesics can be given by a variety of routes and schedules. Little research has examined the relative effectiveness of different strategies. However, there are good reasons to believe that the use of injections and the use of p.r.n. schedules are likely to lead to poorer pain relief. Children frequently report a strong fear of injections as can be seen in Fig. 1. Children may deny pain or at least fail to report pain because they know that pain will result in a needle (Eland and Anderson, 1977; Mather and Mackie, 1983). Similarly, nurses may be reluctant to give children needles because they know how much the needle is feared. Nurses may also wish to avoid being seen as mean or cruel.

p.r.n. schedules, in which medication is administered only when the patient requests it and the nurse agrees when the requisite time is up, are almost

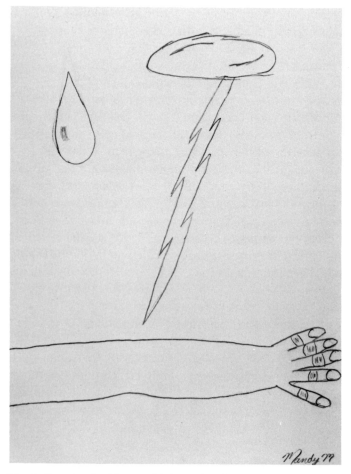

Fig. 1. Drawing by 11-year-old Amanda of how she feels about needles.

guaranteed to result in patients suffering. p.r.n. schedules are also likely to result in reinforcement and exaggeration of pain behavior because the child soon learns that relief is obtained when he/she appears to be in pain. The child must convince the nurse that the medication is needed.

In a randomized trial, Bray (1983) examined the efficacy of morphine infusion compared to p.r.n. intramuscular injections in postoperative pain from major abdominal or thoracic surgery. The results showed clear superiority of the infusion group in controlling pain as estimated by ward nurses. In children over 6 months of age, Bray (1983) reported no respiratory depression or other side effects.

In a recent clinical series, Lynn et al. (1984) described morphine infusion as effective for pain relief after cardiac surgery.

As in many areas, clinical practice has gone far beyond the published research. For example, although intravenous opioid analgesics in the management of postoperative pain in children is not widely recognized, Stevens and Cameron (1987) described the use of intravenous opioid analgesics at the McMaster University Medical Centre in Hamilton, Ontario, Canada. They recommended slow infusion over 30 min and titration of dose based on the child's response to the medication. Titration is necessary to balance the analgesic effects against the side effects. They pointed out that such a strategy is safe (if side effects are monitored), effective and well accepted by the patients, nurses and parents. Similarly, Dilworth and MacKellar (1987) described their success with opioid infusions in postoperative pain at the Princess Margaret Hospital for Children in Perth, Western Australia.

In a recent study in our own lab, we (O'Hara et al., 1987) randomly assigned children undergoing orthopedic surgery to either oral morphine every 4 h or injected meperidine on a p.r.n. schedule. We found that oral morphine q.q.h. was more effective than equianalgesic dosages of injected demerol. As can be seen in Fig. 2, oral morphine resulted in a large percentage of children being maintained pain-free when compared with intramuscular demerol. The study was a management study and could not separate the possible differential effects of the different drugs, different

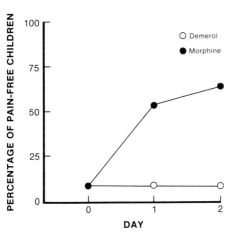

Fig. 2. Percentage of pain-free children on days following surgery. (From O'Hara et al., 1987; used with permission.)

schedules and different routes. Titration of the dosage of oral medication might have produced even more impressive differences.

5.4. *Blocks for postoperative pain relief*

Regional blocks have been widely used and evaluated in reducing postoperative pain, especially the pain due to circumcision, in infants and children. The major advantage of regional blocks is the degree of analgesia. The major disadvantages of blocks are that they require physicians skilled in their usage and they result in sensory blocking and subsequent possible problems of the child contaminating or handling the wound or, in the case of spinal blocks, attempting to walk before the block has resolved. Unfortunately, most studies in this area have suffered from serious design and/or measurement problems.

Davenport (1973) strongly recommended the use of supplemental regional blocks, that is, regional block in addition to general anesthetic, for the postoperative pain of circumcision but he did not present any data to support his recommendation. Kay (1974) reported that of over 300 boys in his series, fewer than a dozen presented the distressed crying upset picture that was characteristic of the typical child who underwent the same procedure without regional blocks. However, no standardized measurement system was used and the person evaluating the pain was aware of what treatment the child had received. The studies by both Davenport (1973) and Kay (1974) can be regarded as only of heuristic value.

In a somewhat more sophisticated study, Shandling and Stewart (1980) studied 156 infants and children who had undergone elective inguinal herniotomy under general anesthetic. Eighty-one of these children also received a regional block using bupivacaine. The authors reported that the blocked patients were able to be managed with less general anesthetic and less postoperative analgesics. As well, the blocked patients were reported to have a more rapid recovery to normal functioning. The major methodological problems in this study were the lack of random assignment of subjects, standardization or description of the outcome measures and blinding of raters. As well, there was no data presented on the exact amount of general anesthetic given to the children.

In a randomized controlled trial, Jensen (1981) found that caudal block with morphine provided longer lasting pain relief than the same block with bupivacaine. No measurement of pain was described.

Martin (1982) randomly assigned 60 boys undergoing circumcision to one of three groups: diamorphine, intravenously and intramuscularly; caudal bupivacaine; and caudal bupivacaine and morphine. He concluded that the use of caudal anesthesia in circumcision was not worth the extra time, risk and expense required for its use. Although Martin (1982) did use random assignment, there were serious measurement problems that cast doubt on the validity of his conclusions. In particular, Martin's major dependent variable was a visual analogue scale in which 'the zero end of the scale represented the anesthetized child and the 10 cm end, a child who was screaming and uncontrollable, with a child who was awake alert and pain-free being recorded near the 50 mm mark' (Martin, 1982, p. 1263). The linear analogue scale actually is an attempt to measure two contructs at once. The 0–50 mm portion of the scale is a measure of the state of the child whereas the 50–100 mm part of the scale is a measure of distress. This can lead to serious measurement problems which can best be illustrated by an example. Consider two pairs of children: one pair, each child rated 5, and one pair in which one child had a rating of 0 and the other a rating of 10. Although each pair would have a mean score of 5, one pair would consist of two alert, calm children; the other pair would be made up of one comatose child and another child who was screaming with pain. In addition, Martin (1982) did not have blinded observers and the inter-rater reliability of the scale was not assessed.

Kay et al. (1982) randomly assigned 44 boys to either caudal bupivacaine or intramuscular buprenorphine. They found that both methods provided good analgesia but that the caudal anesthesia patients had less postoperative vomiting and a faster return to normal activity. Although the design was adequate, the reliability and validity of the scales was not assessed.

Williamson and Williamson (1983) compared 30 newborns, 20 of whom were randomly assigned to receive dorsal penile blocks (1% subcutaneous Xylocaine injection). Ten newborns received no blocks. They found that the blocked infants experienced significantly less stress, as measured by smaller decreases in transcutaneous oxygen levels, less time spent crying, and smaller increases in heart rate than the control group. Interpretation of the data is somewhat clouded by the fact that baseline values were not the same for the two groups. In addition, the control group actually experienced a relative bradycardia during part of the treatment. However, there is little doubt that there was a positive effect of the penile block compared to no intervention. Due to the design of the study (block versus no block), no comparisons were made between different treatments.

In a study in our hospital, we (Johnson et al., 1986) have corrected the previously noted deficiencies in evaluating postoperative pain relief in young children. We compared three groups of randomly assigned patients undergoing circumcision: children receiving general anesthesia alone, children receiving reduced general anesthesia and caudal bupivacaine preceding surgery, and children who received the full amount of general anesthetic and a caudal block following the surgery. Preliminary analyses suggested that the group receiving a block with reduced general anesthetic was superior to the other two groups. A serendipitous finding was that the children, who did not receive blocks but did receive intravenous fentanyl (a synthetic opioid) because of pain in the recovery room, did as well following the administration of fentanyl as the blocked patients.

Vater and Wandless (1985) studied 50 boys (age 1–13 years) in a randomized trial comparing caudal and dorsal nerve block for pain control from circumcision. The dorsal nerve block group micturated earlier, stood unaided earlier, and vomited less than the caudal block group. Pain control was seen as equivalent. The design was appropriate but the pain measurement was weak (the opinion of one observer). Since dorsal nerve blocks are easy to administer, have fewer risks and fewer side effects than caudal blocks, the authors recommended dorsal nerve blocks in circumcision.

In a controlled double blind study of 31 infants, Holve et al. (1983) compared dorsal penile block, mock or placebo block and no block. They found that the dorsal penile block resulted in a 50% reduction in tachycardia during the procedure and a 50% reduction in crying compared to the control groups. The infants were also examined to determine behavioral effects as measured by the Brazelton neonatal assessment scale (Dixon et al., 1984). Infants receiving a block were significantly different from the controls on the orientation, irritability, and motor processes clusters of the Brazelton scale.

In addition, clinical series have suggested the efficacy and safety of lumbar (Glenski et al., 1984) and thoracic (Shapiro et al., 1984) epidural morphine analgesia for major surgeries. No controlled studies have been reported.

Regional blocks have been extensively reported on, compared to most pediatric postoperative pain control but they have not gained widespread use. The need for specialized physicians to administer blocks and the fear for safety may have inhibited their adoption.

5.5. Topical analgesics

Topical analgesic in the form of a spray or jelly has been investigated in one randomized trial. Tree-Trakarn and Pirayavaraporn (1985) randomly assigned 77 healthy boys, aged 1–13 years undergoing outpatient circumcision to six groups: no analgesia, intramuscular morphine, bupivacaine dorsal nerve block, lidocaine spray, lidocaine ointment and lidocaine jelly. The children were circumcised under general anesthesia and then pain was recorded by blinded nurses and subsequently by parents blinded to the group to which their children had been assigned. Results indicated equal pain-free periods (4–5 h) for the five groups receiving analgesia which were superior to the no analgesia condition. Vomiting occurred in 3 of 11 children in the morphine group. One of the 15 nerve blocks failed. The authors recommended the use of topical analgesic because of its simplicity, effectiveness, safety and lack of side effects. They indicated that children appeared to prefer the spray because it could be reapplied without touching the wound. Topical analgesics have the added cost advantage over blocks of not necessitating the specially skilled physicians to administer them which blocks require.

6. Physical methods in postoperative pain

6.1. Transcutaneous electrical nerve stimulation (TENS)

A benign method of enhancing the effectiveness of opioid analgesia in patients with severe postoperative pain is transcutaneous electrical nerve stimulation (TENS) (Wall and Sweet, 1967).

The use of TENS as an adjuvant therapy in controlling postoperative pain has been evaluated in a number of studies. However, most of these studies have suffered from serious methodological flaws such as not using randomized assignment; not using placebo treatment as a control; not measuring pain directly; and not having personnel evaluating symptoms blinded.

In spite of these general deficiencies in the literature, a few better controlled studies of TENS have been completed but no well controlled studies have been done with children.

Issenman et al. (1985) reported a clinical series in which adolescents with idiopathic scoliosis undergoing procedures such as Harrington Rod instrumentation and spinal fusion were treated with supplemental TENS. Although claiming effectiveness, the study was methodologically inadequate. The study was retrospective; patients were not randomly assigned; no placebo control was used; there was no measure of pain; and the major dependent variable, use of p.r.n. medication, may have been influenced by unblinded nurses.

Vibration which might be effective as an adjuvant analgesic method in the same way as TENS has not been evaluated.

6.2. Cognitive/behavioral methods

Cognitive/behavioral methods have not been evaluated for postoperative pain. However, cognitive behavioral methods have been widely used to reduce the distress that has been noted to follow hospitalization of children.

6.2.1. Posthospital distress

The occurrence of posthospital distress is well documented. For example, an early account by Levy (1945) noted regressive behavior, dependency, and disturbed sleep as well as fears of the dark, strange men, men with white coats, nurses and doctors, following hospitalization of children. A landmark paper by Vernon et al. (1966) reviewed the literature up to that point and presented data on the posthospital behavior questionnaire for 387 children. The posthospital behavior questionnaire is a 27 item scale on which parents report changes in their children's behavior following hospitalization by choosing one of five response alternatives. Factor analysis of the scale yielded six factors: general anxiety and regression; separation anxiety; anxiety about sleep; eating disturbance; aggression towards authority; and apathy withdrawal. Children between the ages of 6 months and 4 years were most likely to be upset following hospitalization. Ratings of the likelihood that the child would experience pain based on admission diagnosis and hospital service (at best, an extraordinarily crude index of pain experienced) were not predictive of posthospital upset. Unfortunately, no subsequent research has studied the relationship between pain experienced and posthospital upset.

Cognitive behavioral interventions to reduce posthospital distress have been shown to be effective. For example, Wolfer and Visintainer (1979) randomly assigned 163 children aged 3–12 years, who were hospitalized for tonsillectomy, to one of five groups. The experimental groups consisted of combinations of home preparation with five different types of in hospital preparation and supportive care. Outcome measures included: ratings of behavioral upset and co-operation during procedures; recovery room medications; time to first voiding; posthospital adjustment; and self-ratings for anxiety and satisfaction. Results indicated that children, who were prepared independent of the type of preparation, showed better adjustment than those who were not prepared.

6.2.2. Pain

As previously noted, no studies have examined cognitive behavioral methods in reducing postoperative pain. However, one study evaluated different strategies used to comfort children in hospital, but not necessarily postoperative, who were crying. Crying, of course, may be due to pain, loneliness, fear or boredom. Triplett and Arneson (1979) studied 63 infants and children between 3 days and 44 months of age and intervened 100 times to reduce their distress. They used verbal interventions. If these were not effective then tactile or combined verbal/tactile interventions were used. The tactile interventions included combinations of stroking, patting, repositioning, rocking, holding and offering the pacifier. Only 7 of the 40 verbal interventions were successful. In contrast, 53 of the 60 simultaneous verbal/tactile interventions were successful. Twenty-nine of the 33 unsuccessful verbal interventions were successful when the tactile component was added. The measurement of distress was reliable and it was performed by an independent observer. There were no significant sex differences. However, older children responded better than younger children to verbal intervention. The 13–18-month-old children were the most difficult to comfort by any means.

In spite of the lack of controlled research, common clinical practice in most modern pediatric settings make widespread use of cognitive behavioral methods. For example, at the Children's Hospital of Eastern Ontario, all clinical staff and, in particular, nurses and Child Life staff provide extensive and intensive information, play, distraction, guided imagery, massage, physical comforting and reassurance both before and after surgery. Children, who are experiencing pain, are given analgesics. They are also cuddled, talked to and distracted by play both in their rooms and in specially equipped play rooms.

McCaffery (1977), in a brief instructional article, clearly described non-pharmacological strategies that can and should be used to help children cope with postoperative pain. These included: a caring, accepting, collaborative relationship between nurse, patient and patient's family; teaching about pain; distraction; rhythmic breathing; cutaneous stimulation including massage, rubbing, pressure, vibration, heat and cold; muscle relaxation; imagery and desensitization.

Instruction about what will happen to the child before, during and after surgery should be tailored to the individual. General surgical preparation is not sufficient for complex procedures and specialized material must be developed. For example, Fig. 3 is a page from a booklet about the Luque procedure for idiopathic scoliosis. This booklet is used in preparing children for this type of major surgery so that they know what to expect. Knowing what to expect may well reduce anxiety and pain.

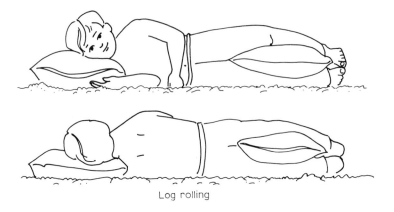

Log rolling

Fig. 3. Page from a booklet for preparing children for back surgery. *Turning*: It is important that you be turned regularly (about every two hours) to protect your skin and keep your lungs clear. The Luque procedure results in a stable spinal column. Turning will not harm the surgical correction. You will be turned in a special manner called 'Log Rolling'. Sheepskin is put on the bed to protect sensitive skin areas from friction with bedclothes etc. (Used with permission of D. Alcock.)

7. Age and personality in postoperative pain

Children differ in their pain reactions at different ages. Leikin et al. (1987) found that older children were perceived by their parents as having more pain following tonsillectomy than were younger children. This may be because the surgery is more traumatic for older children rather than due to developmental differences in children's perception of postoperative pain. However, it is frequently observed that younger children return to play quicker than do older children. Developmental differences in pain perception are discussed in more detail in chapter 2.

Temperament, previous pain experiences, parental reaction and other unknown factors all interact to produce the individual's response to pain. Leikin et al. (1987) found that children, who were high symptom reporters prior to surgery, tended to have more pain (as reported by their mothers) following tonsillectomy than children who were low symptom reporters. However, there was a familial aggregation of symptom reporting and consequently, it is not clear whether it was parental or child factors or a combination of the two that produced the results. Unfortunately, there has been little research in this area (see chapter 2 for a discussion of symptom reporting).

8. Do parents undermedicate in the postoperative period?

No literature has directly examined the question of whether parents undermedicate their children in the postoperative period. Our clinical impression is that parents frequently assess their children as having pain but then do not give analgesic medication such as acetaminophen because they do not want to make their children rely on medication to solve their problems. Leikin (1986) indirectly examined this issue in a study of symptom reporting following tonsillectomy. He found a very low rate of medication use in spite of parental reports of considerable amounts of pain.

9. Clinical guidelines

(1) Insure adequate analgesia during surgery.
(2) Eliminate unnecessary surgery.
(3) Select appropriate analgesic medications. Analgesics should match the level of pain that is expected. Acetaminophen or ASA are unlikely to control pain from major thoracic surgery.
(4) Avoid p.r.n. schedules. p.r.n. schedules guarantee that the child will suffer pain before they get any relief. Regularly scheduled medication can prevent pain from emerging.
(5) Avoid injections. Children fear injections and may deny pain to avoid them. In many circumstances, injections can be substituted by intravenous, sublingual, rectal or oral medication.
(6) Titrate dosage. Dosages of analgesics should begin at a level where pain control can be reasonably expected and then titrated to maximize pain relief and minimize side effects.
(7) Consider the use of regional blocks when possible. The safety, ease and efficacy of penile dorsal blocks in circumcision of infants and children has been clearly established. If circumcision is to be done, it should be done with the benefit of appropriate analgesia.
(8) Provide an interesting and supportive environment. An interesting environment with appropriate play material and skilled facilitation of play for the child following surgery is likely to help reduce pain. Warm, supportive nursing care and parental involvement may reduce anxiety and the reactive component of pain. Although there are no experimental trials to determine the effect of such interventions on pain, play is a normal way for children to distract themselves and to cope with pain.

Many hospitals have Child Life programs which, in close collaboration with nursing and medical departments, develop and implement child-oriented programs.

(9) Provide preoperative teaching. Such teaching prepares the child to know that they may feel pain, that they should report the pain and that measures will be taken to minimize the pain. Children can be taught how to use a self-report scale preoperatively so that they can efficiently communicate their pain postoperatively.

(10) Educate parents to use analgesics when the child goes home. Parents can be taught to use analgesics to prevent pain and not to worry about addiction from analgesics.

10. Future directions

There are a number of directions that should be pursued to develop better perioperative and postoperative pain care.

(1) Further research on perioperative pain in neonates is required. Policies of neonatal anesthesia should change to reflect research findings.

(2) Research on safety of analgesics and their pharmacokinetics in children must be expanded.

(3) Research on efficacy of different analgesic methods, routes and schedules would enable the best analgesic care to be provided. New possibilities of transcutaneous analgesics in the form of 'band-aids' and sublingual analgesics formulated as 'lollipops' may hold promise.

(4) Research on analgesic decision making of nurses and physicians is needed.

(5) Education for physicians and nurses. The level of education for nurses and doctors on pain control is extremely limited. Education about pain control in pediatrics is almost non-existent. Increased knowledge is a prerequisite to better medical care. Information about pediatric pain control should be incorporated into nursing and medical education and should be available in workshops, journal articles and hospital rounds.

(6) Development of quality assurance standards for pain relief. Standard care plans are developed by nursing staff to deal with problems associated with common conditions or diagnoses. In a standard care plan, the nursing care for each problem is detailed. The level of care is that which the hospital expects will be implemented. The management of postoperative pain should be part of the standard care plan for postoperative care.

TABLE 2
Excerpt from standard care plan for pediatric postoperative care. Management of pain. (In conjunction with M. Goodman, Nursing Project Officer, CHEO.)

Nursing diagnosis/problem	Nursing action

I. Alteration in comfort related to surgical trauma.
 	
Objective: Child will experience as little discomfort as possible.
 	
Deadline: Duration of hospital stay.
	I. *Do not* wait until child experiences severe pain
	
	  (a) Assess pain: restlessness or reluctance to move may indicate pain
	
	    – facial expression
	    – crying or whimpering
	    – guarding of site
	    – older children can self-assess using pain scale:
	  No pain 0–1–2–3–4–5–6–7–8–9–10 Severe pain
	  (b) Record nature of pain: note type, location, duration, and severity of pain
	  (c) Administer analgesia as ordered
	  (d) Record effect of analgesia
	
	II. *Plan* nursing care and other treatments to follow analgesia
	
	III. *Initiate* measures to promote comfort and relaxation
	    – use diversional tactics (toys, stories) during painful/aversive procedures
	    – talk to child in soothing voice
	    – encourage parents to hold child
	    – encourage parents to touch and/or stroke child
	    – provide age-appropriate diversional activity
	    – change position at least every 2 h
	    – splint site (abdomen or chest) when moving or assisting with deep breathing or coughing
	    – massage back and pressure areas
	
	IV. *Explain* all procedures to child so he/she knows what to expect

No pain   0--1--2--3--4--5--6--7--8--9--10   Pain as severe as
                                                possible

Date	Time	Activity	Self rating	Nurses rating	Analgesic	Comments (specify effect)

Fig. 4. Proposed flow sheet for postoperative pain.

Table 2 is an example of the pain management component of a standard care plan. Documentation is essential to provide evidence that these measures have in fact been provided. To avoid long and often redundant written nursing notes, flow sheets can be used. Fig. 3 is an example of a postoperative pain flow sheet. Hospitals in North America have, in the past few years, developed quality assurance programs (Donabedian, 1980). These programs are designed to assure an acceptable level of patient care in areas from providing adequate septic procedures to standards of patient physical safety. Quality assurance for postoperative pain control would consist of the standard care plan and an audit procedure to determine if the plan is adhered to. Changes in the standard care plan would be made if the plan did not result in adequate pain control in most patients. The provision of systematic feedback as to the quality of pain control would in itself provide an impetus for better care.

References

American Academy of Pediatrics (1975) Report of the ad hoc task force on circumcision. Pediatrics 56, 610.

Anand, K.J.S. and Aynsley-Green, A. (1985) Metabolic and endocrine effects of surgical ligation of patent ductus arteriosus in the human preterm neonate: Are there implications for further improvements of postoperative outcome? Mod. Probl. Paediatr. 23, 143–157.

Anand, K.J.S., Brown, M.J., Bloom, S.R. and Aynsley-Green, A. (1985a) Studies on the hormonal regulation of fuel metabolism in the human newborn infant undergoing anaesthesia and surgery. Horm. Res. 22, 115–128.

Anand, K.J.S., Brown, M.J., Causon, R.C., Christofides, N.D., Bloom, S.R. and Aynsley-

Green, A. (1985b) Can the human neonate mount an endocrine and metabolic response to surgery? J. Pediatr. Surg. 20, 41–48.

Anand, K.J.S., Sippell, W.G. and Aynsley-Green, A. (1987a) Randomized trial of fentanyl anaesthesia in preterm babies undergoing surgery: Effects on the stress response. Lancet i, 243–247.

Anand, K.J.S., Sippell, W.G. and Aynsley-Green, A. (1987b) Does the newborn infant require anaesthesia during surgery? Answers from a randomised trial of halothane anaesthesia. Vth World Congress on Pain. Hamburg. Pain suppl. 4, S451.

Angell, M. (1982) The quality of mercy. New Engl. J. Med. 306, 98–99.

Barrett, M.J., Hurwitz, E.S., Schonberger, L.B. and Rogers, M.F. (1986) Changing epidemiology of Reye syndrome in the United States. Pediatrics 77, 598–602.

Beyer, J., DeGood, D.E., Ashley, L.C. and Russell, G.A. (1983) Patterns of postoperative analgesic use with adults and children following cardiac surgery. Pain 17, 71–81.

Bray, R.J. (1983) Postoperative analgesia provided by morphine infusion in children. Anaesthesia 38, 1075–1078.

Cole, T.B., Sprinkle, R.H., Smith, S.J. and Buchanan, G.R. (1986) Intravenous narcotic therapy for children with severe sickle cell pain crisis. Am. J. Dis. Child. 140, 1255–1259.

Dahlstrom, B., Bolme, P., Feychting, H., Noack, G. and Paalzow, L. (1979) Morphine kinetics in children. Clin. Pharmacol. Ther. 26, 354–365.

Davenport, H.T. (1973) Paediatric Anaesthesia, 2nd edn. (Heinemann, London) pp. 143–144.

Dilworth, N.M. and MacKellar, A. (1987) Pain relief for the paediatric surgical patient. J. Paediatr. Surg., in press.

Dixon, S., Snyder, J., Holve, R. and Bromberger, P. (1984) Behavioral effects of circumcision with and without anesthesia. Dev. Behav. Pediatr. 5, 246–250.

Donabedian, A. (1980) Methods for deriving criteria for assessing the quality of medical care. Med. Care Rev. 37, 653–698.

Eland, J.M. and Anderson, J.E. (1977) The experience of pain in children. In: A.K. Jacox (Ed.), Pain: A Sourcebook for Nurses and Other Health Professionals (Little Brown, Boston, MA) pp. 453–473.

Fulginiti, V.A., Brunell, P.A., Cherry, J.D., Ector, W.L., Gershon, A.A., Gotoff, S.P., Hughes, W.T., Mortimer, E.A. and Peter, G. (1982) Aspirin and Reye syndrome. Pediatrics 69, 810–812.

Giacomelli, F., Pastore, F., Zangari, M., Marchiori, C. and Soranzo, G.P. (1984) Tonsillectomia: terapia post-operatoria con Tantum Verde nebulizzatore. Gazz. Med. Ital.–Arch. Sci. Med. 143, 639–644.

Glenski, J.A., Warner, M.A., Dawson, B. and Kaufman, B. (1984) Postoperative use of epidurally administered morphine in children and adolescents. Mayo Clin. Proc. 59, 530–533.

Holve, R.L., Bromberger, P.J., Groveman, H.D., Klauber, M.R., Dixon, S.D. and Snyder, J.M. (1983) Regional anesthesia during newborn circumcision. Clin. Pediatr. 22, 813–818.

Issenman, J., Nolan, M.F., Rowley, J. and Hobby, R. (1985) Transcutaneous electrical nerve stimulation for pain control after spinal fusion with Harrington Rods. Phys. Ther. 65, 1517–1520.

Jaffe, J.H. and Martin, W.R. (1985) Opioid analgesics and antagonists. In: A.G. Gilman, L.S. Goodman, T.W. Rall and F. Murad (Eds.), Goodman and Gilman's The Pharmacological Basis of Therapeutics, 7th edn. (Macmillan, New York) pp. 491–531.

Jeans, M.E. (1983) Pain in children: A neglected area. In: P. Firestone, P. McGrath and W.

Feldman (Eds.), Advances in Behavioral Medicine for Children and Adolescents (Erlbaum, Hillsdale, NJ) pp. 23–38.

Jeans, M.E. (1984) Pain in children. Breakfast session. 4th World Congress on Pain, Seattle, WA.

Jensen, B.H. (1981) Caudal block for post-operative pain relief in children after genital operations. A comparison between bupivacaine and morphine. Acta Anaesthesiol. Scand. 25, 373–375.

Johnson, G., McGrath, P., Goodman, J.T. and Schillinger, J. (1987). The evaluation of bupivacaine in pediatric circumcision. Manuscript in preparation.

Kaiko, R.F., Foley, K.M., Grabinski, P.Y., Heidrich, G., Rogers, A.G., Inturrisi, C.E. and Reidenberg, M.M. (1983) Central nervous system excitatory effects of meperidine in cancer patients. Ann. Neurol. 13, 180–185.

Kay, B. (1974) Caudal block for post operative pain relief in children. Anaesthesia 29, 610–614.

Kay, A.E., Wandless, J. and James, R.H. (1982) Analgesia for circumcision in children – A comparison of caudal bupivacaine and intramuscular buprenorphine. Acta Anaesthesiol. Scand. 26, 331–333.

King, L.R. (1982) Commentary – Neonatal Circumcision in the United States in 1982. J. Urol. 128, 1135–1136.

Koren, G., Butt, W., Chinyanga, H., Soldin, S., Tan, Y. and Pape, K. (1985) Postoperative morphine infusion in newborn infants: Assessment of disposition characteristics and safety. J. Pediatr. 107, 63–967.

Leikin, L. (1986) Children's physical symptom reporting and the Type A behavior pattern. Ph.D. dissertation, University of Ottawa, Ottawa, Canada.

Leikin, L., Firestone, P. and McGrath, P. (1987) Symptom reporting and post-operative pain. Manuscript under review.

Levy, D.M. (1945) Psychic trauma of operations in children. Am. J. Dis. Child. 69, 7–25.

Lynn, A.M., Opheim, K.E. and Tyler, D.C. (1984) Morphine infusion after pediatric cardiac surgery. Crit. Care Med. 12, 863–866.

McCaffery, M. (1977) Pain relief for the child: Problem areas and selected nonpharmacological methods. Pediatr. Nurs. 3, 11–16.

McQuay, H.J., Moore, R.A., Glynn, C.J. and Lloyd, J.W. (1985) High systemic availability of oral morphine sulfate solution and sustained-release preparation. In: H.L. Fields, R. Dubner and F. Cervero (Eds.) Advances in Pain Research and Therapy (Raven Press, New York) pp. 719–726.

Mahon, W.A. and DeGregorio, M. (1985) Benzydamine: A critical review of clinical data. Int. J. Tissue React. 7, 229–235.

Martin, L.V.H. (1982) Postoperative analgesia after circumcision in children. Br. J. Anaesth. 54, 1263–1266.

Mather, L. and Mackie, J. (1983) The incidence of postoperative pain in children. Pain 15, 271–282.

Merskey, H. (1970) On the development of pain. Headache 10, 116–123.

Miller, R.R. and Jick, H. (1978) Clinical effects of meperidine in hospitalized patients. J. Clin. Pharmacol. 18, 180–189.

Newburger, P.F. and Sallan, S.E. (1981) Chronic pain: Principles of management. J. Pediatr. 98, 180–189.

O'Hara, M., McGrath, P., D'Astous, J. and Vair, C. (1987) Oral morphine versus injected meperidine (demerol) for pain relief in children after orthopedic surgery. J. Pediatr. Orthop. 7, 78–82.

Paradise, J.C., Bluestone, C.D., Bachman, R.N., Colborn, D.K., Bernard, B.S., Taylor, F.H., Rogers, K.D., Schwarzbach, R.H., Stool, S.E., Friday, G.A., Smith, I.H. and Saez, C.A. (1984) Efficacy of tonsillectomy for recurrent throat infection in severely affected children. N. Engl. J. Med. 310, 674–683.

Peterson, R.G. (1985) Antipyretics and analgesics in children. Dev. Pharmacol. Ther. 8, 68–84.

Peterson, R.G. and Rumack, B.H. (1978) Pharmacokinetics of acetaminophen in children. Pediatrics 62 (suppl.), 877–879.

Porter, J. and Jick, H. (1980) Addiction rate in patients treated with narcotics. N. Engl. J. Med. 302, 123.

Schechter, N.L. (1985) Pain and pain control in children. Curr. Probl. Pediatr. 15, 1–67.

Schechter, N.L., Allen, D.A. and Hanson, K. (1986) The status of pediatric pain control: A comparison of hospital analgesic usage in children and adults. Pediatrics 77, 11–15.

Segre, G. and Hammarstrom, S. (1985) Aspects of the mechanisms of action of benzydamine. Int. J. Tissue React. 7, 187–193.

Shandling, B. and Stewart, D.J. (1980) Regional analgesia for post-operative pain in pediatric outpatient surgery. J. Pediatr. Surg. 15, 477–480.

Shapiro, L.A., Jedeikin, R.J., Shalev, D. and Hoffman, S. (1984) Epidural morphine analgesia in children. Anesthesiology 61, 210–212.

Slotkowski, E.L. and King, L.R. (1982) The incidence of neonatal circumcision in Illinois. Ill. Med. J. 162, 421–426.

Stevens, B. and Cameron, G. (1987) Use of intravenous narcotics in the post-operative pain management of children. Manuscript under review.

Swafford, L.I. and Allan, D. (1968) Pain relief in the pediatric patient. Med. Clin. North Am. 52, 131–136.

Tang, R., Shimomura, S.K. and Rotblatt, M. (1980) Meperidine induced seizures in sickle cell patients. Hosp. Formulary 15, 764–772.

Tree-Trakarn, T. and Pirayavaraporn, S. (1985) Postoperative pain relief for circumcision in children: Comparison among morphine, nerve block and topical analgesia. Anesthesiology 62, 519–522.

Triplett, J.L. and Arneson, S.W. (1979) The use of verbal and tactile comfort to alleviate distress in young hospitalized children. Res. Nurs. Health 2, 17–23.

Vater, M. and Wandless, J. (1985) Caudal or dorsal nerve block? A comparison of two local anaesthetic techniques for postoperative analgesia following day case circumcision. Acta Anaesthesiol. Scand. 29, 175–179.

Vernon, D.T.A., Schulman, J.L. and Foley, J.M. (1966) Changes in children's behavior after hospitalization. Am. J. Dis. Child. 111, 581–593.

Wall, P.D. and Sweet, W.H. (1967) Temporary abolition of pain in man. Science 155, 108–109.

Williamson, P.S. and Williamson, M.L. (1983) Physiologic stress reduction by a local anesthetic during newborn circumcision. Pediatrics 71, 36–40.

Wolfer, J.A. and Visintainer, M.A. (1979) Prehospital psychological preparation for tonsillectomy patients: Effects on children's and parents' adjustment. Pediatrics 64, 646–655.

CHAPTER 5

Medically caused pain

I promise to follow treatment that as best I can will benefit my patients and do them no harm *(from the Hippocratic oath)*.

1. Why medically caused pain is ignored

For the health care professional, one of the most difficult forms of pediatric pain to deal with is pain inflicted on children in the course of their medical treatment. Although physicians are neither callous nor cruel, the most frequent response of physicians to pain which they have inflicted or ordered for children during treatment is a turning away (Neal, 1978). This is a form of denial as if physicians could not be deflected from their main purpose of healing and curing even by acknowledging the pain they caused by a treatment procedure. The denial of pain inflicted on children in medical procedures is made easier for a number of reasons. Children are not routinely asked if they are in pain. Younger children cannot say if they are in pain. Children's pain behavior can be physically controlled by restraint. The measurement of pain in children is not well developed. Children are unable to withdraw consent. They do not write letters of complaint; nor do they sue for medical malpractice; nor do they press charges for assault. In many cases of the most serious medically caused pain, parents are unaware of what is being done to their children.

The most frequent form of medically induced pain is from routine neonatal tests and from immunizations. Virtually all infants will have a heel prick within the first few days of life to collect the few drops of blood required for PKU and adrenal screening. If that were the extent of medically induced pain, one could argue that the failure to adequately assess and control this pain was clinically unimportant. Indeed, for most children, heel pricks and immunization injections are the extent of their exposure to medically caused pain.

2. The victims of medically induced pain

> I pretended I was in a space ship and the pressure was making my ears hurt and I was the only one that could get it back to earth *(girl, aged 9 years about a painful ear procedure, quoted in Ross and Ross, 1984, p. 186)*.

All children are victims of medically induced pain at some time in their lives. However, we can divide children in two groups for our purposes. The first group consists of children who experience pain during routine medical care for the problems of childhood. These children may periodically receive a variety of medical interventions which cause pain such as injections for immunizations or treatment of minor childhood illnesses, suturing for cuts, and surgery and casting for fractures. However, the second group of children consists of those who suffer from, or are suspected to be suffering from a serious and possibly life-threatening condition. For such children, who may require frequent venipunctures, injections, lumbar punctures, bone marrow aspirations and other invasive diagnostic and therapeutic procedures, medically induced pain will become a frequent burden. In our opinion, the weight of this burden is considerable. First of all, there is ample evidence that children undergoing repeated aversive medical procedures do not habituate but actually sensitize (Katz et al., 1980). Repeated procedures become much more distressing for the children. Each procedure causes more suffering. Although there are no studies in infants to see if they sensitize or habituate to painful procedures, it is our impression that habituation does not occur and, even in infants, sensitization may result. Secondly, especially in tiny or ill infants, it may be that amelioration of the pain or distress from aversive procedures enhances the speed of recovery.

In this chapter, we will discuss pain from common procedures such as immunization, heel pricks, intramuscular injections and lumbar punctures followed by pain in intensive care units. Pain from cancer treatment is covered in chapter 10.

3. Pain from immunization

> I counted the tiles on the ceiling till I couldn't count any higher, then I started over and did it again *(girl, aged 6 years, having an injection, quoted in Ross and Ross, 1984, p. 186)*.

The recommended standard schedule for immunization of children in Canada calls for immunization at 2, 4, 6, 12 and 18 months and at 5 years

(Feldman et al., 1987). Other immunizations may be given for specific indications.

Craig et al. (1984) observed 30 children between 2 and 24 months of age and their mothers while the child was receiving routine immunization injections. Using a standardized observational coding system, they documented the reactions of the child, the mothers and the nurse. There was substantial variation in reaction by the children. Some reacted vigorously by crying, screaming, grimacing and writhing but two children did not appear to react at all. In general, the older children cried and screamed for a shorter period of time, oriented toward the injection site, visually tracked their mothers and the nurse, protected and touched their limbs more often and displayed less torso rigidity. The only sex difference was that girls anticipated where the needle was to go whereas boys oriented to that location after the event.

Johnston and Strada (1986) analyzed the response to immunization in 14 infants who were either 2 or 4 months of age. They summarized the response to this pain (Johnston and Strada, 1986, p. 380):

> ... the infant has a response... that lasts for approximately 1 minute, except for the heart rate change which lasts longer. The initial response is characterized by one or two high pitched cries with a period of relative apnea between them, with a brief bradycardic spell, and a rigidity of the body and limbs. This is accompanied by a facial configuration that can be recognized as expressive of pain. There is then a rise in heart rate to a tachycardic level. Then the cries are more tense and grating, although somewhat lower in pitch, and the body has some residual rigidity and occasional thrashing. Finally, the recovery phase is characterized by more rhythmic, rising-falling melodic, lower pitched cries that gradually disappear, facial expression returns to normal, as do body posturing and movements, but the tachycardia is slower to return to the pre-stimulus state.

Older children can rate their pain as well as demonstrate pain behavior in response to immunization. Forty-four pre-operational children aged 4 years 7 months–6 years 8 months rated the pain from DPT (diphtheria, pertussis, tetanus) or DT immunizations in the deltoid muscle of the arm (Hester, 1979). Pain behavior was also observed. Half of the children chose no poker chips (no hurt) to represent their pain. Twenty-five percent of the children represented their hurt by one chip; 11% used two chips; 7% used three chips and 7% used four chips. Just over half the children made no vocal response. Eleven percent of the children screamed; 18% was crying or sobbing; 7% was gasping and 9% was whimpering or whining. Thirty-four percent of the children complained and 2% of them said that it hurt. Sixty-one percent remained quiet during the procedure while the rest moved around. Finally, 86% of the children were observed to be guarded or tense.

In one of the only intervention studies, Eland (1981) studied 40 prekindergarten children (20 of each sex) receiving DPT immunization in the vastus lateralis muscle in the leg. The design was a 2 × 2 randomized design. Children were either treated with Frigiderm (a skin coolant) or a spray of air. They were also either told that the procedure would help or they were not told anything about the procedure. Pain was measured by self-rating using an individually designed four level color scale. Results showed a clear reduction of pain using the skin coolant but no effect for the suggestion.

It is clear that the vast majority of young children have a strong reaction to pain from immunization and that a sizeable proportion continue to experience subsequent immunizations as quite painful. There may be methods, such as a skin coolant, to reduce the pain of immunization.

A second source of pain from immunization is the localized pain and systemic irritability or distress that may result from the immunization. Although, in some quarters, it is standard practice to use acetaminophen as a prophylactic analgesic and antipyretic for immunization in infants, no studies have been reported.

4. Heel pricks

The painful effects of heel pricks used to obtain blood smears for diagnostic purposes was discussed in chapter 3 on measurement of pain. Although there is some diversity in the findings of the various studies (Harpin and Rutter, 1982; Field and Goldson, 1984; Owens and Todt, 1984; Franck, 1986; Grunau and Craig, 1987) an overall pattern emerges of a generalized increase in physiological indices, vocalization and grimacing, when heel pricks are administered to infants.

Technology exists for reducing the pain or distress experienced by infants undergoing heel pricks.

Thirty-six infants were studied by Harpin and Rutter (1983). The 5–6-day-old infants had either a standard heel lance or lancing by means of an autolet, a mechanical device in which the stylet is placed in a spring-loaded cartridge. The cartridge is held against the skin and the spring is released resulting in the stylet piercing the skin 2.4 mm causing bleeding. Physiological reactivity, as measured by emotional sweating, was substantially less in the autolet group. Although crying was not monitored in any standardized way, it appeared to be much less in the autolet group.

Field and Goldson (1984) studied 48 term infants, 48 preterm infants receiving minimal care and 48 infants in the neonatal intensive care unit. Infants were randomly assigned to either receive a pacifier or no soother during heelstick procedures. They found that infants who were given a pacifier were behaviorally less upset. In comparison with infants in the control group, the infants with a pacifier, in each of the samples, spent more time in an alert/quiescent state. The control infants spent more time in fussy/crying states both during and after the heelstick procedure. In the preterm groups, heart rate and respiration were monitored. Treatment effects were noted in the minimal care group but not in the intensive care group. It is not clear but repeated amelioration of pain from aversive procedures might have a cumulative effect on the infant's health.

Grunau and Craig (1987) using facial response and cry discovered that there were important differences in the amount of pain that different technicians produced when doing heel lances.

Heel lances hurt and there are ways of reducing this hurt. However, it appears that methods of reducing the pain of heel pricks are not widely used.

5. Intramuscular injections, venipunctures and finger sticks

For most children who have been hospitalized 'getting the needle' is the most vivid and feared recollection (Eland and Anderson, 1977). As Lewis (1978) emphasized, injection instruments are fearsome looking instruments that are used when the child is fully aware of what is being done. Fernald and Corry (1981) randomly assigned 39 children to an empathic or directive preparation for venipuncture or finger stick. The empathic group had significantly fewer negative behavior responses. No direct measurement of pain was done. No studies have examined the extent of pain from non-immunization intramuscular injections or of ways of reducing the pain of intramuscular injections. Perhaps the most useful way of reducing the pain from injections is to replace regimens requiring injections with alternatives. Unfortunately, only a few studies (e.g., O'Hara et al., 1986) have examined the efficacy of oral, sublingual or intravenous routes as alternatives to injections.

6. Lumbar punctures

Lumbar punctures are a very painful and potentially dangerous diagnostic procedure (Teele et al., 1981). Although lumbar punctures are a valuable tool, they should be used only when required. For example, although many pediatric centers recommend lumbar punctures for all children with febrile seizures in order to rule out meningitis, they may not be necessary. Feldman et al. (1987, pp. 90–91) described how a simple set of decision rules at the Children's Hospital of Eastern Ontario allows 2/3 of children with febrile seizures to avoid the procedure. No cases of meningitis were missed.

7. Pain in the neonatal intensive care unit (NICU)

In a recent study, we (McGrath et al., 1987) asked NICU nurses to tell us what procedures seemed to cause pain in their patients. Table 1 lists those procedures that these nurses felt caused pain. No surveys of aversive procedures in the NICU have been done but it is likely that each day, every child in the NICU is subjected to many of these procedures.

Three major strategies are possible that may reduce pain in the NICU: analgesics; behavioral strategies; and alteration of procedures.

Analgesic usage in tiny sick babies may present unique problems. As Koren et al. (1985) found in one of the few studies on opiate analgesic usage in neonates, the kinetics and safe levels cannot be extrapolated from data on older infants, children or adults. Very little research has examined the kinetics and safety of analgesics in neonates.

Behavioral strategies have the advantage of being low-risk interventions. Field and Goldson (1984) demonstrated that a pacifier was able to reduce the distress of neonates during heelstick procedure. Other types of behavioral procedures which have not been evaluated include: cuddling, rocking, quiet cooing or music and talking to the infant to ameliorate the effects of painful procedures. A second type of behavioral strategy is the signalling of the infant

TABLE 1
Procedures perceived by NICU nurses as causing pain to patients. (Reprinted from McGrath et al. (1987) with permission.)

Injection	i.v.	Intubation	Catheterization
Suctioning	Heel prick	Arterial jab	Positioning for X-ray
Cleaning wound	Venous blood gases	Surgical pain	Suturing
Diaper change	Lumbar puncture	Handling	Feeding
Bathing	Bright lights	Rectal temperatures	Hunger
Electrode removal	Loud noises	Removing sutures	

when aversive procedures will be performed by means of a sound or visual signal. Such signalling might allow the infant to know when they are safe from aversive procedures, to feel more 'in control of' the situation. If neonates have memory from pain, such signalling could allow the neonate to relax when they 'know' they are not about to have a painful procedure.

A new interdisciplinary field of research, Environmental Neonatology (Gottfried and Gaiter, 1985; Wolke, 1987) concerned with the study of the impact of the neonatal intensive care unit on sick infants has recently emerged. For these infants excessive handling and noise may well be frequent pain stimuli that may have serious medical sequelae including intraventricular hemorrhage (Wolke, 1987).

Two final methods of reducing pain in the NICU are to reduce painfulness of procedures and to eliminate unnecessary procedures. We have discussed Harpin and Rutter's (1983) demonstration that the autolet is a less painful method of obtaining heel pricks. Heated transcutaneous gas electrodes may be particularly painful and potentially harmful to the preterm neonate because the skin under the electrode suffers the changes of an early burn and the surface of the skin is stripped when the electrodes are removed (Evans and Rutter, 1986). A spray on dressing (Op-Site Spray Dressing) has been evaluated in ten preterm infants. Although pain was not measured, Evans and Rutter (1986) did find significant differences in skin damage from the electrodes. The use of a single layer of the spray on dressing did not interfere with accurate readings and protected the infant's skin. The authors suggested the use of the spray on dressing with infants less than 30 weeks gestation and less than 1 week old. Grunau and Craig's (1987) finding of individual technician differences might provide a clue for developing better training of technicians in performing less painful heel pricks. It is well known that some procedures require considerable skill and it is reasonable that practice of procedures be conducted on realistic models. The availability of microchip-analyzed input from sensors could make development of models quite feasible.

Some painful procedures, such as lumbar punctures, appear to be generally very poorly done and pain may be inflicted without obtaining a reasonable sample. For example, Schreiner and Kleiman (1979) prospectively analyzed 289 attempts at lumbar punctures in a neonatal intensive care unit. Sixty-one attempts were unsuccessful in that no CSF was obtained. Seventy-six lumbar punctures were traumatic as measured by the presence of more than 5000 red blood cells in the 3rd vial of fluid. In other words, there was a failure rate of 47%. No learning curves were presented to see if the technique is more successful in more experienced hands. Lumbar punctures used in the diagnostic management of cancer are discussed in chapter 10.

It is evident to us that intubation might well be a painful procedure. Intubation of neonates is frequently done without anesthesia. Raju et al. (1980) demonstrated that awake intubation produces much higher rises in intracranial pressure than does intubation under curare. This rise in intracranial pressure increases risk of intraventricular hemorrhage. Waugh and Johnson (1984) reviewed procedures for anesthetized intubation which substantially reduced the rise in intracranial pressure with associated risks and also eliminated pain during intubation. Properly controlled studies are not yet available documenting the effects of different strategies of analgesia for intubation.

Clearly there is a need to do many painful procedures to sick neonates. However, it also is evident that many painful procedures do not have any real use. In a recent paper from our own hospital, Justinich et al. (1986) evaluated the need for lumbar punctures in routine septic workup. They found that upon examination of the results of 317 samples of CSF, only 0.6% yielded positive results. No child had positive CSF with negative blood culture. The authors cautiously recommended that routine lumbar puncture with septic workup has a very low yield and perhaps needs to be done more selectively. Percutaneous drug administration has been suggested by Rutter (1987) to be particularly promising as a pain-free alternative to the intramuscular or intravenous route for preterm infants because of their small size and immature skin. No studies have been completed in this area.

Once one takes the attitude that it is humanitarian and medically indicated to reduce pain in neonates, the possibilities are many.

8. Pain in the pediatric intensive care unit (ICU)

There is virtually no research about the problem of pain for children in a pediatric ICU. A study by Traughber and Cataldo (1983) reviewed the effects of hospitalization in a pediatric ICU. For example, in a series of three studies they have found that much of the interaction between staff and children in the pediatric ICU is emotionally neutral or negative. Specific interventions to increase positive interactions were successful in increasing play and positive social interaction. A negative emotional climate in the pediatric ICU might exacerbate pain experiences.

9. Clinical guidelines

(1) Before each aversive medical procedure, ask 'Is this procedure needed? How will it help this child?'. Each procedure should be justified.

(2) Make each procedure the least painful possible. Psychological methods, improved skill, and improved technology can ameliorate pain. Careful observation of the response of specific babies to caretaking procedures can provide clues of what causes pain for that baby. Problem solving can then be done to try and reduce stress and pain for that infant.

(3) Increasing positive interaction between staff and children in intensive care units may reduce the anxiety contributing to children's experiences of pain.

10. Future directions

(1) Training regimens to decrease the pain of procedures should be developed and evaluated.

(2) The need for routine use of aversive procedures should be evaluated.

(3) Alternatives to painful procedures should be developed and evaluated.

(4) Research on analgesics for painful procedures is needed.

(5) Further research on the possible painful nature of noise and handling on preterm neonates is needed.

References

Craig, K.D., McMahon, R.J., Morison, J.D. and Zaskow, C. (1984) Developmental changes in infant pain expression during immunization injections. Soc. Sci. Med. 19, 1331–1337.

Eland, J.M. (1981) Minimizing pain associated with prekindergarten intramuscular injections. Issues Compr. Pediatr. Nurs. 71, 36–40.

Eland, J.M. and Anderson, J.E. (1977) The experience of pain in children. In: A.K. Jacox (Ed.), Pain: A Sourcebook for Nurses and Other Health Professionals (Little Brown, Boston, MA) pp. 453–473.

Evans, N.J. and Rutter, N. (1986) Reduction of skin damage from transcutaneous oxygen electrodes using a spray on dressing. Arch. Dis. Child. 61, 881–884.

Feldman, W., Rosser, W. and McGrath, P.J. (1987) Primary Medical Care of Children and Adolescents (Oxford University Press, New York).

Fernald, C.D. and Corry, J.J. (1981) Empathic versus directive preparation of children for needles. Children's Health Care 10, 44–47.

Field, T. and Goldson, E. (1984) Pacifying effects of nonnutritive sucking on term and preterm neonates during heelstick procedures. Pediatrics 74, 1012–1015.

Franck, L.S. (1986) A new method to quantitatively describe pain behavior in infants. Nurs. Res. 35, 28–31.

Gottfried, A.W. and Gaiter, J.L. (Eds.) (1985) Infant Stress under Intensive Care: Environmental Neonatology. (University Park Press, Baltimore, MD).

Grunau, R. and Craig, K. (1987) Pain expression in neonates: Facial action and cry. Pain 28, 395–410.

Harpin, V.A. and Rutter, N. (1982) Development of emotional sweating in the newborn infant. Arch. Dis. Child. 57, 691–695.

Harpin, V.A. and Rutter, N. (1983) Making heel pricks less painful. Arch. Dis. Child. 8, 226–228.

Hester, N.K.O. (1979) The preoperational children's reaction to immunization. Nurs. Res. 28, 250–255.

Johnston, C.C. and Strada, M.E. (1986) Acute pain response in infants: a multidimensional description. Pain 24, 373–382.

Justinich, C., Macdonald, N.E., McMurray, S.B. and MacKenzie, A.M.R. (1986) Evaluation of lumbar puncture in neonates with suspected sepsis. Paper presented at the Eastern Ontario Pediatric Association Meeting, Kingston, Ontario, June 1986.

Katz, E.R., Kellerman, J. and Siegel, S.E. (1980) Behavioral distress in children with leukemia undergoing bone marrow aspirations. J. Consult. Clin. Psychol. 48, 356–365.

Koren, G., Butt, W., Chinyanga, H., Soldin, S., Tan, Y.K. and Pape, K. (1985) Postoperative morphine infusion in newborn infants: Assessment of disposition characteristics and safety. J. Pediatr. 107, 963–967.

Lewis, N. (1978) The needle. Child. Today, Jan.-Feb. issue, 18–21.

McGrath, P., Lawrence, J., Martire, H., Vair, C.A. and McMurray, B. (1987) Nurses perceptions of pain in the neonatal intensive care nursery. Manuscript submitted for publication.

Neal, H. (1978) The Politics of Pain (McGraw-Hill, New York), pp. 139–179.

O'Hara, M., McGrath, P.J., D'Astous, J. and Vair, C.A. (1987) Oral morphine versus injected meperidine (Demerol) for pain relief in children after orthopedic surgery. J. Pediatr. Orthop. Surg. 7, 78–82.

Owens, M.E. and Todt, E.H. (1984) Pain in infancy: Neonatal response to a heel lance. Pain 20, 77–86.

Raju, T.N.K., Vidyasagar, D., Torres, C., Grundy, D. and Bennett, E.J. (1980) Intracranial pressure during intubation and anesthesia in infants. J. Pediatr. 96, 860–862.

Ross, D.M. and Ross, S.A. (1984) Childhood pain: the school-aged child's viewpoint. Pain 20, 179–191.

Rutter, N. (1987) Drug absorption through the skin: A mixed blessing. Arch. Dis. Child. 62, 220–221.

Schreiner, R.L. and Kleiman, M.B. (1979) Incidence and effect of traumatic lumbar puncture in the neonate. Dev. Med. Child Neurol. 21, 483–487.

Teele, D.W., Daskofsky, B., Rakusan, T. and Klein, J.O. (1981) Meningitis after lumbar puncture in children with bacteremia. New Engl. J. Med. 305, 1079–1081.

Traughber, B. and Cataldo, M. (1983) Biobehavioral effects of pediatric hospitalization. In: P.J. McGrath and Firestone, P. (Eds.), Pediatric and Adolescent Behavioral Medicine (Springer, New York) pp. 107–131.

Waugh, R. and Johnson, G.G. (1984) Current considerations in neonatal anaesthesia. Can. Anaesth. Soc. J. 31, 700–709.

Wolke, D. (1987) Environmental neonatology. Arch. Dis. Child., in press.

CHAPTER 6

Abdominal pain

Ointments for stomach pain from Thomas Phaer, 1546
Take gallia muscata at the pothecaries .xx. graine weight, myrrhe a verye litle, male it up
in oynmente fourme, with oyle of mastike, and water of roses sufficient, this is a very
good ointment for the stomake.

   Take mastike, franfinsence, and drye redde roses, as muche as is sufficient, make them
in pouder, and temper them up, with the iuyce of mintes, and a sponful of vinegar, and
use it.

   Take wheat floure and parche it on a panne, tyll it begynne to brenne and waxe redde,
than stampe it with vinegar, and adde to it, the yolkes of twoo egges harde rosted,
mastike, gumme, & frankinsence sufficient, make a plaister and laye it to the stomake
(quoted in Ruhrah, 1925, p. 180).

1. Introduction

Abdominal pain is ubiquitous. It can be the prime symptom of a wide variety
of medical conditions. It is a secondary symptom in many disorders or it can
stand alone as a syndrome. Abdominal pain may signal a serious medical
condition or it may be benign. It may be acute or recurrent. Abdominal pain
occurs in almost all children at one time or another and it is frequently of
unknown origin. Abdominal pain is often the cause of considerable distress as
child, parents and doctor struggle to discover what is causing the symptom.
The following is a description of a stomachache from a 6-year-old boy:

> It was like bees in your stomach – stinging your stomach, yellow jackets going ping,
> pong, bop inside – like someone just chopped down your stomach *(quoted in Ross and
> Ross, 1984, p. 184)*.

   This chapter will initially consider abdominal pain due to known medical
conditions and then will deal with the classic recurrent abdominal pain
syndrome (Apley, 1975). Colic, which is thought by some to be a form of
abdominal pain, is discussed in chapter 7 on colic. Our treatment of acute
abdominal pain and abdominal pain due to specific medical conditions will be

cursory and most attention will be paid to an examination of the recurrent abdominal pain syndrome.

2. The acute abdomen

Abdominal pain due to known medical causes can be either acute or recurrent. The acute abdomen is a common reason for a surgical consult that can be due to: constipation, gastroenteritis, polynephritis, renal colic, appendicitis, or ovarian cyst with torsion or twisting. In infants, acute abdominal pain can be due to strangulated inguinal hernia or intussusception. In sexually active girls, lower-quadrant pain can be the result of pelvic inflammatory disease, caused by sexually transmitted disease, or of ectopic pregnancy. The reader is referred to any standard pediatric surgery textbook for further discussion of the acute abdomen.

3. Recurrent abdominal pain due to known medical conditions

Recurrent abdominal pain due to known medical conditions can be due to: gastrointestinal dysfunctions; intake-related pain; musculofascial phenomena; gynecological conditions; acquired non-inflammatory impairments; chronic infections, inflammatory/immune; delayed effects of congenital anomalies; metabolic diseases; late complications of trauma; hematologic diseases; and neurologic disorders (Levine and Rappaport, 1984). As can be seen in Table 1, there are so many possible disorders that only the more common will be discussed.

3.1. Gastrointestinal dysfunctions

Frank constipation or irritable bowel syndrome will result in abdominal pain. Occult constipation, which is more difficult to detect, will be discussed under recurrent abdominal pain syndrome.

3.2. Intake-related pain

Abdominal pain is a common result of overindulgence and is not uncommonly seen with bulimia. Lactose intolerance as a cause of abdominal pain will be discussed in greater detail under recurrent abdominal pain.

TABLE 1
Recurrent abdominal pain: somatic predispositions, dysfunctions and disorders. (Reprinted from Levine and Rappaport, 1984, with permission of the author and publisher.)

Gastrointestinal dysfunctions	*Acquired non-inflammatory impairments*	*Delayed effects of congenital anomalies*
Constipation	Esophagitis	Malrotation
Spastic or irritable colon	Peptic ulcer disease	Duplication
	Gallbladder disease	Congenital stenosis
Intake-related pain	Renal calculi	Recurrent volvulus
Celiac disease		Superior mesenteric artery syndrome
Lead poisoning	*Chronic infections, inflammatory/immune*	Celiac axis compression syndrome
Foreign body	Rheumatic fever	Posterior urethral valves
Aerophagia	Juvenile rheumatoid arthritis	Uretero-pelvic obstruction
Lactose intolerance	Collagen-vascular disease	Hirschsprung's disease
Sucrose intolerance	*Yersinia enterocolitis*	Meckel's diverticulum
Sorbitol intolerance	Hepatitis	Chilaiditis syndrome
Various medications	Pyelonephritis	Bladder neck obstruction
Bulimia	Mesenteric adenitis	Hydronephrosis
Anorexia nervosa	Pancreatitis	Annular pancreas
	Ulcerative colitis	Hematocolpos
Musculofascial phenomena	Crohn's disease	
Inguinal hernia	Giardiasis	*Metabolic diseases*
Internal hernia	Ascariasis	Diabetes mellitus
Hernia of linea alba	Henoch-Schönlein purpura	Porphyria
Asthma	Hereditary angioneurotic edema	Hyperparathyroidism
Exercise	Familial Mediterranean fever	Hyperlipidemia
	Psoas abscess	Multiple endocrine adenomatosis
Gynecological conditions	Pleurodynia	
Ovarian cyst	Cystic fibrosis	*Hematologic diseases*
Ovarian torsion		Sickle cell disease
Endometriosis	*Late complications of trauma*	Thalassemia
Pelvic inflammatory disease	Adhesions	
Mittelschmerz	Pancreatic pseudocyst	
Dysmenorrhea	Abdominal wall strain	
Fitz-Hugh Curtis syndrome	Traumatic hemobilia	
Neoplasias	Subserosal intestinal hemorrhage	
Neurologic disorders		
Abdominal migraine		
Abdominal epilepsy		
Riley-Day syndrome		

3.3. Gynecological conditions

Gynecological conditions with recurrent abdominal pain as a symptom are of importance in the adolescent female. Barr (1983) has carefully described the evaluation of the teenage girl with abdominal pain. The most commonly detected problems are: dysmenorrhea, pelvic inflammatory disease, ovarian cysts, endometriosis and pregnancy.

3.4. Acquired non-inflammatory impairments

Peptic ulcer is the most commonly cited cause of pain in this category. Ulcer disease in adolescents is most frequently primary and duodenal (Barr, 1983). Adolescents with peptic ulcer often do not present the typical picture seen in adults.

3.5. Chronic infections, inflammatory/immune

A common infection causing recurrent abdominal pain is recurrent pyelonephritis (Levine and Rappaport, 1984). Other possible culprits include *Yersinia enterocolitis* (Kohl, 1979), giardiasis (Meyer and Jarroll, 1980), *Dientamoeba fragilis* (Spencer et al., 1979), chronic hepatitis, pancreatitis, or urinary tract infections.

The most common inflammatory/immune diseases are inflammatory bowel disease which include Crohn's disease and ulcerative colitis.

Approximately 2/3 of children with Crohn's disease present with abdominal pain and fully 1/3 have pain as the dominant symptom (O'Donoghue and Dawson, 1977). The pain is frequently in the right lower quadrant beginning as a vague non-specific discomfort (Levine and Rappaport, 1984). Between 18–33% of patients with Crohn's disease present before the age of 20 years. There has been a recent increase in the incidence of Crohn's disease but the reason for this is unknown.

Crohn's disease is characterized by non-caseating granuloma and mucosal, submucosal, transmural and serosal inflammation of the bowel. The most common location is the terminal ileum but the entire gastrointestinal tract including the mouth can be affected. The cause of Crohn's disease is not certain but it is generally agreed that for both Crohn's and ulcerative colitis a genetically determined unusual tissue response to widely present environmental agents is responsible (Sibinga, 1983). Psychological factors are *not* causative, although psychological stress or family pathology may contribute to a remission and may make adherence to the medical regimen difficult.

3.6. Metabolic disorders

Metabolic disorders that have abdominal pain among their symptoms include: hyperlipidemias, porphyria, diabetes and disorders promoting constipation such as hypothyroidism and hypocalcemia.

3.7. Late complications of trauma

Late complications of trauma include pancreatic pseudocyst, splenic trauma and abdominal wall strain.

3.8. Hematologic diseases

Hematologic diseases that can cause recurrent abdominal pain include: sickle cell disease, hemophilia, hemolytic anemias, lymphomas, leukemias and purpuras. Sickle cell disease and hemophilia are discussed in chapter 11. Cancer pain is discussed in chapter 10.

3.9. Neurologic disorders

Abdominal migraine and abdominal epilepsy have been seen as causes of recurrent abdominal pain in children. Children with migraine not infrequently have pain in the abdomen when they have headache. Some children with migraine alternate between headache and abdominal pain. Abdominal epilepsy in which pain in the abdomen is thought to substitute for a seizure is a very controversial diagnosis. We believe the diagnosis of abdominal epilepsy to be unwarranted unless there is loss of consciousness as well as abdominal pain.

4. Recurrent abdominal pain with no known organic cause

4.1. Definition

Recurrent abdominal pain for which no organic cause can be found is usually known simply as recurrent abdominal pain syndrome. Apley's (1975) criteria for recurrent abdominal pain which are universally accepted are:
(a) at least three attacks of pain,
(b) pain severe enough to affect activities,
(c) attacks occurring over a period of 3 months,
(d) no known organic cause.

4.2. Prevalence

Recurrent abdominal pain occurs frequently. The prevalence of the disorder has been estimated in Denmark at 12.1% for boys and 16.7% for girls (Oster, 1972). Apley and Naish (1958) in their study of 1000 unselected British schoolchildren found that 12.3% of girls and 9.5% of boys had recurrent abdominal pain. The prevalence peaked for 9-year-old girls with over one quarter of them affected. In a recently reported study of 6-year-olds in a town in Northern England, Faull and Nicol (1986) determined a prevalence rate of between 24.5% and 26.9% with no significant differences between the sexes. No North American prevalence studies have been done but 19.0% of adolescents in a community survey did report that they worried a lot or some about abdominal pain (Feldman et al., 1984).

4.3. Methodological errors

Two major problems have plagued the recurrent abdominal pain literature. The first (Barr and Feuerstein, 1983) is that clinicians and parents often assume that abdominal pain must be either organic or psychogenic and they conclude that if no organic cause is found for the pain then the pain must be psychogenic (Fig. 1). This error is of major importance because the assignment of an unwarranted diagnosis may lead to failure to discern an organic illness and an unsubstantiated diagnosis of psychogenic pain will frequently lead to patient and family hostility (McGrath et al., 1986).

The second error is that of methodological inadequacy. There is a tendency for subject samples to be the result of a referral filter bias (Sackett et al., 1985). Samples are often drawn from a population such as patients referred to psychiatric services or hospitalized children. The results are then generalized to all children with recurrent abdominal pain. Children admitted to hospital for abdominal pain are likely to be substantially different from children with abdominal pain who see their own physician (Feldman, 1986). As well, most studies in the area have not used control groups nor have standardized measurement techniques been used.

As we discuss in greater detail in chapter 13 on chronic intractable pain and chapter 14 on psychogenic pain, there has been a tendency to confuse the psychological causation or psychogenicity of recurrent abdominal pain with psychological factors involved in coping with the pain. Such factors may exacerbate or maintain the pain or they may influence the reaction to the pain (Barr and Feuerstein, 1983; McGrath and Feldman, 1986). Confusion

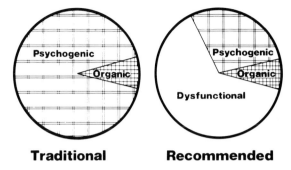

Traditional   **Recommended**

Fig. 1. Alternative clinical models for recurrent abdominal pain syndrome. The presence of cross-hatching indicates an assumption of 'disease' being present. 'Dysfunctional' RAP syndrome refers to children in whom appropriate evidence for organicity or psychogenicity is lacking and no assumption of abnormality is made.

As can be seen the traditional model suggests that recurrent abdominal pain is either psychogenic or organic. We agree with Barr and Feuerstein (1983) that most recurrent abdominal pain is neither organic nor psychogenic but is due not to disease but to some dysfunction. As we have indicated, we believe that, in many cases, this dysfunction is constipation due to problems with gut motility. (Redrawn and reproduced by permission from Stewart Gable (Ed.) (1981) Behavior Problems in Children (Grune & Stratton, New York) p. 237.)

between cause of recurrent abdominal pain and coping with recurrent abdominal pain has slowed development of appropriate understanding of the disorder. Practically, this confusion may lead to inappropriate diagnosis and treatment. For example, a child with obvious psychological problem in coping with recurrent abdominal pain, such as using pain to avoid school, may also be suffering from recurrent abdominal pain caused by lactose intolerance. Similarly, a child with pain due to performance anxiety, may persevere in his tasks in spite of the pain and cope quite well. Moreover, an organically caused disorder may be exacerbated by psychological factors.

4.4. Explanations for recurrent abdominal pain

Explanations for recurrent abdominal pain are usually ad hoc attempts to understand the problems that present in the clinical setting rather than complete theories of causation. Psychological theories that have been utilized to explain recurrent abdominal pain include: operant theories; stress; modelling; depression; family enmeshment; and somatization disorder. Physiological theories include: autonomic instability; lactose intolerance; and constipation/gut motility.

It is a sign of our ignorance that so many diverse explanations can be current without accepted guidelines as to when they may be operative. However, each explanation has some evidence supporting it. Although most researchers would acknowledge that recurrent abdominal pain is likely to be the final common pathway for a number of different problems, no comprehensive attempt to match explanations with patients has yet been attempted. It is important to realize that more than one factor may be operative in any specific case. We will briefly examine each proposed explanation of recurrent abdominal pain.

4.4.1. Operant

The major empirical support for an operant interpretation of recurrent abdominal pain comes from two single case studies and by analogy from work with adults with chronic intractable pain. Sank and Biglan (1974) used a token system with a 10-year-old boy with a 2.5 year history of often severe recurrent abdominal pain and a school attendance rate of 38% for the 72 days preceding treatment. Typically, preceding treatment, the child's mother would stay with him and give him medication and back rubs. When he stayed home from school he would be allowed to read and watch television in bed and to get up when he felt better. With the token system, non-occurrence of severe attacks and attendance at school were rewarded with points which could be exchanged for money and saved for other reinforcers. Attention for being ill was also eliminated. The program was successful in reducing pain by the child's own report and increased school attendance to 86% for 106 school days following treatment.

In a similar study, Miller and Kratchowill (1979) used a multiple baseline across settings design to treat a 10-year-old girl with recurrent abdominal pain. The child had been treated with belladonna and phenobarbital. She had been allowed to stay home and read, watch television and enjoy her mother's company and was reporting an average of 1.5 pain incidents per day. Treatment consisted of reducing the positive aspects of reporting pain. She was made to rest in bed whenever pain occurred. Treatment successfully reduced and eventually eliminated pain at home and at school.

It should be noted that these two children were very different from the average child with recurrent abdominal pain who does not miss excessive amounts of school and reports pain on a much less frequent basis. These children are much more typical of chronic intractable pain syndrome (chapter 13) or what Barr and Feuerstein (1983) have termed 'the extended recurrent abdominal pain syndrome'.

The basic notion is that children express pain because they are reinforced for such pain expression by the environment. Children can be directly reinforced for pain expression by parental attention or special privileges. In addition, aversive events such as a difficult school situation, can be avoided by 'illness'.

The key to tracking down operant factors is to find the link between avoidance behavior or reward and pain incidents. This can be done by a careful history and by use of a prospective pain diary (McGrath, 1983). One concern to keep in mind is that an exclusively operant approach may reduce the report of pain without altering the experience of pain. Teaching children to be reluctant to report may not be in their best interests.

No estimate of the proportion of recurrent abdominal pain that can be explained by operant factors is available.

4.4.2. Stress

Studies have examined the relationship between stress and recurrent abdominal pain. McGrath et al. (1983) found no difference in the amount of life change experienced by children with recurrent abdominal pain and pain-free controls. Similarly, Raymer et al. (1984) in their comparison of children with Crohn's disease, ulcerative colitis, recurrent abdominal pain and pain-free controls found that children with recurrent abdominal pain experienced a similar amount of life stress as did pain-free controls. In sharp contrast with these two studies are the findings of Greene et al. (1985) in their study of 172 adolescents attending an adolescent clinic. They found an average of 13.2 negative life events for children with recurrent abdominal or chest pain or headache and less than four negative life events for adolescents attending for routine examination, acute minor illness or organic pain. They also found elevated life change scores for adolescents with behavior disorders. However, they noted that findings of increased negative life events in patients with non-organic pain appearing at a medical clinic did not prove causation. Crossley (1982) also found an increased rate of stressful life events in children hospitalized for abdominal pain when compared to pain-free controls and children with appendicitis.

Evidence that children with recurrent abdominal pain have anxious personalities that make them prone to the effects of stress is equivocal. Two surveys of children with recurrent abdominal pain which did not use standardized anxiety measures suggest that recurrent abdominal pain children are more anxious (Apley and Naish, 1958; Liebman, 1978). Two case-control studies with outpatients using standardized measures (McGrath et al., 1983; Raymer et al., 1984) suggested that this was not accurate. We (McGrath et al., 1983) compared 30 children seen in the gastroenterology service with recurrent abdominal pain with 30 children matched on age and sex, seen in other clinics for minor problems. Scores on the personality problems subscale and the inadequacy-immaturity subscale of the parent and teacher Quay-Peterson behavior problem checklist yielded no significant differences between the two groups.

Raymer et al. (1984) studied 44 children with organic abdominal pain, 16 children with recurrent abdominal pain and 30 pain-free controls. Using the Rogers personal adjustment inventory and the Coopersmith self esteem inventory, they found no differences between children with organic abdominal pain and classic recurrent abdominal pain. They did find more psychological problems in children who had abdominal pain from any cause than in children who were pain free.

One controlled study (Crossley, 1982) using standard measures with children admitted to hospital with abdominal pain, did find that children with non-specific pain (not specifically following Apley's criteria) were likely to be psychologically abnormal. He found boys were more neurotic at home and school and girls were neurotic at home and antisocial at school. Interestingly, boys with appendicitis also showed serious psychopathology.

In a community survey of all six-year-olds, Faull and Nicol (1986) found that parents rated children with recurrent abdominal pain as more disturbed (both neurotic and antisocial) than children without recurrent abdominal pain. Teachers rated the pain children as more hyperactive than controls. In terms of temperament a case control substudy (Davison et al., 1986) found that the boys with recurrent abdominal pain were more likely to have a slow to warm up temperament whereas girls with recurrent abdominal pain were more likely to have an irregular temperamental style.

A study (Astrada et al., 1981) of 22 children referred to a psychiatry liaison service of which 18 were for recurrent abdominal pain found that four had DSM III (American Psychiatric Association, 1980) diagnoses of separation anxiety and three had overanxious disorder.

It is difficult to reconcile the conflicting findings of these studies. However, some comments are in order. Children, who are hospitalized for recurrent abdominal pain, may be quite different from children who attend as outpatients, who in turn may be different from children who are identified in community surveys. In our own hospital, the only children who would be hospitalized for recurrent abdominal pain would be those with serious psychosocial problems. The vast majority of children with recurrent abdominal pain would not be hospitalized and only those who were thought to be psychiatrically disturbed would be referred for a psychiatric consult. Consequently, extrapolation from hospitalized cases (Crossley, 1982) or cases referred to psychiatry services (Astrada et al., 1981) to the more typical case is unwarranted.

Barr and Feuerstein (1983) have emphasized that stress may be a precipitant of the child not coping well with the pain even if the symptom itself is not causally related to stress. Since Greene et al. (1985) used clinic attenders as controls this should not be a factor. Unfortunately, Greene et al. (1985) did not separate out adolescents with abdominal pain from those with chest pain or headache and did not even indicate how many were in each group.

In the community study by Faull and Nicol (1986), the prevalence rate of recurrent abdominal pain was 2.5 times what is usually reported at this age. Moreover, 96% of their sample was pain free on 6 months follow-up. It may be that for this sample, stress in temperamentally predisposed individuals was important in the genesis of this short-lived recurrent abdominal pain.

4.4.3. Modelling

The role that modelling has in recurrent abdominal pain is difficult to disentangle from constitutional predispositions. Oster (1972), Stone and Barbero (1970) and Apley and Naish (1958) noted that pain problems tend to run in families but the roles of physiologic tendency and psychologic modelling could not be distinguished. Christensen and Mortensen (1975) investigated 34 adults who had been hospitalized as children for abdominal pain approximately 30 years previously. The children of these patients were not more likely to have pain than were controls. However, they did find that children, who had parents currently complaining of pain, were much more likely to have pain. This finding suggests a modelling rather than a biological transmission of stomach pain.

In experimental studies, Craig (1983, 1984) has demonstrated that the reaction to painful stimuli can be modified by modelling. It may be that reaction to pain or coping with pain may be more readily amenable to modelling than causation of pain.

4.4.4. Depression

The role of depression in recurrent abdominal pain is complex. Hughes (1984) found that all 23 of the children hospitalized for recurrent abdominal pain met DSM III criteria for major depressive episode. We (McGrath et al., 1983) found no elevation of depression when measured by self-report or by standardized interviewer assessment in recurrent abdominal pain children. Hodges et al. (1985) found that recurrent abdominal pain children were less depressed than behaviorally disturbed children and not depressed when compared to healthy controls. Raymer et al. (1984) found higher depression in children with recurrent abdominal pain and in children with organic pain. Both Hughes (1984) and Hodges et al. (1985) noted depression in the mothers of the children with recurrent abdominal pain. Hughes (1984) used an unstandardized clinical interview and he did not have a control group. His patients were referred to a psychiatry liaison service in a tertiary care hospital. Subjects in the other three studies (McGrath et al., 1983; Raymer et al., 1984; Hodges et al., 1985) were from pediatric gastroenterology services. The differences may be due to a referral filter bias (Sackett et al., 1985).

Our interpretation is that a high percentage of children with recurrent abdominal pain, who are referred to a mental health service, are depressed but most children with recurrent abdominal pain are not more depressed than controls. It does appear that a long standing problem with abdominal pain may cause depression rather than vice versa. Finally, having a child with recurrent abdominal pain (or any other chronic illness) may trigger maternal depression.

4.4.5. Family enmeshment

Family enmeshment or overinvolvement of parents in the lives of their children have been cited as a cause of abdominal pain in clinical series (Stone and Barbero, 1970; Apley, 1975; Hughes and Zimin, 1978). However, there is no evidence that most children with recurrent abdominal pain have overinvolved or enmeshed families. As discussed in detail in chapter 13, experimental evidence does suggest that children who are not coping with pain, including abdominal pain, have mothers who intrude more in an experimental situation than do mothers of children who are coping with pain (Dunn-Geier et al., 1986). However, it is not clear if parental intrusiveness is a cause of or a result of having a child who is not coping with pain.

4.4.6. Somatization disorder

The essential features of somatization disorder are multiple recurrent somatic complaints of several years duration for which medical attention is sought but which are not due to any apparent physical disorder (American Psychiatric Association, 1980). Ernst et al. (1984) studied the medical charts of 149 children seen in a multispecialty medical clinic for abdominal pain. Children, who had recurrent abdominal pain (108 children), had more symptoms of somatization disorder than children with an organic abdominal pain disorder (21 children) or children with another organic disorder (14 children). They also noted that children with recurrent abdominal pain, who were attending the clinic and who had had pain for several years, had more symptoms of somatization disorder than children with recurrent abdominal pain of more recent onset. They estimated that six of the 36 children who had recurrent abdominal pain for over 1 year would develop into adults with somatization disorder.

Routh and Ernst (1984) compared 20 children with recurrent abdominal pain with 20 children with organic abdominal pain. On interviewing the mothers of the children, they found a higher incidence of alcoholism, conduct disorder, antisocial personality, attention deficit disorder, and somatization disorder in the first and second degree relatives of the recurrent abdominal pain patients. Approximately twice as many relatives of recurrent abdominal pain children had relatives with disorders than did the relatives of controls. The differences between the groups were greatest for somatization disorder which occurred in 14 relatives of the recurrent abdominal pain group and only one of the organic pain group.

The work of this group does suggest that pain problems occur in families that have other problems and a small but important subgroup of children may be at risk for later psychiatric disorders.

4.4.7. Autonomic instability

Four studies have examined aspects of autonomic defect in children with recurrent abdominal pain. Kopel et al. (1967) found that there was increased rectosigmoid motility following subcutaneous injection of prostigmine methyl sulfate in children with recurrent abdominal pain in comparison to controls. This difference suggested an increased sensitivity to parasympathetic stimulation. The authors proposed that children with recurrent abdominal pain have a general autonomic imbalance.

Rubin et al. (1967) found increased recovery time in pupillary response to a cold pressor stress in children with recurrent abdominal pain but no differences in resting levels or response to stress.

Apley et al. (1971) failed to replicate the finding of increased recovery time but did note that children with recurrent abdominal pain were more likely to have an 'unstable' recovery. Unfortunately, the description of what constitutes an unstable recovery is not precise.

In a more recent study using cold pressor stress, Feuerstein et al. (1982)

found no differences in physiological, behavioral or self-report in the stress phase or in the recovery phase between children with recurrent abdominal pain and carefully matched controls.

The data on autonomic instability is difficult to interpret and no firm conclusions can be drawn. The earlier studies are not described clearly enough to be certain of their significance and the latest study by Feuerstein et al. (1982) may be lacking in power because of the small sample size. Autonomic defect is an appealing explanation because it could be the construct that underlies how stress, depression, somatization disorder, and gut motility/constipation might cause recurrent abdominal pain.

4.4.8. Lactose intolerance

Barr et al. (1979a) conducted a prospective study of 80 schoolchildren with recurrent abdominal pain. They detected lactose malabsorption on the basis of a response to a breath hydrogen test (Perman et al., 1978) in 40% of the children. A subsequent dietary trial found that 70% of the children, who reduced their lactose ingestion, had increased pain when they returned to their usual lactose-containing diets. Unfortunately, the diet trial was not blinded. MacLean (1979) has noted that the control period may have predisposed the children to experience symptoms during the lactose-containing experimental period.

Liebman (1979) in a very similar study found that 11 of 38 children with recurrent abdominal pain demonstrated lactose intolerance using a lactose tolerance blood test. Subsequent open dietary trial produced significant pain relief in ten of 11 children.

However, Lebenthal et al. (1981) studying 69 children with recurrent abdominal pain and 61 control subjects did not find any increased prevalence of lactose intolerance in children with recurrent abdominal pain compared with controls. A subsequent diet trial found that the lactose intolerant children did not respond to a lactose-free diet any better than did children who were not lactose intolerant. As well, both Christensen (1980) and McGrath et al. (1983) did not find any differences in lactose intolerance between children with recurrent abdominal pain and pain-free controls.

At this time, the data do not support the notion that lactose intolerance is a major cause of recurrent abdominal pain in children.

4.4.9. Constipation/gut motility

Although obvious constipation is well recognized as a cause of abdominal pain, most children with recurrent abdominal pain are not obviously constipated. Barr et al. (1979b) have shown that many children are constipated without being aware of it or without showing classic signs of constipation. Parents are unlikely to know of their children's bowel habits and children may not remember or may be too shy to discuss their bowel habits.

Dimson (1971) studied transit time measured by the passage of carmine dye in 306 children with recurrent abdominal pain. He described rectal constipation in 22% and delayed transit time in 91% of this group. In the remaining group, transit time was delayed in 44% of the children. Colonic spasm was thought to be responsible for pain in this group.

Feldman et al. (1985) in a double-blind, randomized placebo controlled trial used 10 g of supplementary dietary fiber to treat 52 children with recurrent abdominal pain. There was no attempt to titrate the dose. Minor side effects were equivalent in both groups but these were not problematic. Children were recruited from primary care physicians. We found that 50% of the children on the fiber treatment had a reduction of 50% or more in their pain. Twenty-seven percent of the control group showed a similar response. Although caution is needed in interpreting causation from response to treatment, a constipation/gut motility explanation for recurrent abdominal pain is in keeping with the results of the trial. The best evidence is that a predisposition to constipation is genetically determined (Bakwin and Davidson, 1971) and it may well be that differences in transit time are similarly controlled. Our tentative hypothesis is that a proportion of children with recurrent abdominal pain suffer from occult constipation which can be relieved by dietary manipulation. The results are similar to those when fiber is used in irritable bowel syndrome in adult medicine. Further research will be required to determine the mechanism of action and which children will benefit from increased dietary fiber.

4.5. *Making sense of the various explanations*

It is our belief that recurrent abdominal pain can be the result of many different causes and in some cases may be due to multiple causes. There is in our mind, however, a major difference between 'garden variety' or typical recurrent abdominal pain and what Barr and Feuerstein (1983) have termed the 'extended recurrent abdominal pain syndrome'. The key difference is that the typical recurrent abdominal pain sufferer and his or her family cope well. Consultation may take place with the doctor or even with a specialist if the problem is severe. The child continues to attend school, play with friends and engage in extra-curricular activities. Neither the child nor the family becomes overwhelmed by the symptom. The child with extended recurrent abdominal pain syndrome may not have more severe pain but the reaction is very different. School absence, restriction of social and sports activities is the norm with these children. The children and their families are in a quest for a cure and often visit numerous specialists. They are frequently referred to psychiatrists and psychologists. This type of response can occur with any type of pain and we have termed it chronic intractable pain which is discussed in detail in chapter 13.

No studies have evaluated the relative contribution of different causes for recurrent abdominal pain in children. It is our opinion that the relative contribution of each factor in any given sample of children, will depend to a great extent on the referral pattern. Children seen in psychiatry or psychology clinics will likely have pain due to psychological factors. Children in primary care settings, or in the general population, are much more likely to have pain from physiological causes. Very few children will have abdominal pain from serious organic causes. Finally, as we have emphasized, the finding of one cause does not rule out other causes.

In the individual case, a careful diagnostic evaluation will lead to preferred courses of treatment.

5. Clinical guidelines

(1) Rule out organic illness by means of a thorough physical, history and the following lab tests:
   (a) complete blood count,
   (b) sedimentation rate,
   (c) urinalysis and culture.
   Other lab tests should be ordered only in response to specific indications.
(2) Interview children and parents separately. In this way each party can discuss information they do not wish to disclose in front of the other.
(3) Never doubt that a child is in pain. Doubting that someone is in pain will only encourage increased complaints of pain to prove that the pain is real.
(4) Recurrent abdominal pain should be treated according to those factors thought to be implicated in its cause or in the child's ability to cope with the pain.
   (a) Operant factors contributing to the problem can sometimes be

controlled. For example, parents who are inadvertently encouraging their children to complain (by giving privileges, treats or freedom from responsibility) may respond to suggestions to change their behavior.

(b) Stress situations, such as a single bully who is terrorizing a schoolbus or a teacher who is constantly shouting, may be ameliorated by direct action. In other cases, reduction in stress may be impossible.

(c) If the problem is anxiety and overreaction to stressful situations, stress management (relaxation training, meditative breathing, cognitive restructuring) may be helpful but they are expensive.

(d) Modelling of pain behavior by parents is likely to be very resistant to change and will generally require intensive long term intervention.

(e) Depression can be treated medically or psychologically.

(f) Family enmeshment and somatization disorder are very difficult to treat and treatment is likely to be long term.

(g) Autonomic instability may be treated by stress management methods.

(h) Lactose intolerance is treated by an elimination diet.

(i) Constipation and gut motility contributing to recurrent abdominal pain can be treated benignly by addition of 10 g of fiber to the daily diet. Fiber supplements, high fiber breakfast cereals, fresh fruits and vegetables or a combination of these can be used.

Unfortunately the treatment of the factors involved in recurrent abdominal pain, for the most part, are both largely unproven and very invasive. Psychotherapy, family therapy or intensive behavior therapy are expensive, unpalatable to many families and may do more harm than good.

Consequently, we recommend that a three-step process be used. In the first step, all organic and psychological factors that can be uncovered with relatively innocuous organic and psychological investigations are identified and corrected. Reassurance about the benign nature of the disorder is given. Children, who continue to have abdominal pain of unknown origin, should be tried on a trial of increased fiber in their diet. Six weeks of approximately 10 g of supplementary fiber/day will provide relief for about half of these children with few side effects. Titration of the dose of fiber may be helpful.

Finally, children who fail to improve on this trial should then be considered for more extensive investigation if the pain is severe and frequent enough to warrant the costs and possible iatrogenic effects of the procedures.

Children who are not treated should be followed in order to detect change of symptoms that may lead to clearer diagnosis and also to encourage the family to continue coping.

6. Future directions

(1) Community-based studies are required to determine the correlates of recurrent abdominal pain.

(2) Properly designed randomized trials should evaluate suggested treatments of recurrent abdominal pain. Replicated trials of successful treatments (such as supplementary fiber) are required because of possible differences in clinical populations due to referral filter bias (Sackett et al., 1985).

(3) Studies examining the mechanisms of treatments of recurrent abdominal pain should be undertaken.

(4) Research and public education programs on the explosion of venereal disease in adolescent women is needed.

References

American Psychiatric Association (1980) Diagnostic and Statistical Manual of Mental Disorders, 3rd edn. (A.P.A., Washington DC) pp. 241–252.

Apley, J. (1975) The Child with Abdominal Pains, 2nd edn. (Blackwell, London).

Apley, J. and Naish, N. (1958) Children with recurrent abdominal pains: A field survey of 1000 school children. Arch. Dis. Child. 33, 165–170.

Apley, J., Haslam, D.R. and Tulloch, G. (1971) Pupillary reaction in children with recurrent abdominal pain. Arch. Dis. Childhood 46, 337–340.

Astrada, C.A., Licamele, W.L., Walsh, T.L. and Kessler, E.S. (1981) Recurrent abdominal pain in children and associated DSM-III diagnoses. Am. J. Psychiatr. 138, 687–688.

Bakwin, H. and Davidson, M. (1971) Constipation in twins. Am. J. Dis. Child. 121, 179–181.

Barr, R.G. (1983) Abdominal pain in the female adolescent. Pediatr. Rev. 4, 281–289.

Barr, R.G. and Feuerstein, M. (1983) Recurrent abdominal pain syndrome: How appropriate are our basic clinical assumptions? In: P.J. McGrath and P. Firestone (Eds.), Pediatric and Adolescent Behavioral Medicine: Issues in Treatment (Springer, New York) pp. 13–27.

Barr, R.G., Levine, M.D. and Watkins, J.B. (1979a) Recurrent abdominal pain of childhood due to lactose intolerance. New Engl. J. Med. 300, 1449–1452.

Barr, R.G., Wilkinson, R., Levine, M.D. and Mulvihill, D. (1979b) Chronic and occult stool retention. A clinical tool for its evaluation in school aged children. Clin. Pediatr. 18, 674.

Christensen, M.F. (1980) Prevalence of lactose intolerance in children with recurrent abdominal pain. Pediatrics 65, 681.

Christensen, M.F. and Mortensen, O. (1975) Longterm prognosis in children with recurrent abdominal pain. Arch. Dis. Child. 50, 110–114.

Coleman, W.L. and Levine, M.L. (1986) Recurrent abdominal pain: The cost of the aches and the aches of the cost. Pediatr. Rev. 8, 143–151.

Craig, K.D. (1983) Modelling and social learning factors in chronic pain. In: J.J. Bonica, U. Lindblom and A. Iggo (Eds.), Advances in Pain Research and Therapy (Raven Press, New York) pp. 813–827.

Craig, K.D. (1984) Emotional aspects of pain. In: P.D. Wall and R. Melzack (Eds.), Textbook of Pain (Churchill Livingstone, Edinburgh) pp. 153–161.

Crossley, R.B. (1982) Hospital admissions for abdominal pain in childhood. J. Roy. Soc. Med. 75, 772–776.

Davison, I.S., Faull, C. and Nicoll, A.R. (1986) Research note: Temperament and behavior in six-year-olds with recurrent abdominal pain: A follow up. J. Child Psychol. Psychiatr. 27, 539–544.

Dimson, S.B. (1971) Transit time related to clinical findings in children with recurrent abdominal pain. Pediatrics 47, 666–674.

Dunn-Geier, J., McGrath, P.J., Rourke, B., Latter, J. and D'Astous, J. (1986) Chronic pain in adolescents: The ability to cope. Pain 26, 23–32.

Ernst, A.R., Routh, D.K. and Harper, D.C. (1984) Abdominal pain in children and symptoms of somatization disorder. J. Pediatr. Psychol. 9, 77–86.

Faull, C. and Nicol, A.R. (1986) Abdominal pain in six-year-olds: An epidemiological study in a new town. J. Child Psychol. Psychiatr. 27, 251–260.

Feldman, W. (1986) Response to Christensen. Am. J. Dis. Child. 140, 739.

Feldman, W., Hodgson, C., Corber, S. and Quinn, A. (1984) Health concerns and health-related behaviours of adolescents. Can. Med. Assoc. J. 134, 489–493.

Feldman, W., McGrath, P.J., Hodgson, C., Ritter, H. and Shipman, R.T. (1985) The use of dietary fiber in the management of simple childhood idiopathic recurrent abdominal pain: Results in a prospective double blind randomized controlled trial. Am. J. Dis. Child. 139, 1216–1218.

Feuerstein, M., Barr, R.G., Francoeur, T.E., Houle, M. and Rafman, S. (1982) Potential biobehavioral mechanisms of recurrent abdominal pain in children. Pain 13, 287–298.

Greene, J.W., Walker, L.S., Hickson, G. and Thompson, J. (1985) Stressful life events and somatic complaints in adolescents. Pediatrics 75, 19–22.

Hodges, K., Kline, J.J., Barbero, G. and Flanery, R. (1985) Depressive symptoms in children with recurrent abdominal pain and in their families. J. Pediatr. 107, 622–626.

Hughes, M.C. (1984) Recurrent abdominal pain and childhood depression: Clinical observation of 23 children and their families. Am. J. Orthopsychiatr. 54, 146–155.

Hughes, M.C. and Zimin, R. (1978) Children with psychogenic abdominal pain and their families: Management during hospitalization. Clin. Pediatr. 17, 569–573.

Kohl, S. (1979) *Yersinia enterocolitica* infections in children. Pediatr. Clin. North Am. 26, 433–443.

Kopel, F.B., Kim, I.C. and Barbero, G.J. (1967) Comparison of rectosigmoid motility in normal children, children with recurrent abdominal pain, and children with ulcerative colitis. Pediatrics 39, 539–545.

Lebenthal, E., Rossi, T.M., Nord, K.S. and Branski, D. (1981) Recurrent abdominal pain and lactose absorption in children. Pediatrics 67, 828–832.

Levine, M. and Rappaport, L.A. (1984) Recurrent abdominal pain in school children: The loneliness of the long distance physician. Pediatr. Clin. North Am. 31, 969–991.

Liebman, W.M. (1978) Recurrent abdominal pain in children: A retrospective study of 119 patients. Clin. Pediatr. 17, 149–153.

Liebman, W.M. (1979) Recurrent abdominal pain in children: Lactose and sucrose intolerance, a prospective study. Pediatrics 64, 43–45.

McGrath, P.J. (1983) Psychological aspects of recurrent abdominal pain. Can. Fam. Phys. 29, 1655–1659.

McGrath, P.J. and Feldman, W. (1986) Clinical approach to recurrent abdominal pain in children. Dev. Behav. Pediatr. 7, 56–61.

McGrath, P.J., Goodman, J.T., Firestone, P., Shipman, R. and Peters, S. (1983) Recurrent abdominal pain: A Psychogenic disorder? Arch. Dis. Child 58, 888–890.

McGrath, P.J., Dunn-Geier, B.J., Cunningham, S.J., Brunette, R., D'Astous, J., Humphreys, P., Latter, J. and Keene, D. (1986) Psychological guidelines for helping children cope with chronic benign intractable pain. Clin. J. Pain 1, 229–233.

MacLean, W.C. (1980) Lactose intolerance. New Engl. J. Med. 302, 177–178.

Meyer, E.A. and Jarroll, E.L. (1980) Giardiasis. Am. J. Epidemiol. 111, 1–12.

Miller, A.J. and Kratchowill, T.R. (1979) Reduction of frequent stomach-ache complaints by time-out. Behav. Ther. 10, 211–218.

O'Donoghue, D.P. and Dawson, A.M. (1977) Crohn's disease in childhood. Arch. Dis. Child. 52, 627–632.

Oster, J. (1972) Recurrent abdominal pain, headache and limb pain in children and adolescents. Pediatrics 50, 429–436.

Perman, J.A., Barr, R.G. and Watkins, J.B. (1978) Sucrose malabsorption in children: Non-invasive diagnosis by interval breath hydrogen determination. J. Pediatr. 93, 17–22.

Raymer, D., Weininger, O. and Hamilton, J.R. (1984) Psychological problems in children with abdominal pain. Lancet i, 439–440.

Ross, D.M. and Ross, S.A. (1984) Childhood pain: The school-aged child's viewpoint. Pain 20, 179–191.

Routh, D.K. and Ernst, A.R. (1984) Somatization disorder in relatives of children and adolescents with functional abdominal pain. J. Pediatr. Psychol. 9, 427–437.

Rubin, L.S., Barbero, G.J. and Sibinga, M.S. (1967) Pupillary reactivity of children with recurrent abdominal pain. Psychosom. Med. 29, 111–120.

Ruhrah, J. (1925) Pediatrics of the Past (Paul B. Hoeber, New York) p. 180.

Sackett, D.L., Haynes, R.B. and Tugwell, P. (1985) Clinical epidemiology: A Basic Science for Clinical Medicine (Little Brown, Toronto) pp. 162–164.

Sank, L.I. and Biglan, A. (1984) Operant treatment of a case of recurrent abdominal pain in a 10-year-old boy. Behav. Ther. 5, 677–681.

Sibinga, M.S. (1983) The gastrointestinal tract. In: M.D. Levine, W.B. Carey, A.C. Crocker and R. Gross (Eds.), Developmental-Behavioral Pediatrics (Saunders, Philadelphia, PA) pp. 482–487.

Spencer, M.J., Garcia, L.S. and Chapin, M.R. (1979) *Dientamoeba fragilis*: An intestinal pathogen in children? Am. J. Dis. Child. 133, 390–393.

Stone, R.T. and Barbero, G.J. (1970) Recurrent abdominal pain in childhood. Pediatrics 45, 732–738.

CHAPTER 7

Colic

The colike ... ingendreth in a gutte named colon *(definition of colic in 1528, Oxford Dictionary, 1973, p. 366)*.

Colic is a common problem in the first year of childhood and it causes considerable distress for parents. In this chapter, we will discuss the definition of colic, its prevalence and theories of what causes colic. We will also examine various treatments of colic and what is known of the long-term sequelae of colic. Finally, we will review clinical guidelines and directions for future research.

1. What is colic?

The word colic is derived from the French 'colique' which in turn comes from the late Latin 'colicus' and from the Greek 'κωλικός' (kolikos) meaning pertaining to the colon. Although the term implies that there is something wrong with the baby's colon, there is no evidence that babies with colic do not have a perfectly normal colon.

Carey has pointed out that:

> ... for most infants who are 'colicky' it is not at all clear that they are experiencing pain. They do appear distressed but infants look much the same when they are sufficiently tired, hungry or frightened. They cannot tell us whether they are experiencing pain; they can only report their distress by crying *(Carey, 1984, p. 994)*.

Careful studies will be required to throw light on the question of whether colic causes pain. Such studies might use measurement techniques such as those of Grunau and Craig (1987) and Johnston and Strada (1986), which we described in chapter 2 to examine the behavior of colicky babies, especially at the beginning of bouts of colic.

Colic has been used to describe a very wide variety of symptoms but the most widely accepted operational definition of colic is:

> Inconsolable crying for which no physical cause can be found, which lasts more than three hours a day, occurs at least three days a week and continues for at least three weeks *(Wessell et al., 1954)*.

The most typical story is that of an apparently healthy baby between 3 days and 3 weeks who develops violent screaming attacks usually in the evening (Illingworth, 1954). The baby cannot be comforted and appears to be suffering from abdominal pain. Colic can occur with greater or lesser ferocity and, in less severe cases, the crying may be more of a whimper or may be less than daily. In terms of the observed behavior, there is nothing qualitative to mark colic as different from 'normal' fussing.

Babies with colic develop normally and do not appear to be different in any significant way from their peers who cry less. They cry at the same times (mostly in the evening) as babies without colic but simply cry more often and cannot be as easily stopped.

Colic can be seen as an extreme of 'normal' crying in infancy or it can be seen as the result of some as yet undetermined non-pathological variation of normal functioning.

If colic is an extreme of normal crying then: 'What is normal?'. Brazelton in his classic paper (Brazelton, 1962) studied 80 mothers and their babies and had the mothers keep daily logs of their babies' crying. He found that there was a gradual increase in the median amount of crying from 1.75 h/day at 2 weeks of age to a median of 2.75 h at 6 weeks with a steady decrease thereafter. Brazelton's (1962) findings have been widely replicated and are accepted as norms for industrialized cultures.

2. Theories of the cause of colic

Over 30 years ago Illingworth (1954), in a still relevant paper, evaluated and summarized the numerous etiological theories of colic. These etiological theories are listed in Table 1. He concluded that:

> ...Colic is not caused by underfeeding, overfeeding, errors of feeding technique, mismanagement, allergy, substances taken by the mother or swallowing air. I do not think it is due to an excess of wind in the intestines. I have never seen any evidence that colic is associated with hypertonicity or with any particular type of baby or parent. The outstanding impression given by the colicky baby is that he is a well, happy, thriving, well fed and well managed baby with nothing wrong with him. His stools are normal; he may posset, but he does not posset more than any other baby. He grows up to be a nice normal child in no way different from other children *(Illingworth, 1954, p. 173)*.

TABLE 1
Reputed causes of colic (after Illingworth, 1954).

Overfeeding; underfeeding; excessively frequent feeds; too infrequent feeds; food too rich; food too weak; food too hot; food too cold; too much fat; too much carbohydrate; too much protein; allergy to cow's milk; allergy to cod liver oil; allergy to orange juice; sensitivity to feathers; sensitivity to horsehair; allergy as manifested by hiccoughs in utero; hypertonicity as manifested by: exaggerated Moro reflex, sharp response to sudden light, vigorous crying when having a bath, tenseness; wakefulness, pylorospasm, vomiting, spastic constipation, diarrhea, abdominal distension, visible peristalsis, cardiospasm, tetany, over-reaction of the involuntary muscles, general spasticity, unusual alertness, pruritus ani, poor weight gain; picking up baby too much; bouncing baby; overpermissive and anxious mothers; mishandling; overstimulation; excess wind in the bowel; wind trapped in a loop of the bowel; air swallowing; immaturity of the intestine; spasm of the bowel; vagogenic gastroenterospasm; excessive propulsive activity of the colon; congenital malformation of the alimentary tract; lead poisoning; anal fissure; imperforate anus; peptic ulcer; disease of the gall bladder; disease of the respiratory tract; disease of the osseous system; congenital syphilis; volvulus; intussusception; renal colic; nasopharyngitis; otitis; pyelitis; tension developed in utero from a uterine handicap; hyperacidity; exposure to cold; chilling of the extremities; abdominal binders; fatigue toxins from the mother; tension due to lack of oral satisfaction; acidosis; introversion; accumulation of uric acid in the kidneys.

Illingworth (1954) concluded that colic was probably due to the baby's inability to adequately pass gas, perhaps because it becomes blocked in the loops of the bowel. No direct evidence was presented for this conclusion. Since Illingworth's paper, several key studies have discounted a number of causes of colic.

Wessel et al. (1954) investigated the longitudinal records of 98 infants who were involved in the Yale rooming in project and found that contented babies and fussy babies were equally likely to have allergy in themselves or in their family members. The results tended to discount allergy as a cause of colic.

Paradise (1966) critically reviewed the existing literature and also examined the occurrence of colic in 146 normal newborns. He found that colic was unrelated to family economic class, maternal age, birth order, sex, weight gain, type of feeding, family history of allergic or gastrointestinal disorder or maternal psychological characteristics.

Carey (1968) prospectively investigated 103 mothers and their newborns. Carey interviewed the mothers before they went home and rated each mother's anxiety using a structured six item author-developed anxiety interview. The reliability and validity of this interview is unknown. Forty mothers were defined as being anxious. Using Wessel et al.'s (1954) criteria, each baby was classified as having or not having colic. Of the 103 infants, 13 had colic. Anxious mothers were about nine times more likely to have colicky babies than non-anxious mothers. Carey's study suffered from a lack of blindness and reliance on retrospective reports of crying by parents. In the same vein, Ames and Bradley (1983) used questionnaires to study 267 first-time parents and their babies. Measures taken before the birth of the baby indicated that both mothers and fathers, who identified their babies as colicky, were more likely to be anxious, worried and subject to negative moods. Unfortunately, the determination of colic was based on a single question ('Is your baby colicky?') to the parents at each time frame.

Some indirect evidence for the role of anxiety in fussiness was provided by Smith and Steinschneider's (1975) finding that mothers who had slower heart rates tended to have babies who were more easily consoled.

It is not clear if anxious parents are more likely to give birth to babies who are colicky or if anxious parents engender colic in their babies. As well, both of these studies can be interpreted as indicating that anxious parents perceive their babies as crying more, rather than indicating that the babies of anxious parents actually cry more.

Weissbluth (1984) has argued that colic is a neurological and developmental problem which he hypothesized is closely associated with disordered sleep. He speculated that colic may be the result of disordered biological rhythms which prevent babies from being able to breathe regularly enough to allow themselves to remain asleep. According to this speculation, the crying of colic is the way the baby has of getting enough oxygen into the lungs to compensate for the disordered breathing. Alternatively, Weissbluth (1984) argued, colic attacks may in fact be periods of rapid eye movement (REM) sleep in which the typical muscle inhibition is not in place (uncoupled REM storms). Weissbluth (1984) suggested that temperament may be another manifestation of the underlying problem. No direct test of Weissbluth's theory has been presented.

Carey (1972) examined the relationship between temperament and colic in a sample of 200 babies. He found that a significantly high proportion of colicky babies were later rated as having a very difficult or rather difficult temperament. He also found that almost all colicky babies were rated as having a low sensory threshold. Weissbluth et al. (1984) also found many colicky babies to have a difficult temperament. The temperament did not change in spite of successful drug treatment of the colic.

Barr et al. (1983) examined 286 healthy breast-fed and 93 healthy formula-fed babies in terms of prediction of cry/fuss behavior at 6 weeks of age. They found significant but small ($r = 0.19$ for cry and $r = 0.21$) correlations between temperament, as measured by parents when their infants were 2 weeks of age, and crying and fussing, as measured by a well validated diary method.

Recently, Carey (1983) has suggested an interaction model in which colic develops when a physiologically predisposed infant is cared for by an anxious caregiver whose soothing behaviors are ineffective. No test or assessment of this model has been undertaken at this time.

The potential role of invasive medical procedures in labor and birth as a cause of colic has been highlighted by Thomas (1981) who studied 130 consecutively born babies. He found that prolonged labor, forceps delivery, and epidural anesthesia as well as primiparity were related to colic.

In a well publicized study, Jacobsson and Lindberg (1978) reported that colic remitted when mothers of breast-fed colicky babies eliminated milk from their diet. The study was poorly described and was not blinded. To correct these difficulties, Evans et al. (1981) did a double-blind placebo-controlled crossover study involving 20 breast-feeding mothers and their colicky babies. Mothers were placed on a milk-free diet and then challenged with cow's milk or soy milk that was flavored to taste the same. Mother's milk was assessed for milk antigens. No relationship between milk ingestion, milk antigens and colicky behavior was found. However, the diversity of the mother's diet was related to colicky behavior, with more varied diets resulting in more colic. In a related study, Liebman (1981) prospectively evaluated intolerance to lactose and cow's milk protein in 56 infants with apparent colic. He found no evidence of intolerance in the colicky babies. On the other hand, Lothe et al. (1982) claimed that cow's milk was a major cause of colic. 60 colicky babies were blindly sequentially assigned to cow's milk-containing formula and a soy-based formula. Recovery occurred in 29% of infants on cow's milk formula. Soy formula resulted in 18% of infants being colic free. 53% of the sample had not improved on either formula but all of these did respond within 48 h to an open trial of a hydrolyzed casein-based formula. Blind trials of hydrolyzed casein have not been reported. The report is somewhat confused; the definition of colic was not explicit; and others have not yet replicated the work of this group.

At this time, the cause of colic has not been determined. Gastrointestinal, neurological, psychological and interactionist theories exist, but none have been firmly established. Colic may well be multidetermined or caused by different factors in different babies.

3. Prevalence of colic

Colic has been estimated to occur in 13% of babies (Carey, 1968); 23% of babies (Paradise, 1966); 35% of babies (Thomas, 1981) or 49% of babies (Cobb, 1956). The prevalence of colic in low birth weight babies has been estimated at 11.4% (Meyer and Thaler, 1971). Interestingly the colic in these babies begins within 2 weeks of the expected birth date regardless of gestational age at birth. There are major difficulties in comparing estimates of the occurrence of colic. The definition of colic is not uniformly agreed upon. In most studies, the estimates are retrospective. Finally, the methods of measuring components such as length of crying and consolability of the baby are not standardized.

4. Treatment of colic

The parent and the physician confronted with what appears to be colic must exclude both normal crying and crying that is secondary to another problem. The best way of determining if the baby is crying more than normal is to have the parent keep a diary of the length of time and the circumstances in which the crying occurred. Global retrospective reports such as: 'How much did your baby cry last week?', are likely to be unreliable.

Ruling out pathological causes of excessive crying is best done by history and physical examination. A healthy infant, who is gaining at least 150 g/week, in whom all obvious causes of excessive crying have been eliminated and who meets the criteria mentioned earlier in our discussion, can be said to have colic.

No one can understand better the need for effective treatment of colic than a bleary-eyed parent suffering from severe sleep deprivation having repeatedly tried to comfort a crying baby. The stress experienced by the parent who has a child with colic cannot be underestimated. Time provides a sure cure for colic since almost all colic will spontaneously remit by the age of 9 months.

Several behavioral strategies have been suggested to be effective in short-circuiting colic. Two types of research have been developed. The first, which has predominated, is research on soothing strategies. This research examines short-term interventions on crying in normal infants. The research is usually carefully controlled with stimuli delivered in a laboratory. This type of research is helpful in determining the effects of specific soothing strategies but adds little to the therapeutic armamentarium in the war against colic.

The second type of research is on the clinically meaningful issue of long-term reduction of crying. The subjects are sometimes normal babies and sometimes colicky babies. The interventions generally occur in the infants' homes and are usually less well controlled than in the soothing studies.

We will discuss the research on the different types of short- and long-term interventions in turn.

4.1. Rocking

Rocking is the most widely studied strategy to reduce crying and has been used since the dawn of time. Experimental studies have usually been short term and have shown that rocking soothes babies immediately following the rocking. For example, Van den Daele (1970) examined the effects of having an infant in a rockerbox that oscillated with a standard horizontal displacement of 3 in, 30 times or 60 times/min. The rockerbox treatment had a marked effect on activity and distress. Ter Vrugt and Pederson (1973) showed that increasing the frequency of rocking decreased crying. Pederson (1975) demonstrated that the direction of rocking was not important.

Khazaie (1981) calculated acceleration in order to compare rocking studies and found that a g of between 0.5 and 1.5 lowers the arousal level of infants who are not crying or fussing at the time rocking is beginning and that a g of over 1.5 quiets even a crying baby.

No studies have examined the long term effectiveness of rocking in calming babies or the effects of rocking on colicky babies.

4.2. Swaddling

Swaddling is an ancient practice with a wide variety of meanings and forms. Lipton et al. (1965) in their excellent treatise, detail the history and varieties of swaddling. They also described two experimental studies that demonstrated that the effects of swaddling were due to motor restraint. Although there were large individual differences, swaddling increased sleeping, reduced motor responsivity and startle responses.

The authors cautioned that extreme swaddling combined with sensory deprivation may cause problems with development. Similarly, very tight swaddling may contribute to hip dislocation in predisposed infants. Ames (personal communication) has noted that swaddling initiated after the first few weeks of life often results in distress rather than calming.

No uncontrolled or controlled trials have been done in which swaddling was used as a treatment for colic.

4.3. Non-nutritive sucking

Non-nutritive sucking refers to having the baby suck without feeding. The use of a pacifier for a fussing baby has a very long history. As discussed in chapter 5, non-nutritive sucking has been shown effective in soothing babies undergoing heel prick (Field and Goldson, 1984) and in calming neonates who were being tube fed in a neonatal intensive care unit (Field et al., 1982).

Non-nutritive sucking may also result in more quiet alert rather than fussy periods for the baby. Anderson (1983) reported on a study of 20 fussy but healthy infants in the newborn nursery who were randomly assigned to either routine care or non-nutritive sucking. Infants given a soother each sucked an average of 60 min after each feeding. There followed a lengthy period of settling and a quiet alert state. Infants, who did not receive a soother slept less, were less alert and cried significantly more.

Levine and Bell (1950) described a clinical series in which 28 colicky babies were given a pacifier. Twenty-five of the babies were reported by their parents to have overcome their colic. At follow up, when the children were over 18 months of age, only two were thumb-sucking. Thus, the only study of non-nutritive sucking on colicky babies was uncontrolled and no clear diagnostic or measurement procedures were used.

4.4. Auditory stimulation

It is a curious observation that otherwise unconsolable colicky infants are frequently comforted by exposure to various sounds such as a vacuum cleaner or a washing machine (Paradise, 1966). Bench (1969) conducted two short-term studies investigating the effects of pure tones and noise bands of 1 min duration. He found that babies became more quiet in response to auditory stimuli and that the effectiveness of the sound was in inverse relation to frequency.

Salk (1962) has suggested that the fetus imprints in utero on the repetitive sound of the mother's heartbeat and that the infant is later calmed by this sound. However, it appears that any sound will calm babies more than no sound. Heartbeat similar to mother's is no more effective than heart-beat dissimilar to that of the infant's mother (Smith and Steinschneider, 1975).

Heartbeats and intra-uterine sounds and pure tones are all effective in the short term, but a limiting factor of the use of sound as a treatment of colic is that increasing volume may be required as the baby habituates to the sound.

No studies have examined the long term effect of auditory stimulation or the effects of sound on colicky babies.

4.5. Warmth

Warmth has been investigated in few studies. Birns et al. (1966) found that immersing the infant's foot in water at 42°C was as effective a calming stimulus as a 250 cps continuous tone, gentle rocking, or a sweetened pacifier. Clearly, putting a baby's foot in warm water is not a clinically useful strategy. However, swaddling and carrying may owe part of their effectiveness to increasing the infant's warmth.

4.6. Changing feeding, especially removing milk

As previously indicated, it is our opinion that changes in feeding have not been clearly shown to be effective in treating colic. However, changing feeding remains the most commonly used intervention. No clear suggestions can be given at this time to guide changes in feeding.

4.7. Problem solving

Taubman (1984), in a non-randomized trial, compared six colicky babies whose parents were advised to decrease excessive stimulation and leave babies who cry in their cribs. A second group of 20 parents were given instructions to try never to let the baby cry and to try and problem solve what was wrong. The problem solving group was found to resolve their crying more quickly than those who were left to cry. The mechanism of action is not known but it could be increased carrying which is discussed below.

A properly designed randomized trial has not yet been done to confirm or repudiate Taubman's findings.

4.8. Visual distraction

Visual distraction may be a component of problem solving or carrying treatment for colic but visual distraction has not been investigated independently.

4.9. Carrying

In industrialized societies, infants are carried much less frequently than in non-industrialized societies. There is some evidence that colic is less of a problem in non-industrialized cultures. Based on these findings, Hunziker and Barr (1986) examined the role of supplemental carrying in reducing crying in 99 breast-fed, first born healthy infants. The randomized controlled trial demonstrated that babies in the carrying group were carried an average

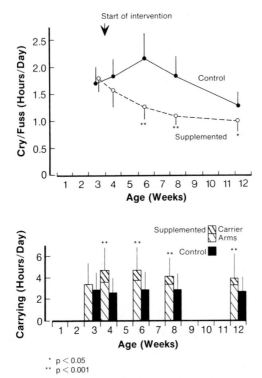

Fig. 1. Effects of supplemental carrying on crying. Daily duration of infant crying/fussing in response to change in parental carrying. Top: Means and SD of crying/fussing behavior in h/day averaged over each week of parental recording for supplemented (○–○) and control (●–●) infants, respectively. Intervention for both groups started at beginning of week 4 after 1 week of baseline recording (week 3). Bottom: Means and SD of carrying in h/day averaged over each week of parental recording for supplemented and control groups. Carrying during intervention in supplemented group is represented by method of holding in parent's arms or in infant carrier. (Reprinted from Hunziker and Barr, 1986, with permission of the authors and the publisher.)

of 1.8 h more than the control group and cried less than the children who were not carried (Fig. 1). Fig. 1 shows that the pattern of the amount of crying among the control group is the same as has been reported by Brazelton (1962) for infants; the experimental group cried significantly less at 6 weeks and at 8 weeks. The experimental group also showed an increase in quiet alert time.

The mechanism of action might be that carrying promotes a number of soothing behaviors such as rhythmic repetitive movement, auditory stimulation, visual distraction, warmth and postural changes. In addition, supplemental carrying may have increased the sensitivity and immediacy of the mothers' response to their infants. The authors speculated that early infant crying is an adaptive response that tends to promote mother-infant proximity and to provide opportunities for mother-infant social interaction. Increased carrying reduces crying and promotes social interaction both because of increased proximity but also because of the increase in quiet alert time. No studies with colicky babies have been done.

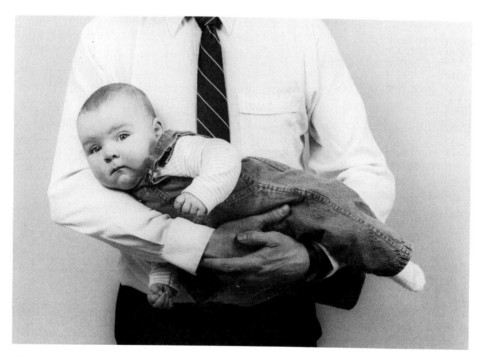

Fig. 2. The colic hold.

LaLeche League International (1981) suggested the use of a 'colic hold' which involves holding the baby astraddle one's arm (Fig. 2).

Studies of this method of holding with colicky babies remain to be done.

4.10. Drug treatment

Dicyclomine hydrochloride (Merbentyl syrup, Merrell Dow Pharmaceuticals) has been demonstrated to be effective in three randomized controlled trials. Dicyclomine is a synthetic tertiary amine, antimuscarinic agent with moderate antispasmodic activity and the major action is thought to be a non-specific direct relaxant activity on smooth muscle. In recommended dosages, it will relieve spasm of the gastrointestinal tract, biliary tract, ureter and uterus without typical atropine-like side effects (Dupuis, 1985). The trial of Illingworth (1959) compared the efficacy of 5 mg dicyclomine given before the early evening feeding with placebo. Sixty percent of the dicyclomine group versus 25% of the placebo group were judged greatly improved. Grunseit (1977), using doses of 5 mg dicyclomine or placebo administered before four feedings (including the early evening feed), found superiority for dicyclomine. Both of these studies used subjective evaluation of success and did not rigorously define entry criteria for their patients. Recently, Weissbluth et al. (1984), using specified entry criteria and objective outcome measurement, demonstrated the superiority of dicyclomine over placebo. Parents titrated the dose of dicyclomine according to specific directions over the first 4 days of the study from 3.75 mg/day up to a maximum of 10 mg/day. Weissbluth et al. (1984) found that colic was eliminated in 65% of the babies receiving dicyclomine and 25% of the placebo babies.

Concern has been expressed about a possible relationship between dicyclomine and sudden infant death syndrome. These concerns have been based on approximately 16 anecdotally reported cases of the occurrence of apnea or respiratory difficulties with dicyclomine. As Dupuis (1985) has emphasized:

> At the present time there are insufficient data to conclude that dicyclomine causes apnea or to propose a mechanism for the reaction. It is also difficult to determine the incidence of the reaction *(Dupuis, 1985, p. 3)*.

However, as a result of the reports of apnea, the manufacturer has removed its indication for infant colic and has contraindicated its use for children under 6 months of age.

Gripe water, alcohol and phenobarbital-atropine combinations are not recommended and have no evidence for effectiveness. There are no other medications of demonstrated effectiveness in infantile colic (O'Donovan and Brenstock, 1979).

Although dicyclomine has been withdrawn for colic, it remains the only validated treatment for this condition.

4.11. Reassurance

A major effort must be made to insure that parents realize that colic is a benign self-limiting disorder of unknown physical origin. Parents need reassurance that they are not the cause of colic. Mobilization of family and friends as resources to help parents through this difficult time will be beneficial. It is our opinion that maternal anxiety and overstimulation do not cause colic but might be the result of colic and may exacerbate the condition.

Although colic is a benign disorder, the impact of colic on the family should not be minimized. Weissbluth's (1984) book 'Crybabies: Coping with Colic' or Kirkland's (1985) book 'Crying and Babies: Helping Families Cope' are excellent resources to recommend to parents.

5. Long-term sequelae of colic

5.1. Recurrent abdominal pain

In a follow-up of 30 infants followed yearly for 13 years, no relationship between colic and recurrent abdominal pain of childhood was found (Joseph and Lupu, 1984).

5.2. Child abuse

Frodi (1985) has summarized much of the literature on the relationship between crying and child abuse. She noted that a majority of abusive mothers reported that 'incessant crying', 'the grating sound of the cry', and 'whining for a prolonged period of time' were precipitants to the abuse. Similarly, Weston (1968) found that excessive crying was given as a reason for battering by 80% of parents who battered infants less than 1 year old. Both the aversive sound of the cry and the helplessness that parents may feel when faced by the colicky baby have been suggested as the mechanism linking colic and abuse.

5.3. Sleep problems

As previously described, Weissbluth (1984) has argued that colic may well be a type of sleep disorder. He has noted that even after successful drug treatment, babies with colic have shorter sleep durations than usual (Weissbluth et al., 1984). Moreover, the constant attempts by parents to use soothing strategies with colicky babies may teach them to fuss and expect entertainment when they awake at night. Learned postcolic sleep problems have been reported by Weissbluth (1984). No long-term studies have been done to confirm that sleep problems continue with colicky babies.

5.4. Parent-child interactions

An inconsolable crying baby could interfere with the later relationship between the baby and the parent. Shaw (1977) compared ten previously colicky babies and their mothers with ten more contented controls and their mothers in a play situation. She found that the previously colicky babies, at the age of 9–14 months, were less likely to be responded to by their mothers. In effect, the mothers had learned to ignore their fussy babies and this ignoring continued even after the fussiness had abated. Children who have had colic may also have learned that parents are not beneficent but rather frustrated and irritable. It is possible that the interaction observed by Shaw (1977) might be the result of both the parent and the child learning from the aversive experience of colic. In addition, if colicky babies are temperamentally more difficult and parents more anxious, the long-term relationship between the child and the parent may be affected. It is unlikely that these different strands can be readily untangled.

5.5. Parental stress

Parental stress with resulting psychological sequelae including loss of self-esteem (especially about competence as a parent), anxiety and depression may result from colic. Mothers, who are most frequently the primary caregiver, may be most vulnerable to colic-induced parental stress. The role of colic in marital distress may also be important. No research has yet examined these issues.

6. Clinical guidelines

(1) Listen. Provide a sympathetic ear. Colic although benign can be a serious strain. Reassurance is necessary but facile reassurance not to worry is not likely to be helpful.

(2) Assist mother to mobilize resources. External resources may include the family, friends, self-help or social service agencies. Internal resources may include helping the mother to view the colic as a difficult but not impossible challenge. Encouraging the mother to talk to herself in more helpful ways such as: 'The baby is OK', 'All I can do is my best', 'It is tough but I can cope', may be helpful.

(3) Have parents keep a log of crying and fussing to get a clear idea of how much the child is crying. This will show the effectiveness of any strategies and will also put the amount of crying into perspective.

(4) Problem solve and try systematic use of carrying, rocking and soother. Avoid frequent changes in feeding and unproven medications.

(5) Encourage the father to provide relief and support.

7. Future directions

(1) Proper evaluation by means of randomized controlled trials of behavioral interventions such as carrying, rocking and problem solving need to be done with colicky babies. Careful epidemiologic review of the evidence linking dicyclomine to apnea may show no real relationship, thereby allowing an efficacious medicine to be used.

(2) Self-help support groups such as CrySOS (Kirkland, 1985) and LaLeche League (for breast-fed babies) need to be more available to families with colicky babies.

(3) Much more research is needed on the causes of colic. Specific promising areas include: direct examination of Illingworth's hypothesis of gas in the loops of the bowel; delineation of subgroups of colicky babies; examination of Carey's interaction hypothesis.

(4) More research on the long-term sequelae of colic is needed. If negative long-term sequelae are found, strategies designed to mitigate these effects should be developed and evaluated.

References

Ames, E.W. and Bradley, C.F. (1983) Infant and parent characteristics related to parental reports of colic in one-month-old and three-month-old infants. Paper presented at the Canadian Psychological Association Meeting, Winnipeg.

Anderson, G.C. (1983) Infant colic: A possible solution. Matern. Child Nurs. 8, 185.

Barr, R.G., Kramer, M.S., Pless, I.B., Boisjoly, C. and Leduc, D.G. (1983) Feeding and temperament predispose to cry/fuss behavior at six weeks. Am. J. Dis. Child. 137, 541.

Bench, J. (1969) Some effects of audio-frequency stimulation on the crying baby. J. Audit. Res. 9, 122–128.

Birns, B., Blank, M. and Bridger, W.H. (1966) The effectiveness of various soothing techniques on human neonates. Psychosom. Med. 28, 316–322.

Brazelton, T.B. (1962) Crying in infancy. Pediatrics 29, 579–588.

Carey, W.B. (1968) Maternal anxiety and infantile colic: Is there a relationship? Clin. Pediatr. 7, 590–595.

Carey, W.B. (1972) Clinical applications of infant temperament measurements. J. Pediatr. 81, 823–828.

Carey, W.B. (1983) 'Colic' or excessive crying in young infants. In: M.D. Levine, W.B. Carey, A.C. Crocker and R.T. Gross (Eds.), Developmental-Behavioral Pediatrics (Saunders Philadelphia, PA), pp. 518–521.

Carey, W.B. (1984) 'Colic' – Primary excessive crying as an infant-environment interaction. Pediatr. Clin. North Am. 31, 993–1005.

Cobb, J.C. (1956) Family tension as a cause of colic in infants. Pediatrics 18, 835–836.

Dupuis, L. (1985) Dicyclomine: A recent orphan. Drug Inf. Bull. (The Hospital for Sick Children, Toronto) 2, 1–3.

Evans, R.W., Fergusson, D.M., Allardyce, R.A. and Taylor, B. (1981) Maternal diet and infantile colic in breast-fed infants. Lancet i, 1340–1342.

Field, T. and Goldson, E. (1984) Pacifying effects of nonnutritive sucking on term and preterm neonates during heelstick procedures. Pediatrics 74, 1012–1015.

Field, T., Ignatoff, E., Stringer, S., Brennan, J., Greenberg, R., Windmayer, S. and Anderson, G.C. (1982) Nonnutritive sucking during tube feedings: Effects on preterm neonates in an intensive care unit. Pediatrics 70, 381–384.

Frodi, A. (1985) When empathy fails: Aversive infant crying and child abuse. In: B. Lester and C.F.Z. Boukydis (Eds.), Infant Crying: Theoretical and Research Perspectives (Plenum, New York) pp. 263–277.

Grunau, R. and Craig, K.D. (1987) Pain expression in neonates: Facial action and cry. Pain 28, 395–410.

Grunseit, F. (1977) Evaluation of the efficacy of dicyclomine hydrochloride (Merbentyl) syrup in the treatment of infantile colic. Curr. Med. Res. Opin. 5, 258–261.

Hunziker, U.A. and Barr, R.G. (1986) Increased carrying reduces infant crying: A randomized controlled trial. Pediatrics 77, 641–648.

Illingworth, R.S. (1954) Three months colic. Arch. Dis. Child. 29, 165–174.

Illingworth, R.S. (1959) Evening colic in infants. A double blind trial of dicyclomine hydrochloride. Lancet ii, 1119.

Jacobsson, I. and Lindberg, T. (1978) Cow's milk as a cause of infantile colic in breast-fed infants. Lancet ii, 437–439.

Johnston, C.C. and Strada, M.E. (1986) Acute pain response in infants: A multidimensional description. Pain 24, 373–382.

Joseph, A.Y. and Lupa, G.H. (1984) Recurrent abdominal pain and infantile colic. Am. J. Dis. Child. 138, 990–991.

Khazaie, S.M.G. (1981) The effect of rocking on infant state and visual behaviour. Unpublished thesis, Simon Fraser University, Vancouver, Canada.

Kirkland, J. (1986) Crying and Babies (Croom Helm, Beckenham, Kent, England).

LaLeche League International (1981) The Womanly Art of Breastfeeding (LaLeche League International, Franklin Park, IL).

Levine, M.I. and Bell, A.I. (1950) The treatment of 'Colic' in infancy by use of the pacifier. J. Pediatr. 37, 750–755.

Liebman, W.M. (1981) Infantile colic: Association with lactose and milk intolerance. J. Am. Med. Assoc. 245, 732–733.

Lipton, E.L., Steinschneider, A. and Richmond, J.B. (1965) Swaddling, a child care practice: Historical, cultural and experimental observations. Pediatrics 35, 521–567.

Lothe, L., Lindberg, T. and Jacobsson, I. (1982) Cow's milk formula as a cause of infantile colic: A double blind study. Pediatrics 70, 7–10.

Meyer, J.E. and Thaler, M.M. (1971) Colic in low birth weight infants. Am. J. Dis. Child. 122, 25–27.

O'Donovan, J.D. and Brenstock, A.S. (1979) The failure of conventional drug therapy in the management of infantile colic. Am. J. Dis. Child. 133, 999–1001.

Oxford University Press (1973) The Shorter Oxford English Dictionary on Historical Principles (Oxford University Press, Oxford) p. 366.

Paradise, J.L. (1966) Maternal and other factors in the etiology of infantile colic: Report of a prospective study of 146 infants. J. Am. Med. Assoc. 197, 123–199.

Pederson, D.R. (1975) The soothing effect of rocking as determined by the direction and frequency of movement. C. J. Behav. Sci. 7, 237–243.

Salk, L. (1962) Mother's heartbeat as an imprinting stimulus. Trans. N.Y. Acad. Sci. 24, 753.

Shaw, C. (1977) A comparison of the patterns of mother-baby interaction for a group of crying, irritable babies and a group of more amenable babies. Child Care, Health Dev. 3, 1–12.

Smith, C.R. and Steinschneider, A. (1975) Differential effects of prenatal rhythmic stimulation on neonatal arousal states. Child Dev. 46, 574–578.

Taubman, B. (1984) Clinical trial of the treatment of colic by modification of parent-infant interaction. Pediatrics 74, 998–1003.

Ter Vrugt, D. and Pederson, D.R. (1973) The effects of vertical rocking frequencies in the arousal level in two-month-old infants. Child Dev. 44, 205–209.

Thomas, D.B. (1981) Aetiological associations in infantile colic: an hypothesis. Aust. Paediatr. J. 17, 292–295.

Van den Daele, L. (1970) Modification of infant state by treatment in a rockerbox. J. Psychol. 74, 161–165.

Weissbluth, M. (1984) Crybabies: Coping with Colic (Arbor House, New York).

Weissbluth, M., Christoffel, K.K. and Davis, A.T. (1984) Treatment of infantile colic with dicyclomine hydrochloride. J. Pediatr. 104, 951–955.

Wessel, M.A., Cobb, J.C., Jackson, E.B., Harris, G.S. and Detwiler, A.C. (1954) Paroxysmal fussing in infancy, sometimes called colic. Pediatrics 14, 421–434.

Weston, J. (1968) The pathology of child abuse. In: R. Helfer and C. Kempe (Eds.) The Battered Child (University of Chicago Press, Chicago, IL) pp. 77–100.

CHAPTER 8

Headache

For headache take the root of peony mixed with oil of roses. When thoroughly mixed soak a piece of linen in it and apply constantly to the place where the pain is. Without doubt it will help *(11th century A.D., prescription quoted in MacKinney, 1937, p. 35)*.

1. Introduction

Headache is the commonest indisposition of mankind *(Barlow, 1984, p. 1)*.

It is a rare individual, child or adult who has not suffered from headache at one time or another. Seven types of headache will be discussed in this chapter: headache due to a transient illness; headache secondary to head trauma; pathological headache; migraine and its variants; muscle contraction headache; sinus headache; and psychogenic headache.

2. Headache due to a transient illness

Headache is a common symptom accompanying flu or a cold and in these circumstances, it is usually transient and benign. The exception is headache accompanying acute brain infection including meningitis and encephalitis.

Treatment for headache due to flu or a cold is symptomatic and usually effective. Acetaminophen or ASA are the drugs of choice because they are both antipyretic and analgesic. ASA should be avoided in children with flu because of the association with Reye syndrome (see chapter 4 for a discussion of Reye syndrome). Distinguishing innocent infections from serious, life-threatening infections depends on the age of the child and is detailed in pediatric texts (e.g., Feldman et al., 1987). Treatment of headache due to serious infection such as meningitis is focussed on treatment of the underlying infection.

3. Pathological headache

Pathological headache refers to headache due to organic pathology. Table 1 outlines some of the very wide range of organic pathology that can cause headache.

The principal task facing the clinician dealing with childhood headache is to distinguish children who have headache as a symptom of underlying systemic, head, face, neck or central nervous system pathology and those who have benign headache. The most important tools for making this distinction are a careful history and a thorough physical examination. Table 2 outlines aspects of the history that are important in giving clues to the differentiation of types of headaches. Table 3 lists those items which should be done routinely in the physical examination for headache. Routine laboratory tests should not be done. However, specific symptoms should trigger further laboratory investigations.

TABLE 1
Pathological causes of headache.

Infectious (viral or bacterial), chemical or allergic meningitis
Subarachnoid hemorrhage
Arteritis
Cellulitis
Increased intracranial pressure
Hypoxia
Carbon monoxide poisoning
Primary or metastatic tumors of meninges, vessels or brain
Intracranial mass lesion
Epidural, subdural or parenchymal hematoma
Increased intraocular pressure, excessive contraction of ocular muscles
Trauma, new growth or inflammation of ocular structures
Trauma, new growth or inflammation of nasal or sinus structures
Trauma, new growth or inflammation of dental structures
Aneurysm
Intracranial hypertension
Arteriovenous malformation
Multiple sclerosis
Postictal state
Acute hypertension

TABLE 2
Narrowing down: recurrent headache.
(Reprinted from Feldman et al., 1987, with permission of the authors and Oxford University Press.)

History item	Suspect migraine	Suspect muscle contraction	Suspect pathological headache
Family history of migraine	×		
Completely normal physical examination	×	×	
Pain getting worse			×
Headaches last 2–3 h	×		
0.5 h prodrome	×		
Nausea or vomiting	×		×
History of motion sickness, breath holding spells or syncope	×		
Constant pain		×	×
Band-like pressure		×	
Related to 'stress'		×	
Intellectual decline			×
Personality change			×
Pain in face			×
Waking at night with pain			×
Motor or perceptual difficulties during pain-free intervals			×
Changes in fundi			×
Localizing CNS findings			×

4. Headache secondary to head trauma

The sequelae of head trauma in children may include behavioral and cognitive changes (Rutter et al., 1983). It is often not recognized that post-traumatic headache may also result. For example, in their excellent review of head injury Rutter et al. (1983) do not even mention headache. Two forms of post-traumatic headache have been described. Immediate post-traumatic headache and late post-traumatic headache.

TABLE 3
Physical examination for headache.

Height
Weight
Head circumference
Blood pressure
Complete neurological exam
Percussion of sinuses
Listening for bruits
Examination of skin for neurocutaneous stigmata
Examination of fundi

Immediately following any head trauma, headache can occur. Such headaches may occur after even a minor blow and be migrainous with severe vascular headache and vomiting. Given the life style of some children, bumps on the head may be quite common and in some children may be the trigger of frequent headache (Barlow, 1984). More typical is the very frequent generalized headache accompanied by lethargy and irritability that occur for a few days to a week following a concussion in children.

Much more dramatic is the phenomenon reviewed by Haas et al. (1975). They described hemiparesis, hemianopsia, somnolence, irritability, vomiting, cortical blindness, brainstem signs and confusional state following minor head trauma, usually without loss of consciousness. Their 25 patients reported 50 incidents. Repeated incidents in the same patient were not necessarily the same. Barlow (1984) suggested that head trauma triggered transient vasospasm causing the symptoms or alternatively, that the stress and anxiety of the trauma call forth humoral and vasoactive substances that cause the symptomatology.

Also of interest is late post-traumatic headache. Lanzi et al. (1985a) evaluated the incidence and clinical characteristics of headache which arise 12–18 months after head injury. Of the 138 patients in their study, 29% had headaches. They concluded that an increased headache frequency was associated with average to severe trauma but that children with minor head trauma did not have increased rate of headaches. Patients, who did not have a loss of consciousness and/or focal neurological signs, were not at greater risk to have headaches. The nature of the late post-traumatic headache varies and the mechanism is unclear. Some post-traumatic headaches appear to be migrainous and some appear to be more akin to muscle contraction headaches. However, as discussed in the following section on migraine headache, the distinction between migraine and muscle contraction head-aches is frequently not clear. According to the traditional models of migraine and muscle contraction headache, migraine may be triggered by vascular changes in response to trauma. On the other hand, trauma to the head and neck may lead to changes in muscle tension and resultant muscle contraction headache. Rarely, headache may be due to local scalp or nuchal injury (Ad Hoc Committee, 1962).

5. Migraine and its variants

> Like there's this big monster in there, see, and he's growing like crazy and there's no room and he's pulling the two sides of my head apart he's getting so big *(boy, age 7, quoted in Ross and Ross, 1984, p. 189)*.

5.1. Are migraine and muscle contraction headache the same?

The Ad Hoc Committee on Classification of Headache's (1962) nosology has dominated both clinical understanding and research of migraine in North America. This classification specified that migraine headaches are paroxysmal and usually described as throbbing. Migraines are typically unilateral and they may be associated with systemic symptoms such as anorexia, nausea, vomiting, and sensory and motor disturbances. Migraine is contrasted with tension or muscle contraction headache which is not paroxysmal and is marked by band-like tension and pressure with a lower level of pain than is typical of migraine. The International Association for the Study of Pain, Subcommittee on Taxonomy (Merskey, 1986) has followed this convention in their recently published Classification of Chronic Pain. Pediatric and adult patients with clinically significant headache frequently do not comfortably fit into the categories defined by the Ad Hoc Committee (1962). In particular, the distinction between common migraine and muscle contraction or tension headache in the clinic is frequently unclear. As well, many patients have a mixture of both types of headaches. In spite of the fact that official classifications clearly separate the two disorders, a large number of clinicians and researchers (e.g., Raskin and Appenzeller, 1980; Bakal, 1982; Saper, 1986) are questioning whether migraine (especially common migraine) and muscle contraction headache are separate disorders. Evidence for the unitary nature of migraine and muscle contraction headache comes from several sources: clinical observation; vascular studies; muscle tension studies;

psychopathology studies; and treatment studies. Only one study has examined this issue in pediatric migraine. Joffe et al. (1983) examined the headache diaries of 47 children who had problem headaches. They found that children did not experience distinct patterns of muscle contraction or migraine but that most experienced both. As the number of headache hours increased so did the extensiveness of the symptoms. The authors interpreted these findings as supporting a unitary model of headache.

In spite of serious reservations about the distinction between migraine and muscle contraction headache, we will maintain the distinction because the research is organized in this way and, at this time, alternative classification systems are not well developed.

5.2. Types of migraine

There are a number of different types of migraine including: classic migraine; common migraine; complicated migraine; and cluster headache.

5.2.1. Classic migraine

> First I get this sticky feeling in my stomach and I see all these spots and then it starts, always on the left side, and it pounds and pounds and my eye on that side is burning red hot *(girl, aged 10, quoted in Ross and Ross, 1984, p. 185)*.

Classic migraines are preceded by an aura which is usually visual, typically a scintillating scotoma or fortification spectrum, but may be sensory in the form of a paresthesia or an olfactory aura. In rare cases, the aura may be in the form of a motor ataxia. The headache itself is characterized by unilateral pounding pain in a sharply defined location. Occasionally, the migraine aura may occur in the absence of a headache. Fig. 1 is a drawing by a child with classic migraine detailing the visual disturbance, a scotoma.

5.2.2. Common migraine

Common migraines which are the most frequent type of migraine in children, do not have prodromal auras and are more typically frontal and bilateral. Fig. 2 is a drawing by a child of the more frequent common migraine.

5.2.3. Complicated migraine

Complicated migraine includes: basilar artery migraine; confusional migraine; hemiplegic migraine; ophthalmoplegic migraine; and the 'Alice in

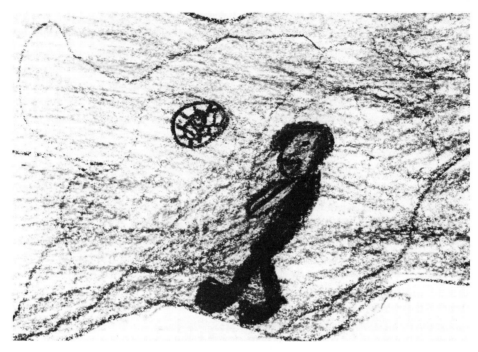

Fig. 1. Drawing of the headache by a child with classic migraine.

Wonderland' syndrome. They are characterized by sensory and motor defects that persist during and after the headache which may not be a prominent feature of the migraine attack.

5.2.3.1. Basilar artery migraine Basilar artery migraine was described by Bickerstaff (1961) and has a wide variety of expressions that is often constant within the same patient across attacks. The common presentation is the development of signs and symptoms of multiple cranial nerve malfunctioning including dimming of vision, hemianopsia, diplopia or even almost complete blindness; vertigo; alternating hemiparesis; muscle weakness; ataxia; and loss of consciousness and syncope. Typically the signs and symptoms are short-lived much like the prodrome of classic migraine. However, on occasion, the basilar-vertebral symptoms may persist for hours or days. The disorder is thought to be caused by transient ischemia or edema in the brainstem. The prevalence of basilar artery migraine has been estimated as occurring in about 2.3% (Barlow, 1984) to 3.7% (Jay and Tomasi, 1981) of children with migraine.

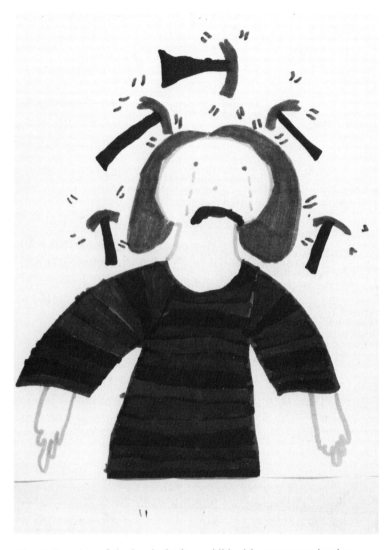

Fig. 2. Drawing of the headache by a child with common migraine.

5.2.3.2. Confusional migraine   Migraine presenting as an acute confusional state is not typical but by no means is it unusual. Gascon and Barlow (1970) described four cases of children admitted to hospital in acute confusion. The mental disturbance lasted from 4 to 24 h and following the attack each child had normal mental state and normal neurological exam. The mechanism is thought to be cerebral edema of deep midline subcortical structures (Gascon and Barlow, 1970; Barlow, 1984).

5.2.3.3. Hemiplegic migraine Hemiplegic migraine results in a transient hemiplegia that may last from a few hours to several days. The hemiparesis may be accompanied by aphasia, paresthesia of one half of the body or even motor tics on the affected side. The symptoms suggest involvement of the internal carotid area (Barlow, 1984).

5.2.3.4. Ophthalmoplegic migraine Ophthalmoplegic migraine is a rare disorder characterized by a third nerve palsy that develops during or after a headache. The symptoms are ptosis, dilation of the pupil on the affected side, paresis of the extraocular muscles, vomiting and pain. Van Pelt and Andermann (1964) and Robertson and Schnitzler (1978) both reported on ophthalmoplegic migraine beginning in the first year of life. The pathogenesis is not known but thought to be pressure from a swollen carotid artery on nearby cranial nerves. Long-term sequelae are not unusual following re-peated attacks. Propranolol has been recommended as a prophylactic treatment and prednisone has been used to treat specific attacks. Recently, a debate has been underway about the differential diagnosis of ophthalmo-plegic migraine vis-à-vis Tolosa-Hunt syndrome (inflammation of the caver-nous sinus characterized by: often steady, gnawing or boring pain behind the eye; involvement of nerves passing through the cavernous sinus; symptoms for days or weeks; spontaneous remissions sometimes with residual deficits; attacks at intervals of months or years; and exhaustive studies excluding involvement outside the cavernous sinus) (Kandt, 1986; Reeves, 1986).

5.2.3.5. 'Alice in Wonderland' syndrome 'Alice in Wonderland' syndrome is a rare phenomenon characterized by complex impairments of the sense of time, and of consciousness, body image and visual analysis of the environment, much like those described by Lewis Carroll in Alice in Wonderland (Golden, 1979). These symptoms often provoke anxiety in these children. The pathophy-siology is unclear but it is thought to be similar to basilar artery migraine.

5.2.4. Cluster headache
Cluster headache (also known as Horton's cephalalgia) are extremely painful, brief, unilateral (always the same side) headaches that occur in periodic clusters. The face usually becomes flushed on the same side, and there may be unilateral nasal congestion and tearing. Ipsilateral ptosis and miosis some-

times develop. Cluster headaches are usually associated with middle-aged men and seldom described in the pediatric age group. However, Curless (1982) has described adolescent cases.

5.3. Prevalence of migraine

Headache is the most common reason for consultation with a pediatric neurologist (Sillanpaa, 1976). The prevalence of migraine headache has been established in a number of epidemiologic surveys. The most widely cited study is that of Bille (1962) who surveyed 9059 children aged 7–15 years. Questionnaires were sent to the parents of all children who were attending regular schools in Uppsala, Sweden, in 1955 and 99.3% of the questionnaires were returned properly completed. The prevalence of migraine at the age of 7 years was 1.4% increasing progressively to 5.3% at 15 years of age. Gender was not related to the prevalence of migraine below age 10. In the 10–12-year-olds, girls (5.4%) were more likely to have migraine than boys (3.9%). This preponderance of girls increased with age so that in the 13–15-year-old group, 6.4% of the girls and 4% of the boys were afflicted. Other estimates of prevalence of migraine have been higher. Sillanpaa (1976) reported on a survey of 4235, 7-year-old children who were beginning school in two Finnish cities (Tampere and Turku) in 1974. Using the same criteria as Bille (1962), Sillanpaa diagnosed 3.2% of the children as having migraine. In a follow-up 7 years later, Sillanpaa (1983a) contacted 2921 of the original participants and found that the prevalence of headache increased markedly to 6.4% for boys and 14.8% for girls.

In a related study, Sillanpaa (1983b) examined a sample of 3784, 13-year-old schoolchildren in the same two cities. The survey revealed that 8.1% of boys and 15.1% of girls had migraine (either classic or common). The prevalence of classic migraine was 1.9% for boys and 6.5% for girls. The comparable rates for common migraine were 6.2% and 8.0%. In a study of Neapolitan children, the prevalence of migraine in 11- and 12-year-olds was found to be about 8% (Sorge and Dipietro, 1981). Oster (1972) reported an overall incidence of 5.5% with girls and boys showing similar incidence until age 11 when girls showed predominance. Oster's criteria were not specified.

5.4. Onset of migraine

Cross-sectional studies such as those of Bille (1962) indicate that for many children, especially girls, migraine begins in the early teenage years. Longitudinal studies such as Sillanpaa (1983a) have confirmed these findings. For some children, however, migraine begins much earlier. In an early series, Vahlquist and Hackzell (1949) described 31 cases in which migraine first appeared between 1 and 4 years of age. They noted that the symptom picture is similar to older children except that diagnosis is more difficult because of the difficulty in communicating symptoms. They also noted that the attacks are generally shorter, the prodrome less marked and the nausea more intense than in adults. The authors suggested that the prognosis for early onset migraine is not unfavorable.

Using a very different approach, Guidetti et al. (1983a) followed up 102 full-term newborn healthy infants, who were 'hyperreactive' in infancy, and 80 similar infants, who were not hyperreactive, for over 8 years. Hyperreactivity was measured during neurological examination by: reaction to light, sound, manipulation, heat or nociception; feeding behavior; behavior during the day; night sleep and skin reactivity. Of the 102 children who were 'hyperreactive', 78 (76%) developed headache or periodic syndrome. Of the 80 control children, only 15 (19%) developed headache or periodic syndrome. The average age of onset of headache was 7 years. These data suggested that early detection of some children at high risk for migraine is possible. The measures used in the study are not clearly described and the results have not been replicated.

5.5. Child versus adult migraine

As previously mentioned, the presentation of children's migraine is frequently different from adult migraine. Nausea, vomiting and abdominal pain are often a prominent component of migraine in children especially in younger children. In some children, headache plays a relatively minor role in the syndrome. As well, although classic migraine is less frequent in adults than is common migraine, this predominance of common migraine is more marked in children.

The predominance of females suffering from migraine is not evident prior to puberty. In the younger years, the prevalence of migraine in males is equivalent to the prevalence in females.

Finally, the use of medication for migraine is markedly less in children than adults. Because of the low level of drug usage in pediatric migraine, researchers have been unable to use amount of medication as an outcome measure in treatment studies. In our own lab, we have found it impossible to complete a trial of prophylactic medication because of the reluctance of parents and children to take daily medication even though the children were suffering frequent severe headache.

5.6. *Pathogenesis of migraine headache*

Virtually no research on the pathogenesis of migraine has used pediatric subjects and speculations about the cause of migraine are based on research with adults. The lack of studies of migraine headache mechanisms with children is understandable because of the relative lack of research of pediatric headache. Most adult migraineurs have been subjected to years of taking very powerful pharmaceuticals and years of repeated migraine, both of which may have caused changes in vascular immunological and biochemical reactivity. Research with pediatric migraineurs could avoid these potential difficulties. However, as we discuss in chapter 15, there are specific ethical problems in research with children, especially if the research does not have the possibility of helping the child directly.

There is no agreement as to the pathogenesis of migraine or even agreement about whether migraine is a unitary disorder or a set of disorders. We will only briefly cover this area.

Most clinicians and the official classification systems of both the Ad Hoc Committee (1962) and the International Association for the Study of Pain (Merskey, 1986) presume that migraine is a vascular disorder. However, neurogenic or central theories have been gaining strong support in recent years.

Most theoretical models have good evidence supporting them but all are unable to account for other data. Commenting on this phenomenon and on the growth of high tech in headache research, Edmeads (1986, pp. 434–435) editorialized:

> Clearly we are not discovering any new worlds. But we are exploring and re-exploring the terrain we know, and maybe learning just a little more about it each time. As long as we keep in mind that we are orbiting rather than advancing in a straight line, we can even derive a little comfort from knowing that in headache, as in all else, 'the more things change, the more they stay the same'.

5.6.1. *Neurogenic theories*
Neurogenic theories suggest that vascular changes in migraine are epipheno-mena or of secondary importance to the primary defect which involves some form of neurological dysfunction. Several different neurological theories have been suggested.

5.6.1.1. Spreading cortical depression   Olesen and his colleagues (Olesen et al., 1981, 1982; Olesen and Lauritzen, 1984) have measured regional cerebral blood flow with xenon 133 intra-arterial injection and monitoring of 254 areas of the hemisphere. They found that during classic migraine but not during common migraine, focal hyperemia was followed by spreading oligemia. Most of the patients studied have been adults, however Olesen et al. (1981) do report on a 14-year-old boy studied during a classic headache accompanied by paresthesia in the left hand ascending to the left side of the chin. There was also mild paresis of the left hand. There was a gradual spread of oligemia concomitant with accompaniments and headache. A preceding frontal hyperemia was also detected. This group has hypothesized that an alteration in neuronal function in the blood-brain barrier or other brain process triggers a reaction that is akin to the spreading cortical depression described originally by Leão. This neuronal event then triggers vascular reactions via vasoactive neurotransmitters.

This model does not attempt to explain common migraine.

5.6.1.2. Serotonin   Sicuteri et al. (1961) originated the major interest in serotonin when they found elevated levels of a metabolite of serotonin in the urine of migraineurs during the headache attacks. The exact role of serotonin is not known but serotonin is a potent vasoactive amine which tends to constrict large arteries and to dilate smaller arterioles and capillaries (Raskin and Appenzeller, 1980). The relationships among the roles of serotonin, platelets and the prostaglandins in the pathogenesis of migraine is not clear.

5.6.1.3. Focal cerebral hypoxia   Amery (1982) has marshalled an impressive array of evidence to argue that a migraine attack is a particular reaction pattern in susceptible individuals to a localized imbalance between energy supply and energy use in specific areas of the brain (focal hypoxia). The hypoxia theory suggests that common and classic migraine are basically the same phenomenon and that the visual aura is an epiphenomenon.

5.6.2. Vascular theories

For more than 200 years, migraine has been assumed to be a vascular phenomenon (Dalessio, 1984). In the modern era, the research of Wolff (Dalessio, 1984) has been seminal. According to Wolff's hypothesis, both classic and common migraine are due to painful vascular engorgement resulting from cephalic vasodilation. In classic migraine, it was hypothesized that prodromal symptoms were due to cerebral vasoconstriction. Vasoconstriction in different blood vessels cause different prodromes. Although Wolff's hypothesis is in disfavor in many quarters there are current supporters. In a recent study, Meyer et al. (1986) did serial xenon inhalation regional cephalic blood flow studies on 60 patients during both a headache and a headache-free period. Hyperemia (defined as regional blood flow more than two standard deviations above normal values) occurred in 53% of the classic migraines and 58% of the common migraines. If less stringent criteria are used the hyperemia rates rise to 67% and 74% respectively. The authors argued that the exceptions to the hyperemia may be due to relatively mild headaches, cerebral hemodynamic effects of prodromes, misdiagnosis and increased blood volume without increased blood flow.

5.6.3. Immunological theories

Complement studies have examined the hypothesis that immunological mechanisms are involved in the pathogenesis of migraine and that activation of the complement system is a pathogenetic factor in at least some cases of migraine. Lord et al. (1972) found evidence of activation of the complement system during migraine headaches. On the other hand, Behan et al. (1981) were unable to replicate these findings. Visintini et al. (1986) had similar difficulty in their study of 32 subjects with common migraine, 12 with classic migraine and two with reputed milk allergic migraine. They found that the migraineurs did not differ from controls on immunoglobulin concentrations, complement components or immune complex assays.

5.6.4. Platelet theories

The hypothesis that migraine is fundamentally a blood disorder and specifically a platelet disorder has been controversial since its origin in 1978 (Hanington, 1978). The evidence for platelet abnormality in migraineurs has been recently summarized by Hanington (1986) who began with the premise that if migraine was caused by a primary abnormality of the platelets then one might reasonably expect that the platelets of migraineurs did differ from non-migraine sufferers at all times. Specifically, Hanington (1986, p. 414) has emphasized that:

> These differences include a significant increase in spontaneous aggregation, highly significant differences in its manner of 5-HT release and significant differences in platelet composition. These differences are so inextricably linked with the onset and recurrence of migraine attacks that it is reasonable to conclude that migraine attacks occur because of this basic difference in platelet behaviour.

Others (e.g., Steiner et al., 1985; Rajiv et al., 1986) have argued that the platelet disorder may be a marker for migraine but do not serve a primary causal role.

5.7. Genetic factors

A strong genetic component has been suggested in the origin of migraine. The identification of a parent, who has migraine, is often used as a factor in the diagnosis of migraine. This fact would artificially increase the concordance for migraine. As well, problems commonly arise because diagnosis of family members is usually not on the basis of clinical examination. Bille (1981) reported on the only longitudinal study of the inheritance of childhood migraine. He did a 23 year follow-up study on 73 persons who had been diagnosed as having severe migraines. Forty-seven individuals (19 men and 28 women) had a total of 90 children who were then 4 years of age or more. Two of the 19 fathers each had a girl with migraine and 13 of the 28 mothers had a total of four boys and nine girls with migraine. Migraine seems to be inherited more frequently by way of the mother and more often by girls.

Other researchers have also found a strong genetic component. For example, Friedman and Merritt (1959) found that 65% of the nearest relatives of their migraine patients also had migraine. Selby and Lance (1960) found that 55% of their 464 patients had relatives with migraine. Finally, Dalsgaard-Neilsen (1965) demonstrated a family incidence of 90%.

Although it is clear that there is some genetic component in migraine, the lack of an unequivocal marker for migraine and the resultant variability in diagnosis makes it difficult to determine the exact contribution of heredity to migraine. Moreover, the possibility that migraine and muscle contraction headache are merely ends of the same continuum would mean that the determination of genetic contribution would be all the more difficult.

5.8. Psychological factors

Operant conditioning, stress, depression, and personality factors have been implicated in causing migraine headache. The following provides a brief discussion of the research related to each of these factors.

5.8.1. Operant factors

The notion that children usually complain about headache to avoid unpleasant events or to receive special privileges and attention appears prevalent.

However, it is our clinical impression that this is usually not the case. An important diagnostic test of operant pain is to assess what contingencies surround the occurrence of pain. If pain does not lead to special privileges, excuse from duties, or escape from an unpleasant situation, it is unlikely to be operant. Unfortunately, pain that is not operantly driven also often leads to special privileges, excuse from duties and, in some cases, escape from an unpleasant situation. One single case study has been reported (Ramsden et al., 1983) and is discussed in the treatment section of this chapter.

Operantly driven pain may be quite important in cases of chronic pain and will be discussed in greater detail in chapter 13.

5.8.2. Stress

Although most researchers and clinicians agree that there is a biological predisposition to migraine, many operate on the assumption that migraine is triggered by either psychological or physiological stress. However, the mechanism of stress has not been well investigated. Some argue that stress causes a cognitive shift which mediates autonomic arousal (Bakal, 1982) whereas others suggest a muscular mediation. The physiological impact of psychological states has not been adequately investigated.

There is a limited amount of research that has been concerned with the relationship between pediatric migraine and stress. Vahlquist (1955) found that among 55 children, 87% reported that mental stress was a trigger for migraine attacks. Bille (1962) reported that of the 61 children, who were able to identify factors that would lead to migraines, 28 children mentioned schoolwork and seven children mentioned mental stress. A recent survey of 2181 schoolchildren in Amsterdam (Passchier and Orlebeke, 1985) found that 30% of the elementary school students and 40% of the secondary school students attributed their headaches to stress. Maratos and Wilkinson (1982) reported in their study of 47 consecutive referrals to a specialist migraine clinic compared with dental clinic referrals, that 86% of the children with migraine reported that emotional upset triggered their headaches. However, all of these studies were retrospective in nature. That is, stress was not recorded before the headache and therefore stress may just be a convenient, but erroneous, way to explain headache. As well, no controls were used and as a result there is no evidence that non-migraineurs do not experience as much stress.

5.8.3. Depression

The role that depression may play in triggering migraine has also received some consideration. Ling et al. (1970) reported that 40% of a sample of 25 children presenting with headache to a child neurology clinic could be retrospectively diagnosed as suffering from depression. The study is suspect for several reasons. First of all, the study was retrospective and based on a review of charts and thus open to serious errors. As well, the reliability and validity of the diagnostic code used has not been established. Finally, the sample is unusual. The headache sample was only 3% of the patients seen in the clinic. Given the high prevalence of pediatric migraine, it appears that this sample was a very select group and likely a particularly disturbed group. Other research has used better methodology. For example, Andrasik et al. (1987) found that children with migraine were more depressed than pain-free controls. Similarly, we (Cunningham et al., 1987) showed that migraineurs were more depressed than controls. However, the amount of pain, that a child had, was related to the level of depression regardless of whether the pain was migraine or musculoskeletal pain. These findings suggest that depression may be the result of, rather than the cause of, a severe pain disorder.

5.8.4. Personality

There has been strong suggestion that children with migraine have a specific personality type that predisposes them to migraine. This view was espoused by Wolff (Anderson, 1980) who reported on the recall of his adult migraine patients as to what they were like as children. More than half were described as being children who were delicate, shy, withdrawn, sober, polite, well-mannered, conscientious, responsible, unusually thoughtful and extremely obedient to parental wishes. These sterling but submissive qualities were said to coexist with unusual obstinacy, stubbornness and inflexibility (Anderson, 1980). They were also described as being very neat and clean as children and, as adolescents, unusually concerned with moral and ethical issues. Methodological problems with this study include: only people who had migraine as adults and who consulted a world famous specialist for their migraines were studied; the reliance on memory of what the patients were as children might have been biased; the unstructured clinical interview used to gather the information may have allowed the interviewer's biases to intrude; and the lack of a control group prevents meaningful comparisons with headache-free individuals.

There have been a number of poorly designed studies since Wolff's observations that have tended to support the image of childhood migraineurs being withdrawn, over-achieving and anxious. For example, Koch and Melchior (1969) found that 39 of their 136 pediatric migraineurs exhibited some degree of mental symptoms related to stress. Similarly, Krupp and

Friedman (1953) found that superior intelligence, sensitivity, thoroughness, high need for approval, seriousness, orderliness, reliability, feelings of inadequacy, excessive guilt, strong superego, and psychogenic symptoms characterized their pediatric migraine patients.

Three well controlled studies (Bille, 1962; Andrasik et al., 1987; Cunningham et al., 1987) have also examined the personality of pediatric migraineurs. Bille tested 73 children with migraine occurring at least once a month and 73 headache-free controls matched on age, sex, social class and school grade. A comprehensive battery of tests including self-reports, parent reports, direct observations, as well as sensory-motor, perceptual and intelligence tests were administered. Migraineurs described themselves as more anxious, fearful, tense and nervous, while parents described them as more anxious, sensitive, vulnerable to frustration, more tidy and less physically enduring than did the parents of children without migraine. Children with migraine were observed as being less confident and tending to block on some test items. They also displayed more deliberateness, caution and less active effort. The rating scales used in the study were not normed or validated and no group of children with pain from sources other than migraine were used. In a similar study, Andrasik et al. (1987) compared 32 childhood migraineurs with 32 children matched on age, sex and demographic variables. Standardized, validated scales of psychological functioning were administered. These researchers found that headache sufferers were more depressed, expressed a greater number of somatic complaints and experienced more internalizing behavior disorders. Adolescent migraineurs in the study were more anxious and the male adolescents had poorer overall psychological adjustment. The migraineurs although suffering some psychological problems were not clinically maladjusted.

Andrasik et al. (1987) noted that one of the limitations of their study was the lack of a group of children who had pain from causes other than migraine. Therefore, the possibility that the personality differences could have been the result of having a long-standing pain disorder could not be eliminated.

In a recently published study, from our lab, Cunningham et al. (1987) examined 20 migraineurs (ten boys, ten girls) and two control groups matched on age and sex. One control group was pain-free and one group was suffering from chronic musculoskeletal pain including juvenile rheumatoid arthritis and patellofemoral knee pain. The State-Trait Anxiety Inventory (Spielberger, 1973), the Children's Depression Rating Scale (Poznanski et al., 1979), the Birleson Self-rating Scale (1981) and both the parent and teacher version of the Child Behavior Checklist (Achenbach and Edelbrock, 1983) were used in this study. When the amount of pain experienced by children was statistically controlled, the only variable that discriminated between the three groups was that of somatic complaints which included vomiting, nausea, and perceptual disturbance, all migraine-related phenomena. The inclusion of a pain control group in this study yielded results which indicated that the behavioral and personality features thought to be characteristic of childhood migraine are common to other long-standing pain disorders. These characteristics correlate with the amount of pain experienced and suggest that they are the result of rather than the cause of the pain.

5.9. Migraine and cognitive/learning ability

Some have suggested that children with migraine are generally academically superior to their peers (Krupp and Friedman, 1953; Vahlquist, 1955). These assertions were based on clinical observations. On the other hand, learning problems could be associated in a number of ways with pediatric migraine. First of all, migraine might be triggered by the stress from a learning disability. Secondly, repeated absence from school because of migraine might lead to problems with missed instruction and learning difficulties. Finally, learning problems might arise from the pathophysiology of migraine itself. Repeated ischemia might lead to specific or diffuse brain damage and resultant learning disabilities.

Bille (1962) has done the best work in this area. He analyzed the schoolmarks for the spring term of the fourth class of 6313 children of whom 196 had migraine. In Sweden, at the time of the study, the fourth class marks were used to determine whether a child could enter secondary school. The total marks for seven subjects were compared for migraineurs and non-migraineurs. He found that children with migraine were no more likely to have marks above or below their peers.

In a second portion of his study, Bille (1962) compared 73 children with 'pronounced' migraine with 73 headache-free children matched on age, sex, social class and type of school-class. The children were compared on a battery of cognitive and intellectual tasks. All analyses were repeated deleting the four pairs of boys in classes for 'backward' children. Bille (1962, pp. 102–103) concluded:

> ...tests related to complex cognitive functioning and/or 'general intelligence' did not yield any differences between the two groups.

In contrast, Ferguson and Robinson (1982) have reported on a single case of a child who had developed learning problems following the onset of migraine. As well, Guidetti et al. (1983b) reported that migraineurs were deficient on memory and perceptual tasks.

5.10. Migraine and motion sickness

Motion sickness has long been seen as a frequent correlate of pediatric migraine. Bille (1962) found that 54.8% of the migraine children and 31.5% of other children had nausea or vomiting on car, train or boat trips or on swings and roundabouts. More recently, Barabas et al. (1983) compared children attending clinic with a diagnosis of migraine, non-migraine headaches, seizure disorders or learning disabilities. Forty-five percent of the children with migraine had motion sickness. They were between six-and-a-half and nine times more likely to have motion sickness than the other children.

The mechanism by which migraineurs are more likely to have motion sickness than controls is not known but it may be either of peripheral or central origin. Children with migraine may have suffered from repeated vasoconstriction of the cranial arteries especially the basilar artery. It would result in ischemia in the region of the labyrinth arteries potentially leading to hypersensitivity of the peripheral receptors to body and head movements (Barabas et al., 1983). As well, if migraine is a disorder of intermittent serotonin depletion, this decrease could result in a predominance of the cholinergic pathways that stimulate central medullary chemoceptive and emetic areas. This could result in a proclivity to motion sickness.

5.11. Migraine and diet

Many parents feel that their children's migraine headaches are due to allergies. Not surprisingly, this belief has received attention in the headache literature. Much of the evidence for a link between migraine and allergies comes from uncontrolled clinical observation that many children with migraine have allergies. Since both migraine and allergy are common and a child with multiple problems is more likely to be seen in the doctor's office, it is not surprising to find that some children with migraines also suffer from allergies.

Adult studies have addressed this issue. For example, in a well designed epidemiological study, Waters (1972) found an association between migraine and eczema which is a known allergic disorder. The association between eczema and migraine was evident even when the degree of neuroticism was held constant. Unfortunately, the definition of eczema was based on a single question: 'Have you ever had skin trouble?'

Histamine, which is a product of allergic reaction, does provoke migraine headache in migraineurs (Aebelholt and Olesen, 1980) but the contribution of histamine to the clinical syndrome of migraine appears to be simply that it is involved in the local reaction rather than being causally significant (Amery, 1982).

Three research strategies have been used to examine the link between food allergy and migraine. These are: analysis of food consumed before spontaneous attacks, food challenges and diet trials.

Analysis of food consumed before an attack was done by Dalton and Dalton (1979) who collected retrospective food diaries from 77 children for the 24 h prior to the occurrence of a migraine attack, and also for a control period of 24 h 1 week later. They noted that specific foods (cheese, chocolate and citrus fruit) occurred more frequently before headache days than before control days for 38% of the children. Missing meals or fasting were also related to headache days in 41% of the children. The use of retrospective rather than prospective report and the lack of subject blindness reduce the validity of this study. Other studies with adults (Dexter et al., 1978) have also found that missing meals and fasting may trigger migraine.

The best designed diet trials have focussed on Hanington's (1967) oral tyramine hypothesis which was based on a series of observations: (1) a small number of migraine sufferers report that they reliably get a headache if they eat specific foods; (2) patients, who were not migraineurs but who were being treated by monoamine oxidase inhibitors (MAOIs), a type of antidepressant, react to certain foods with headaches and high blood pressure; (3) the foods that trigger dietary migraine and MAOI headaches are similar; and (4) most of the foodstuffs contain tyramine, a naturally occurring vasoactive amine.

A review by Kohlenberg (1982) noted that of the 11 published reports of the tyramine hypothesis, six conducted by Hanington supported the hypothesis, four did not support the hypothesis and one was equivocal. Kohlenberg (1982) reported that patients in Hanington's studies, which supported the tyramine hypothesis, were rigorously selected and were tested in the natural environment. Patients in the negative trials were not as carefully selected. Patients in the equivocal trial were carefully selected but were tested in a hospital environment. Kohlenberg (1982) concluded that a small group (approximately 5%) of migraineurs are tyramine-sensitive.

The tyramine studies were all done on adults and have not been replicated on children. However, Egger et al. (1983a) have used a dietary trial in pediatric migraine. They reported that 93% of 88 children with severe frequent migraine recovered on oligoantigenic diets. The oligoantigenic diet consisted of one meat (lamb or chicken), one carbohydrate (rice or potato), one fruit (banana or apple), one vegetable (brassica), water and vitamin supplements. The offending foods were identified by sequential reintroduction of foods. The role of the foods in provoking migraine was established in a double-blind controlled trial in 40 of the children. Although the design appeared appropriate and the results extraordinarily impressive, many commentators have questioned this study. Leviton (1984) and Wilkinson and Blau (1983) for example, noted that the subjects in the Egger et al. (1983a) study were not typical pediatric migraineurs. The subjects had headaches at least once a week for the previous 6 months even though some were on medication. Seven percent had complicated migraine; 16% had 'fits'; and 47% had behavior disturbance (mostly hyperkinetic) at other times. This was clearly a very unusual sample. The 'trigger foods' noted Leviton (1984) and Peatfield (1983) were ingested for 2–7 days before the patients developed abdominal symptoms (not necessarily headache). This response was not typical for individuals with dietary migraine who usually respond within 1 h.

Other researchers (Cook and Joseph, 1983) have pointed out that the measurement and design of the study by Egger et al. (1983a) were confusing in that no definition of a reaction to the reintroduced food was given; changes in the diet were mentioned but not detailed; and the length of the different sequences in the study were not clear. Compliance to the oligoantigenic diet was not discussed and because the diet was so demanding compliance was likely to be problematic.

The oligoantigenic diet as a treatment for pediatric migraine remains an interesting hypothesis. We do not consider the Egger et al. (1983a) study to provide sufficient evidence for its effectiveness.

5.12. Stroke and migraine

Stroke in an adolescent is a rarity. The relationship between migraine and risk for premature stroke is not completely clear. However, in a recent critical review of 64 cases of young adult migraineurs suffering stroke, Featherstone (1986, p. 131) concluded:

> ...the risk of thrombotic stroke for classic and/or complicated migraine is more than fifty times that for the three-fourths of migraineurs with common migraine, who have the same risk for stroke as normal individuals without migraine.

Featherstone (1986) also suggested that the risk of stroke for complicated migraine is approximately 750 times greater than the risk for a person without migraine. The prevalence of stroke, even in complicated migraine, is still low but the effects of stroke are serious and thus the issue warrants attention. The mechanism is unclear but three possible candidates have been suggested: ischemia, lipids and mitral valve prolapse.

5.12.1. Ischemia

The traditional vascular theory of migraine suggests that the vasoconstrictive phase produces a transient ischemia. The work of Olesen et al. (1981, 1982) also posits a diffuse oligemia in classic migraine. Amery's (1982) notion of focal hypoxia is also in keeping with an ischemia factor in migraine-related stroke.

5.12.2. Lipids

One of the potential links between stroke and migraine could be abnormal lipids. Glueck and Bates (1986) studied lipids and lipoprotein cholesterols in 39 children between the age of 4 and 20 years with severe migraine. In 9 of the 26 boys (three times what was expected), low-density lipoprotein cholesterol levels were greater than the appropriate 90th percentile values. As well, six boys (twice expected values) had bottom decile levels of high-density lipoprotein cholesterol. The authors pointed out that lipoproteins track over time and that these children may be a higher risk for cardiovascular disease. They suggested that boys with migraine be routinely evaluated for lipids and lipoprotein cholesterols.

5.12.3. Mitral valve prolapse

In mitral valve prolapse one or both of the mitral valve leaflets balloon back into the left atrium during left ventricular systole. Mitral valve prolapse can be diagnosed by auscultation (one or more non-ejection clicks and a late systolic murmur), imaging techniques (M-mode electrocardiography revealing abnormal late systolic or pansystolic posterior motion of the mitral leaflets) or pathologic examination (thickening and elongation of the leaflets). The diagnostic criteria are not universally agreed upon and depend on subjective interpretation and the method used. Mitral valve prolapse is an autosomal dominant condition which has been thought to predispose to cerebral ischemic attacks and has been correlated with pediatric migraine, especially complicated migraine (Lanzi et al., 1986). The clinical meaningfulness of mitral valve prolapse in migraine has been sharply debated. One might argue that diagnosis of mitral valve prolapse, if there are no symptoms, has no advantage to the patient and carries the potential for creating unnecessary anxiety and cardiac non-disease (Bergman and Stamm, 1967). On the other hand, it may be wiser to warn any family that has a child with mitral valve prolapse that the disorder is benign so that future, less experienced clinicians do not unnecessarily frighten the patient and order unnecessary tests should the phenomenon be later discovered (Feldman et al., 1987).

5.13. Migraine and EEG

There is an extensive literature on the EEG in migraine. For example, Bille (1962) compared the EEGs recorded during rest and during activation by hyperventilation and by photic stimulation of 73 children with frequent migraine and controls. He found that abnormal records occurred in 22% of the migraine group and 15% of the controls. The difference was not significant. Other researchers have found a higher incidence of abnormality. For example, Froelich et al. (1960) found 44% of the records of childhood migraineurs to be abnormal. Similarly, Prensky and Sommer (1979) reported that of the 64 patients that had EEGs only 17 were normal. The most common abnormality (24 patients) was diffuse slowing with random sharp waves.

The findings of EEG abnormality in migraine is well summarized by Barlow (1984) who concluded:
(1) There is no specific EEG abnormality in juvenile migraine.
(2) Incidence of unusual migraine is higher in children with migraine than in adults with migraine or in headache-free children.
(3) Paroxysmal discharges, benign mid temporal or Rolandic spikes are encountered with greater frequency in childhood migraine.
(4) Both slowing and paroxysmal discharges are seen in normal children.
(5) EEG recording during complicated migraine is usually abnormally slow with high amplitude. It may be asymmetrical or focal and if focal it is often consistent with the expected areas of cerebral dysfunction.

Barlow (1984) does not recommend routine use of the EEG in juvenile migraine.

5.14. Migraine and epilepsy

The relationship between migraine and epilepsy is controversial. Some authors such as Kellaway et al. (1959), Whitehouse et al. (1967), and Jay

(1982) have argued that a specific EEG pattern characterized by 14 and 6/s positive spikes, especially during sleep, is a marker for a seizure equivalent migraine disorder. Jay (1982) has suggested this pattern may be a marker of autonomic instability deriving from an abnormal central nervous system electrical discharge. This discharge induces excessive discharge in the hypothalamic autonomic nervous system outflow, resulting in the typical migraine symptoms. Alternatively, Jay (1982) argued that cycles of 14 and 6 positive spikes may indicate an incident of spreading cortical depression. However, the findings of Lombroso et al. (1966) of this pattern in 58% of 212 normal children aged 13–15 years casts serious doubt on the 14 and 6/s spikes as any sort of meaningful marker for migraine (McGrath, 1983; Barlow, 1984).

5.15. Prognosis of childhood migraine

The short-term prognosis of childhood migraine is excellent. Prensky and Sommer (1979) found that half of the children with migraine were substantially improved within 6 months of a visit to a neurologist and that this remission was independent of the treatment given. Similar findings have been reported by Forsythe et al. (1984) and Noronha (1985).

However, contrary to popular opinion, children often do not outgrow headache. Bille (1981), for example, found that after 23 years, approximately 60% of his more severe migraine headache sufferers were continuing to experience headache. Prognosis was better for males (52% remitting) than for females (30% remitting). Sillanpaa (1983a) reported on a 7 year follow-up of 2921 children who were first assessed at the age of 7 years. Migraine had entirely disappeared in 22% of these children. It had been alleviated in 37% of children but remained unchanged or became more severe in 41% of the children. There was a poorer prognosis for girls than for boys who had migraine beginning before school entrance and the reverse for migraine beginning at school entrance.

5.16. Treatment

Treatment of pediatric headache can be pharmacological, environmental or psychological (behavioral).

5.16.1. Pharmacological treatment
Pharmacological treatment can be abortive, palliative, or prophylactic. Abortive medication which frequently consists of ergotamine preparations is

not commonly used with children but is appropriate for occasional use with adolescents with particularly disabling migraine. However, no evaluations of abortive medications in this age group have been done.

The most common type of pharmacological treatment for children with migraines is palliative medication (i.e., analgesics, sedatives, and antiemetics). Acetaminophen and ASA are the most frequently used. However, our clinical impression is that children are frequently not appropriately medicated for headache. Typically, analgesics are either not taken or they are taken only after the headache becomes severe. Parents and children frequently have a strong anti-drug bias that interferes with appropriate analgesic usage. No evaluations of palliative medication have been done in pediatric headache, although clinical reports indicate that early use of palliative medication reduces the severity and duration of the headaches but not the frequency.

Prophylactic medication refers to drugs which are taken daily to prevent the occurrence of migraines. Several types of prophylactic medication are used with children including propranolol, tricyclic antidepressants especially amitriptyline; antiepileptics especially phenytoin, methysergide; and calcium channel blockers. However, very little well controlled research has been done.

5.16.1.1. Anecdotal reports   The following drugs have been recommended for prophylaxis of childhood migraine on the basis of anecdotal reports: pizotifen (Bille et al., 1977); amitriptyline (McCarthy and Mehegan, 1982); methysergide (McCarthy and Mehegan, 1982); cyproheptadine (Bille et al., 1977); phenytoin and phenobarbital (Buda and Joyce, 1979); ergonovine maleate (Barlow, 1978), the ergotamine derivatives and isometheptene preparations (Gascon and Barlow, 1984).

5.16.1.2. Open trials and clinical series   Buda and Joyce (1979) reported on a series of 62 patients with migraine who were treated with anticonvulsants (either phenobarbital or phenytoin). They reported that 94% of the patients were at least 75% improved. The trial was unblinded and uncontrolled. Measurement was simply on the basis of global patient report of decrease of headache.

In an uncontrolled trial, Bille et al. (1977) studied 19 children aged 6–16 years, who were used to evaluate cyproheptadine for migraine. Only two children were not improved.

5.16.1.3. Properly controlled trials   In a double-blind placebo-controlled crossover study involving 32 migraineurs between 7 and 16 years of age,

Ludviggson (1974) found that propranolol resulted in a substantial reduction in headaches compared to responses to a placebo. Propranolol was credited with an excellent improvement in 20 of the 28 children who completed the trial. In three children the effect was good and in another three children a moderate effect was noted. Only two children were not helped on propranolol. In contrast, 21 children showed no response to a placebo. However, a recently published double-blind crossover study with 53 pediatric migraineurs between 9 and 15 years of age (Forsythe et al., 1984) has failed to show that propranolol is more effective than placebo. In fact, there was some indication that headaches lasted longer and were more frequent with propranolol.

A second beta-blocker timolol has also been evaluated in a randomized double-blind crossover study (Noronha, 1985). Seventeen patients completed the trial. There was a progressive reduction in headache irrespective of the treatment. Timolol was not more effective than placebo.

In a brief abstract Salmon (1985) reported that pizotifen was effective in a double-blind parallel group study with 37 migraineurs aged 6–15 years.

The only study to compare psychological and pharmacological treatment was that of Olness et al. (1987) who randomly assigned children aged 6–12 years with classic migraine to receive either propranolol or placebo for 3 months and then crossed over into the other treatment. Following drug treatment, the migraineurs were treated by self-hypnosis. The mean number of headaches experienced by each child during the 3 month placebo condition was 13.3. During the propranolol condition, children averaged 14.9 headaches, whereas the self-hypnosis condition resulted in an average of 5.8 headaches for the 3 month period. There were no differences in the severity or duration of headaches that did occur across the three conditions. The failure of the propranolol treatment to show any effect compared to placebo is in keeping with the Forsythe et al. (1984) finding. Although the self-hypnosis condition was not randomly assigned (all subjects received the self-hypnosis) and as a result this element of the study is a pre-post study, the data provide a good indication that a self-hypnosis procedure may be effective in treating classic migraine in children.

Sorge and Marano (1985) compared flunarizine, a calcium channel blocker, and placebo in a randomized double-blind trial with 48 children suffering from migraine. They noted that the children, who took 5 mg of flunarizine at bedtime, had significant reduction of headache frequency compared to the children on placebo. Sixteen of the 24 children in the flunarizine group experienced a greater than 50% reduction in both intensity and frequency of headache. Side effects were important in only three children.

The major drawback with flunarizine was that its major effect occurred in the third month of treatment.

Sillanpaa (1977) did a randomized double-blind trial of clonidine, a central sympatholytic antihypertensive agent, which has been used in adult migraine. Clonidine was not found to be superior to placebo.

5.16.2. Psychological treatment

Although pharmacological treatments are available, the most commonly researched treatment for migraine in children and adolescents follows a psychological orientation. Psychological or behavioral treatment for pediatric headache has focussed on relaxation, biofeedback or cognitive interventions.

5.16.2.1. Anecdotal reports

Olness and MacDonald (1981) used self-hypnosis both with and without skin temperature biofeedback and relaxation exercises in the treatment of 15 children with migraine. Based on global judgements of headache improvement, all children were reported to have improved.

Similarly, impressive results were reported by Werder and Sargent (1984) in a retrospective uncontrolled report of 31 children, 19 of whom had migraine. They reported that all the migraine subjects had a reduction of greater than 50% in headaches.

5.16.2.2. Uncontrolled trials, single subject designs and clinical series

Andrasik et al. (1982) reported on two subjects in a single subject design. They found that skin temperature biofeedback was effective in reducing headache frequency by 57% and 86% and headache severity by 62% and 85% in two female children. Similar results were reported by Houts (1982), who found that relaxation increased headache in an 11-year-old boy, but that thermal biofeedback decreased headache. Gains were maintained at follow-up.

The only report of blood volume pulse (BVP) biofeedback in the childhood migraine literature is that of Feuerstein and Adams (1977), who used a single subject design with baseline and EMG biofeedback preceding the BVP biofeedback. BVP biofeedback was the only effective treatment.

In an uncontrolled single group outcome study, Diamond and Franklin (1975) treated 32 childhood migraineurs. Twenty-six of the children were reported to have been improved with autogenic feedback.

In a very different approach, Ramsden et al. (1983) demonstrated by means of a single subject design across settings the efficacy of contingency management in treating a 6-year-old girl with migraine.

Mehegan et al. (1986) evaluated a combination of EMG biofeedback, relaxation training and operant pain behavior management using a multiple baseline across subjects. They demonstrated significant effects of treatment.

Mention should be made again of the study by Olness et al. (1987) who found that self-hypnosis was better than a previous trial of propranolol or placebo.

5.16.2.3. Properly controlled trials Four randomized trials have been reported. Labbe and Williamson (1984) randomly assigned 28 childhood migraineurs to either a wait-list control or autogenic biofeedback. Autogenic biofeedback was superior to the control condition with 93% of the children in the biofeedback group reporting a reduction of 50% or more in headache activity. There was no improvement in the control group. Improvements were maintained at 6 month follow-up.

In our lab, Richter et al. (1986) randomly assigned 51 children with migraine to one of three groups: relaxation training, cognitive coping therapy and a placebo treatment. The two active treatments were superior to the placebo treatment, with those children who suffered the more severe headaches doing particularly well. Gains were maintained at 16 week follow-up.

Similarly, a group at the Children's Hospital in Boston (Fentress et al., 1986) randomly assigned 18 pediatric migraineurs between the ages of 8 and 12 years to one of three groups: relaxation-response, relaxation-response plus biofeedback and waiting-list control group. They found the two active treatment groups to be superior to the control condition and equivalent to each other. Treatment effectiveness was maintained at 1 year follow-up. The researchers noted that both active treatment groups did receive brief pain management suggestions that could be construed as a confound and that future studies should include an attention control condition.

A second randomized trial from our lab (McGrath et al., 1987) studied 92 children with migraine and compared relaxation training, placebo therapy and a minimal contact 'own best efforts' therapy. All groups of children were significantly improved after treatment as compared to before. However, there were no differences between the three groups.

Finally in a yet unpublished study from our lab (Davies, 1987), we compared a comprehensive psychological treatment that included relaxation, problem-solving and cognitive therapy given individually or in a group format. A control condition consisting of group discussions about headaches was also included. The 48 participants in the study were adolescent female migraineurs. Results indicated that both treatments were superior to the control condition and that the individual treatment was superior to the group condition for adolescents with more severe migraine.

We are currently evaluating a detailed manual and set of tapes which teach relaxation and cognitive strategies for adolescents with migraine.

In summary, there is good indication that behavioral strategies including thermal biofeedback, relaxation, self-hypnosis and cognitive restructuring may be effective in treatment of juvenile migraine. However, in research in this area, care must be taken to control for expectancy effects and simple problem-solving strategies that are often part of a more complex (and expensive) psychological treatment. Such simple expectancy manipulations and problem-solving strategies may be a viable alternative when the more extensive psychological treatments are not available.

6. Muscle contraction headache

> ... mostly they're (headaches) from all the hurrying. See, I have competitive swimming every (school) day so I have to leave right on the bell. And 3 days a week I get drama and tournament tennis so I have to ride (bicycle) like crazy not to be late. And I'm in the Gifted Minor Program so I have all this extra reading and stuff ... *(girl, aged 9, quoted in Ross and Ross, 1984, p. 185).*

6.1. What is muscle contraction headache?

Muscle contraction headaches in children have not been as extensively investigated as have migraine headaches.

In contrast to the vascular origin of migraine, muscle contraction headaches are thought to arise from prolonged muscle tension in the head and neck. These headaches tend to be more constant, tend to occur in response to specific stressors and present as a band-like tightness.

As we have previously discussed many view migraine and muscle contraction headaches as overlapping disorders and many children with a serious headache disorder report both types of headaches.

6.2. Prevalence

The prevalence of muscle contraction headache in childhood is unknown.

6.3. Mechanisms

The mechanism of muscle contraction headache is thought to be that of increased muscle tension in the head and neck. However, as discussed previously, there is substantial debate about the mechanisms that may be operative in both migraine and muscle contraction headache. Although no studies have been done with children or adolescents, studies with adults have failed to show increased muscle tension in muscle contraction headache sufferers. The overlap in symptomatology between children with muscle contraction and migraine headache is considerable. As previously mentioned, Joffe et al. (1983) found that the presence of both muscle contraction and migraine symptoms increased with the number of hours of headache reported per day.

6.4. Genetic factors

There is not thought to be a strong genetic component in muscle contraction headache.

6.5. Psychological factors

There are no studies on stress, personality or depression in muscle contraction headache in children but clinical lore about the relationship of stress and personality to muscle contraction headache is similar to that of the relationship between stress and personality and migraine. Children with muscle contraction headache are thought to be anxious children under stress.

6.6. Treatment

6.6.1. Medical
The most common medical treatment of muscle contraction headaches is palliative medication such as ASA or acetaminophen. Occasionally muscle relaxants are prescribed but these are rarely indicated. No trials of medical treatment of childhood muscle contraction headaches have been published.

6.6.2. Psychological
Attanasio et al. (1984) provided a preliminary report (ten subjects only) of a randomized trial using both EMG biofeedback and progressive relaxation in

comparison to a wait list control. The two active treatments were both superior to the control.

Larsson and Melin (1986) conducted an experimental trial of relaxation on 33 adolescent students. After a 4 week baseline, adolescents with tension and mixed tension-migraine headache were randomly assigned to either relaxation or an information-contact condition. Relaxation training resulted in a greater than 50% reduction in headache activity in nine of 11 relaxation subjects post-treatment and six of 11 at 6 months follow-up. Only one of 13 information-contact subjects reported 50% or greater reduction after treatment and five of 13 reported such improvement at follow-up.

In a second study by this group, Larsson et al. (1987) reported on a trial in which 46 high school students were randomly assigned to therapist-assisted relaxation, a self-help condition and a self-monitoring condition. Thirty-four of the subjects were suffering from tension headache, ten had mixed headache and two had migraine. The students were treated at school. The therapist-assisted relaxation was done over nine 45 min sessions augmented by two booster sessions 2 months later. These sessions were conducted in small groups by senior graduate students in clinical psychology. The self-help treatment was administered by school nurses. The self-monitoring group received no treatment but completed diaries. Both the self-help and the therapist-mediated treatment were superior to the self-monitoring group. Sixty-four percent of the therapist-assisted group, 50% of the self-help group but none of the self-monitoring group had at least a 50% reduction in headache at the 5 month follow-up. The authors concluded that a self-help regimen is an inexpensive but effective treatment for chronic headache in adolescents.

7. Sinus headache

Sinus headaches are caused by pressure in the sinus cavities. Sinus headaches can be the result of acute or chronic problems in any of the sinus cavities and may be frontal, maxillary, behind the eyes, and over the vertex of the skull (Stevenson, 1980). The pain is of a deep, dull, aching, non-pulsatile quality. The pain is seldom associated with nausea and is increased by shaking the head, the head-down position or by procedures such as straining, coughing or wearing a tight collar (Stevenson, 1980).

Sinus headache is most often because of infection but can occur with allergic, irritant or vasomotor causes (Solomon, 1967). The primary infection is usually viral but secondary bacterial infection is not infrequent. Symptomatic treatment by decongestants will usually abolish the symptoms. Underlying causes should be treated.

8. Psychogenic headache

Psychogenic headache usually refers to a persistent and intractable headache of the muscle contraction type. Psychogenic headache can arise from:
(1) Avoidance or escape from unpleasant events.
(2) Direct reward of pain behavior.
(3) Anxiety, especially performance anxiety.
(4) Depression.
(5) Psychosis.
   Psychogenic pain is discussed in more detail in chapter 14 'Psychogenic pain'.

9. Impact of headaches on child and family

Some children and their families are almost totally consumed by problems associated with headaches. They are constantly seeking a cure for the headache problem, restrict their lives because of the child's headaches and focus much of their energies on headaches. Medical and mental health professionals are frequently stymied in their attempts to help them. This small group of headache sufferers and their families consume a disproportionate amount of professional time and have been frequently reported on in the psychiatric and psychological literature. In contrast, the vast majority of children, even children with severe and frequent headaches, cope well. They take appropriate measures when they do have severe headache but they minimize the impact on their academic, social and family life.
   There has been little well-designed research on the impact of ordinary headache on the lives of children. Collin et al. (1985) examined the amount of time missed from school in two small town school populations in England. They recorded absence from school and attendance at sick bay during two, 12 week periods in children 5–14 years of age. School absence was 0.05% representing about 1% of all school absences. Absence for headache was recorded for 3.7% of children. On 85% of the occasions, absence was for less than 1 day. Attendance at sick bay was also very low and only rarely resulted in leaving school early. Although the prevalence of headache was very high, most children coped without missing school.

10. *Clinical guidelines*

(1) Children with suspected migraine should be evaluated by a physician experienced with childhood migraine prior to treatment.

(2) The first line of treatment in childhood migraine is simple prophylactic measures such as identifying and eliminating potential triggers combined with simple palliative procedures such as rest, appropriate use of ASA and acetaminophen.

(3) Psychological treatments for migraine and muscle contraction headache may be effective.

(4) Although the effectiveness of prophylactic medication for childhood migraine is unproven, some children will respond well to propranolol. Calcium blockers should also be considered.

(5) If a child is missing school because of headaches, suspicion should be aroused that the problem is chronic intractable pain (see chapter 13) rather than simple migraine or muscle contraction headaches.

11. *Future directions*

(1) Evaluations of palliative medication such as ASA and acetaminophen with pediatric migraine should be undertaken.

(2) Further evaluations of prophylactic medications including the calcium blockers are needed.

(3) Factors predicting the spontaneous remission of headache and the development of more severe headache need to be investigated.

(4) The possibility of cognitive deficits as the result of repeated bouts of complicated migraine should be investigated.

References

Achenbach, T.M. and Edelbrock, C.S. (1983) Manual for the Child Behavior Checklist and Revised Child Behavior Profile (Queen City Printers, Burlington, VT).

Ad Hoc Committee on Classification of Headache (1962) Classification of headache. J. Am. Med. Assoc. 179, 127–128.

Aebelholt, A.K. and Olesen, J. (1980) Headache provocation by continuous intravenous infusion of histamine: Clinical results and receptor mechanisms. Pain 8, 253–259.

Amery, W.K. (1982) Brain hypoxia: The turning point in the genesis of the migraine attack. Cephalalgia 2, 83–109.

Anderson, R.W. (1980) The relation of life situations, personality features and reactions to the migraine syndrome. In: D.J. Dalessio (Ed.), Wolff's Headache and Other Head Pain, 4th edn. (Oxford University Press, New York).

Andrasik, F., Blanchard, E.B., Edlund, S.R. and Rosenblum, E.L. (1982) Autogenic feedback in the treatment of two children with migraine headache. Child Fam Behav. Ther. 4, 13–23.

Andrasik, F., Burke, E.J., Attanasio, V. and Rosenblum, E.L. (1985) Child, parent and physician reports of a child's headache pain: Relationships prior to and following treatment. Headache 25, 421–425.

Andrasik, F., Kabela, E., Quinn, S., Blanchard, E.B. and Rosenblum, E.L. (1987) Psychological functioning of children who have recurrent migraine. Manuscript under review.

Attanasio, V., Andrasik, F., Blanchard, E.B., Burke, E., Kabela, E., McCarran, M., Blake, D. and Rosenblum, E.L. (1984) Behavioral treatment of pediatric tension headache. Paper presented at the annual meeting of the Association for Advancement of Behavior Therapy, Philadelphia, PA.

Bakal, D.A. (1978) Headache: A biopsychological perspective. Psychol. Bull. 82, 369–382.

Bakal, D.A. (1982) Chronic Headache: A Psychobiological Perspective (Springer, New York).

Barabas, G., Matthews, W.S. and Ferrari, M. (1983) Childhood migraine and motion sickness. Pediatrics 72, 188–190.

Barlow, C.F. (1978) Migraine in children. Res. Clin. Stud. Headache 5, 34–46.

Barlow, C.F. (1984) Headaches and Migraine in Childhood, Clinics in Developmental Medicine, Vol. 91 (Lippincott, Philadelphia, PA) pp. 1–13, 46–75, 93–125, 181–197.

Behan, W.M.H., Behan, P.O. and Durward, W.F. (1981) Complement studies in migraine. Headache 21, 55–57.

Bergman, A.B. and Stamm, S.J. (1967) The morbidity of cardiac non-disease in schoolchildren. New Eng. J. Med. 276, 1008–1013.

Bickerstaff, E.R. (1961) Basilar artery migraine. Lancet i, 15–17.

Bille, B. (1962) Migraine in school children. Acta Paediatr. 51 (suppl. 136), 1–151.

Bille, B. (1981) Migraine in childhood and its prognosis. Cephalalgia 1, 71–75.

Bille, B., Ludvigsson, J. and Sanner, G. (1977) Prophylaxis of migraine in children. Headache 17, 61–63.

Birleson, P. (1981) The validity of depressive disorder in childhood and the development of a self-rating scale: A research report. J. Child Psychol. Psychiatr. 22, 73–78.

Buda, F.B. and Joyce, R.P. (1979) Successful treatment of atypical migraine of childhood with anticonvulsants. Mil. Med. 144, 521–523.

Collin, C., Hockaday, J.M. and Waters, W.E. (1985) Headache and school absence. Arch. Dis. Child. 60, 245–247.

Cook, G.E. and Joseph, R. (1983) Food allergy and migraine. Lancet ii, 1256–1257.

Cunningham, S.J., McGrath, P.J., Ferguson, H.B., D'Astous, J.D., Latter, J., Goodman, J.T. and Firestone, P. (1987) Personality and behavioral characteristics in pediatric migraine. Headache 27, 16–20.

Curless, R.G. (1982) Cluster headaches in childhood. J. Pediatr. 101, 393–395.

Dalessio, D.J. (1980) Wolff's Headache and Other Pain, 4th edn. (Oxford University Press, New York).

Dalessio, D.J. (1984) Headache. In: P.D. Wall and R. Melzack (Eds.), Textbook of Pain (Churchill Livingstone, Edinburgh) pp. 277–292.

Dalsgaard-Neilsen, T. (1965) Migraine heredity. Arch. Neurol. Scand. 41, 287.

Dalton, K. and Dalton, M.E. (1979) Food intake before migraine attacks in children. J. R. Coll. Gen. Pract. 29, 662–665.

Davies, K. (1987) Group versus individual behavioral treatment in adolescent migraine. Dissertation, University of Manitoba, Winnipeg.

Dexter, J.D., Roberts, J. and Byer, J.A. (1978) The five hour glucose tolerance test and migraine. Headache 18, 91–95.

Diamond, S. and Franklin, M. (1975) Autogenic training with biofeedback in the treatment of children with migraine. In: W. Luthe and F. Antonelli (Eds.), Therapy in Psychosomatic Medicine, Vol. 4, Autogenic Therapy (Rome), pp. 190–192.

Edmeads, J. (1986) Headache and déjà vu. Headache 26, 434–435.

Egger, J., Carter, C., Soothill, J.F., Turner, M.W. and Wilson, J. (1983a) Controlled trial of diet in migraine. Arch. Dis. Child. 58, 648.

Egger, J., Carter, C., Wilson, J., Turner, M.W. and Soothill, J.F. (1983b) Is migraine food allergy? A double-blind controlled trial of oligantigenic diet treatment. Lancet ii, 865–869.

Featherstone, H.J. (1986) Clinical features of stroke in migraine. Headache 26, 128–133.

Feldman, W., Rosser, W. and McGrath, P.J. (1987) Primary Medical Care of Children and Adolescents (Oxford University Press, New York).

Fentress, D.W., Masek, B.J., Mehegan, J.E. and Benson, H. (1986) Biofeedback and relaxation-response training in the treatment of pediatric migraine. Dev. Med. Child Neurol. 28, 139–146.

Ferguson, K.S. and Robinson, S.S. (1982) Acquired learning problems secondary to migraine. J. Dev. Behav. Pediatr. 3, 247–248.

Feuerstein, M. and Adams, H.E. (1977) Cephalic vasomotor feedback in the modification of migraine headache. Biofeedback Self-Regul. 2, 241–254.

Forsythe, W.I., Gillies, D. and Sills, M.A. (1984) Propranolol ('Inderal') in the treatment of childhood migraine. Dev. Med. Child Neurol. 26, 737–741.

Friedman, A.P. and Merritt, H.H. (1959) Headache Diagnosis and Treatment (Davis, Philadelphia, PA).

Froelich, W.A., Carter, C.C., O'Leary, J.L. and Rosenbaum, H.E. (1960) Headache in childhood. Neurology 10, 639–642.

Fulop-Miller, R. (1938) (translated by Eden and Cedar Paul) Triumph over Pain (Literary Guild of America, New York), pp. 1–4.

Gascon, G. and Barlow, C.F. (1970) Juvenile migraine, presenting as an acute confusional state. Pediatrics 45, 628–635.

Glueck, C.J. and Bates, S.R. (1986) Migraine in children: Association with primary and familial dyslipoproteinemias. Pediatrics 77, 316–321.

Golden, G.S. (1979) The Alice in Wonderland syndrome in juvenile migraine. Pediatrics 63, 517–519.

Guidetti, V., Ottaviano, S. and Pagliarini, M. (1983a) Children headache risk: Warning signs and symptoms presenting during the first six months of life. Presented at the First International Headache Congress, Munich.

Guidetti, V., Ottaviano, S., Pagliarini, M., Paolella, A. and Seri, S. (1983b) Psychological peculiarities in children with recurrent primary headache. Cephalalgia 3 (suppl. 1), 215–217.

Haas, D.C., Pineda, G.S. and Lourie, H. (1975) Juvenile head trauma syndromes and their relationship to migraine. Arch. Neurol. 32, 727–730.

Hanington, E. (1967) Preliminary report on tyramine headache. Br. Med. J. 1, 550–551.

Hanington, E. (1978) Migraine: A blood disorder? Lancet ii, 501–503.

Hanington, E. (1986) Viewpoint: The platelet and migraine. Headache 26, 411–415.

Houts, A. (1982) Relaxation and thermal feedback treatment of child migraine headache: A case study. Am. J. Clin. Biofeedback 5, 154–157.

Jackson, A.C. (1986) Neurologic disorders associated with mitral valve prolapse. Can. J. Neurol. Sci. 13, 15–20.

Jay, G.W. (1982) Epilepsy, migraine, and EEG abnormalities in children: A review and hypothesis. Headache 22, 110–114.

Jay, G.Y. and Tomasi, L.G. (1981) Pediatric headaches: A one year retrospective analysis. Headache 21, 5–9.

Joffe, R., Bakal, D.A. and Kaganov, J. (1983) A self-observation study of headache symptoms in children. Headache 23, 20–25.

Kandt, R.S. (1986) Can we reliably differentiate Tolusa-Hunt syndrome from ophthalmoplegic migraine? Headache 26, 436.

Kellaway, P., Crawley, J.W. and Kagawa, N. (1959) A specific electroencephalographic correlate of convulsive equivalent disorder in children. J. Pediatr. 55, 582–592.

Koch, C. and Melchior, J.C. (1969) Headache in childhood: A five year material from a pediatric university clinic. Dan. Med. Bull. 16, 109–114.

Kohlenberg, R.J. (1982) Tyramine sensitivity in dietary migraine: A critical review. Headache 22, 30–34.

Krupp, G.R. and Friedman, A.P. (1953) Migraine in children. Am. J. Dis. Child. 53, 146–150.

Labbe, E.L. and Williamson, D.A. (1983) Temperature biofeedback in the treatment of children with migraine headaches. J. Pediatr. Psychol. 8, 317–326.

Labbe, E.L. and Williamson, D.A. (1984) Treatment of childhood migraine using autogenic feedback training. J. Consult. Clin. Psychol. 52, 968–976.

Lanzi, G., Balottin, U., Borgatti, R., De Agostini, G., Pezzotta, S. and Spanu, G. (1985a) Late post-traumatic headache in pediatric age. Cephalalgia 5, 211–215.

Lanzi, G., Balottin, U., Fazzi, E. and Gamba, N. (1985b) Psychopathology of migraine in childhood. Cephalagia 5 (suppl. 3), 158–159.

Lanzi, G., Grandi, A.M., Gamba, G., Balottin, U., Barzizza, F., Longoni, P., Fazzi, E. and Venco, A. (1986) Migraine, mitral valve prolapse and platelet function in the pediatric age group. Headache 26, 142–145.

Larsson, B. and Melin, L. (1986) Chronic headaches in adolescents: Treatment in a school setting with relaxation training as compared with information-contact and self-registration. Pain 25, 325–336.

Larsson, B., Daleflod, B., Hakansson, L. and Melin, L. (1987) Therapist-assisted versus self-help relaxation treatment of chronic headaches in adolescents: A school based intervention. J. Child Psychol. Psychiatr. 28, 127–136.

Leviton, A. (1984) To what extent does food sensitivity contribute to headache recurrence? Dev. Med. Child Neurol. 26, 542–545.

Ling, W., Oftedal, G. and Weinberg, W. (1970) Depressive illness in childhood presenting as severe headache. Am. J. Dis. Child. 120, 122–124.

Lombroso, C.T., Schwartz, I.H., Clark, D.M., Meunch, H. and Barry, J. (1966) Ctenoids in healthy youths: Controlled study of 14 and 6 per second positive spiking. Neurology 16, 1152–1158.

Lord, G.D.A., Duckworth, J.W. and Charlesworth, J.A. (1972) Complement activation in migraine. Lancet i, 781–782.

Ludvigsson, J. (1974) Propranolol used in prophylaxis of migraine in children. Acta Neurol. Scand. 20, 109–115.

McCarthy, A.M. and Mehegan, J. (1982) Migraine headaches in children: Treatm. Pediatr. Nurs. 8, 173–176.

McGrath, P.J. (1983) Migraine headaches in children and adolescents. In: P. Firestone, P.J. McGrath and W. Feldman (Eds.), Advances in Behavioral Medicine for Children and Adolescents, (Lawrence Erlbaum, Hillsdale, NJ) pp. 39–57.

McGrath, P.J., Humphreys, P., Goodman, J.T., Keene, D., Firestone, P., Jacob, P. and Cunningham, S.J. (1987) Relaxation prophylaxis of childhood migraine: A randomized placebo controlled trial. Manuscript under review.

MacKinney, L. (1937) Early Medieval Medicine (Johns Hopkins Press, Baltimore, MD) p. 35.

Maratos, J. and Wilkinson, M. (1982) Migraine in children: A medical and psychiatric study. Cephalalgia 2, 179–187.

Mehegan, J.E., Masek, B.J., Harrison, R.H., Russo, D.C. and Leviton, A. (1986) A multicomponent behavioral treatment for pediatric migraine. Clin. J. Pain 2, 191–196.

Merskey, H. (Ed.) (1986) Classification of chronic pain: Description of chronic pain syndromes and definition of pain terms. Pain suppl. 3, S58–S79.

Meyer, J.S, Zetusky, W., Jonsdottir, M. and Mortel, K. (1986) Cephalic hyperemia during migraine headaches: A prospective study. Headache 26, 388–397.

Noronha, M.J. (1985) Double blind randomised cross-over trial of timolol in migraine prophylaxis in children. Cephalalgia 5 (suppl. 3), 174–175.

Olesen, J. and Lauritzen, M. (1984) The role of vasoconstriction in the pathogenesis of migraine. In: W.K. Amery, J.M. Van Neuth and A. Wasuquitr (Eds.), The Pharmacological Basis of Migraine Therapy (Pitman, Bath) pp. 7–19.

Olesen, J., Larsen, B. and Lauritzen, M. (1981) Focal hyperemia followed by spreading oligemia and impaired activation of rCBF in classic migraine. Ann. Neurol. 9, 344–352.

Olesen, J., Lauritzen, M., Tfelt-Hansen, P., Henricksen, L. and Larsen, B. (1982) Spreading cerebral oligemia in classical and normal cerebral blood flow in common migraine. Headache 22, 242–248.

Olness, K. and MacDonald, J. (1981) Self hypnosis and biofeedback in the management of juvenile migraine. J. Dev. Behav. Pediatr. 2, 168–170.

Olness, K., MacDonald, J.T. and Uden, D.L. (1987) Comparison of self hypnosis and propranolol in the treatment of juvenile classic migraine. Pediatrics 79, 593–597.

Oster, J. (1972) Recurrent abdominal pain, headache and limb pains in children and adolescents. Pediatrics 50, 429–436.

Passchier, J. and Orlebeke, J.F. (1985) Headaches and stress in schoolchildren: An epidemiological study. Cephalalgia 5, 167–176.

Peatfield, R.C. (1983) Is migraine food allergy? Lancet ii, 1082.

Poznanski, E.O., Cook, G.E. and Carroll, B.J. (1979) A depression rating scale for children, Pediatrics 64, 442–450.

Prensky, A.L. (1980) Migraine and migrainous variants in pediatric patients. Pediatr. Clin. North Am. 23, 461–471.

Prensky, A.L. and Sommer, D. (1979) Diagnosis and treatment of migraine in children. Neurology 29, 506–510.

Rajiv, J., Welch, K.M.A., D'Andrea, G. and Levine, S. (1986) ATP hyposecretion from platelet dense bodies – Evidence for the purinergic hypothesis and a marker of migraine. Headache 26, 403–410.

Ramsden, R., Friedman, B. and Williamson, D. (1983) Treatment of childhood headache reports with contingency management procedures. J. Clin. Child Psychol. 123, 202–206.

Raskin, N.H. and Appenzeller, O. (1980) Headache (Saunders, Philadelphia, PA) pp. 84–110.

Reeves, A.G. (1986) Reply to Dr. Kandt. Headache 26, 436–437.

Richardson, G.M., McGrath, P.J., Cunningham, S.J. and Humphreys, P. (1983) Validity of the headache diary for children, Headache 23, 184–187.

Richter, I.L., McGrath, P.J., Humphreys, P.J., Goodman, John T., Firestone, P. and Keene, D. (1986) Cognitive and relaxation treatment of pediatric migraine. Pain 25, 195–203.

Robertson, W.C. and Schnitzler, E.R. (1978) Ophthalmoplegic migraine in infancy. Pediatrics 61, 886–888.

Ross, D.M. and Ross, S.A. (1984) Childhood pain: the school-aged child's viewpoint. Pain 20, 179–191.

Rutter, M., Chadwick, O. and Shaffer, D. (1983) Head injury. In: M. Rutter (Ed.), Developmental Neuropsychiatry (Guilford Press, New York) pp. 83–111.

Salmon, M.A. (1985) Pizotifen (BC.105. Sanomigran) in the prophylaxis of childhood migraine. Cephalalgia 5 (suppl. 3), 178–179.

Saper, J.R. (1986) Changing perspectives on chronic headache. Clin. J. Pain 2, 19–28.

Selby, G. and Lance, J.W. (1960) Observations on 500 cases of migraine and allied vascular headache. J. Neurol. Neurosurg. Psychiatry 23, 23–32.

Sicuteri, F., Testi, A. and Anselmi, B. (1961) Biochemical investigations in headache: Increase in hydroxyindole acetic acid excretion during migraine attacks. Int. Arch. Allergy Appl. Immunol. 19, 55–58.

Sillanpaa, M. (1976) Prevalence of migraine and other headache in Finnish children starting school. Headache 15, 288–290.

Sillanpaa, M. (1977) Clonidine prophylaxis of childhood migraine and other vascular headache. Headache 17, 28–31.

Sillanpaa, M. (1983a) Prevalence of headache in prepuberty. Headache 23, 10–14.

Sillanpaa, M. (1983b) Changes in the prevalence and other headaches during the first seven school years. Headache 23, 15–19.

Solomon, W.R. (1967) Hay fever, allergic rhinitis and asthma. In: J.M. Sheldon (Ed.), A Manual of Clinical Allergy (Saunders, Philadelphia, PA) pp. 78–88.

Sorge, F. and Dipietro, G. (1981) Headache in children: An epidemiological study. Acta Neurol. 2, 414–419.

Sorge, F. and Marano, E. (1985) Flunarizine, v. placebo in childhood migraine: A double-blind study. Cephalalgia suppl. 2, 145–148.

Spielberger, C.D. (1973) State-Trait Anxiety Inventory for Children (Consulting Psychologists Press, Palo Alto, CA).

Steiner, T.J., Joseph, R. and Rose, C.F. (1985) Migraine is not a platelet disorder. Headache 25, 434–440.

Stevenson, D.D. (1980) Allergy, atopy, nasal disease and headache. In: D.J. Dalessio (Ed.), Wolff's Headache and Other Head Pain, 4th edn. (Oxford, University Press, New York) pp. 256–286.

Vahlquist, B. (1955) Migraine in children. Int. Arch. Allergy 7, 348–355.

Vahlquist, B. and Hackzell, G. (1949) Migraine of early onset – A study of thirty-one cases in which the disease first appeared between one and four years of age. Acta Paediatr. 38, 622–636.

Van Pelt, W. and Andermann, F. (1964) On the early onset of ophthalmoplegic migraine. Am. J. Dis. Child. 107, 628–631.

Visintini, D., Trabattoni, G., Manzoni, G.C., Lechi, A., Bortone, L. and Behan, P.O. (1986) Immunological studies in cluster headache and migraine. Headache 26, 398–402.

Waters, W.E. (1972) Migraine and symptoms in childhood: Bilious attacks, travel sickness and eczema. Headache 12, 55–61.

Werder, D.S. and Sargent, J.D. (1984) A study of childhood headache using biofeedback as a treatment alternative. Headache 24, 122–126.

Whitehouse, D., Pappas, J.A., Escala, P.H. and Lingston, S. (1967) Electroencephalographic changes in children with migraine. New Engl. J. Med. 276, 23–27.

Wilkinson, M. and Blau, N. (1983) Is migraine food allergy? Lancet ii, 1082.

CHAPTER 9

Musculoskeletal pain

1. Introduction

This chapter will focus on musculoskeletal pain of which the most numerous are the arthritic diseases and benign limb pain. Musculoskeletal pain is common. Approximately 15.5% of school-age children have recurrent musculoskeletal pain and 4.5% of children are estimated to have pain that is sufficient to interfere with activities for more than 3 months (Passo, 1982).

2. Juvenile arthritis

> I never do some things I'd like to do, and if I start slipping and doing them I just give myself a terrible lecture. And I never, ever let myself get sad about it. If I start getting sad I make myself think what are all the things I can do. I have to have a lot of talks with myself all the time *(boy, aged 10 years, quoted in Ross and Ross, 1984, p. 1870).*

In 1897, George Still, in a clinical series of 22 patients published the first English language description of chronic arthritis of childhood. At that time, he noted that all children with arthritis were not the same and that there were probably a number of different diseases. Now it is recognized that chronic arthritis in children, which is known as juvenile chronic arthritis (JCA) in Europe and juvenile rheumatoid arthritis (JRA) in North America, represents a set of disorders. Schaller (1984) includes the following: systemic onset JRA; rheumatoid factor-negative polyarticular JRA; rheumatoid factor-positive JRA; pauciarticular JRA I; pauciarticular JRA II; and spondylarthropathy.

2.1. Types of juvenile arthritis

Systemic onset JRA is characterized by high intermittent fever and a characteristic rash for a number of weeks at onset. These children almost always have rather severe pain in numerous joints during the initial period of the disease and during remissions. Factor-negative polyarticular JRA is characterized by symmetric arthritis in the small joints of the hands. Most patients also have involvement of knees, ankles, elbows and feet.

Rheumatoid factor-positive JRA appears to be the childhood equivalent of classic adult rheumatoid arthritis.

Pauciarticular JRA I usually occurs in children before 5 years of age. They have involvement of only a few joints, hence the term 'pauci' for few and 'articular' for joints. Pain may be long lasting but ultimate prognosis is good. These children may develop eye pain from iridocyclitis.

Pauciarticular JRA II patients have onset after 8 years of age. They usually have lower limb involvement and frequently hip girdle involvement.

Finally, the spondylarthropathies include ankylosing spondylitis, Reiter's syndrome, childhood enthesopathy syndrome, arthritis of inflammatory bowel disease, reactive arthritis, and psoriatic arthritis.

The epidemiology of childhood arthritis is not well understood and incidence and prevalence studies are not numerous. There are no good studies of the occurrence of specific subtypes of the disease. The best estimate of prevalence is between 0.6 and 1.1‰ (Schaller, 1984).

The prognosis of childhood arthritis depends, to some extent, on the type. The prognosis is poor for rheumatoid factor-positive JRA with about 50% suffering severe arthritis into adulthood. Ten to 15% of rheumatoid factor-negative polyarticular JRA and 25% of children with systemic onset JRA have continuing severe arthritis. Children with pauciarticular JRA I seldom have arthritic problems in later life but about 10–20% do develop ocular damage. Children with pauciarticular JRA II and spondylarthropathies may be at risk for adult spondylarthropathies.

2.2. Pain in juvenile arthritis

Five studies have specifically examined the pain due to juvenile rheumatoid arthritis.

The two earlier studies (Laaksonen and Laine 1961; Scott et al., 1977) both found that pain reports by children were markedly lower than those given by adult arthritics. Both groups of researchers suggested that, in some way, reaction to the pain is a learned phenomenon.

In a study designed to elucidate some of the factors influencing rating of pain, Beales et al. (1983) interviewed 39 consecutive attenders with juvenile arthritis to an outpatient clinic. Twenty-four children were in the 6–11 year age group and 15 children were aged 12–17 years. Joint sensation was assessed by asking children to indicate how their joints felt by choosing from a list of alternative responses. The alternatives, developed in a previous study, were: cut, bumped or banged, burning, grazed, pricked, pinched, smacked, shocked, squeezed, pulled and aching. Children were then asked to indicate what the sensations meant to them. Finally, children were asked to rate the unpleasantness of the joint sensations and the severity of joint pain using 10 cm visual analogue scales.

All children reported some sensations from their joints and each of the 11 items were chosen by some children. All of the children said their joints ached and 53% of the 12–17 year olds and 50% of the 6–11 year olds indicated some form of sharp pain (cut, pricked, smacked or pinched). Burning sensation was described by 53% of the older group in contrast to 37% of the younger group.

There were marked differences between the two age groups in terms of the meaning they ascribed to the sensations. The younger group appeared to experience their joint sensations in a vacuum. They did not perceive the sensations as representing joint pathology. The older subjects unanimously reported that the sensations they experienced reminded them of their disabling condition.

Older children also interpreted their sensations as much more unpleasant, with 80% of them scoring the visual analogue scale for unpleasantness above the midpoint. Eighty-three percent of the younger group scored unpleasantness below the midpoint. In terms of pain, 42% of the younger children scored above the midpoint, whereas 80% of the older group scored above the midpoint.

Beales et al. (1983) concluded that the meaning that patients attributed to their joint sensations may have an important influence on the extent to which the sensations are experienced as unpleasant or as pain. Many of the older children had unrealistically negative views of their disease and in some cases, horrific fantasies of what was happening to them. The authors noted that appropriate counselling might be able to promote a less pessimistic view in older children and thus reduce their joint pain. This study highlights the possibility that the reactive component of pain may be at least a partially learned phenomenon.

Varni et al. (1987) investigated 25 children (19 females and 6 males) using the Varni/Thompson pediatric pain questionnaire (described in detail in chapter 3). The children's version measures the intensity, sensory, affective and evaluative qualities and location of pain. The parents' version also asks for a number of socioenvironmental, family and child background items. Results indicated that the children, parents and the doctor agreed in their estimate of the child's current pain. Correlations ranged from 0.65 for the parent and child to 0.85 for the parent and doctor. Parents and children also agreed on the worst pain experienced in the last week ($r = 0.54$). Adults tended to rate the child's pain higher than did the child. Red was the most frequently selected color for severe pain but orange, blue, black, green were also selected for severe pain. Children used the following pain descriptors most frequently (percentage of children using that word in parentheses): sore (70); aching (65); uncomfortable (65); miserable (52); tiring (48); horrible (48); pins and needles (48).

In a second study by this research group on this population, Thompson et al. (1987) examined relationships between pain perception, family environment, child psychosocial adjustment and disease parameters in 23 families who had a child with JRA. Pauciarticular JRA was rated as least painful with polyarticular JRA next and systemic JRA deemed to be the most painful. Present pain activity was significantly correlated to physician's ratings of disease activity. Multiple regression analyses of present pain and worst pain in the preceding week were undertaken against family environment scores, disease activity, arthritis subtype, and the behavior and social scales of the child behavior checklist. Thirty-three percent of the variance in present pain was accounted for by the dependent variables with the externalizing scale of the child behavior checklist contributing the greatest increase in percentage of variance (10.7%). Over 70% of worst pain experienced was predicted in the multiple regression with disease activity and the family relationship index each contributing to a 23% increase in variance accounted for. Comparisons were made between the families studied and norms for the family environment scale and the child behavior checklist. No clear results were found on the child behavior checklist except that of raised levels on the somatic complaints subscale. The family environment scales showed elevated cohesion and expressiveness subscale scores and lower conflict scores. These findings suggested enhanced family closeness.

The multiple regression results may not be stable because of the small sample size. Moreover, comparisons with norms are less robust than the use of a control group because of possible variations due to the differences in administration. As a result, the findings of this study must be viewed with caution.

2.3. Analgesics in juvenile arthritis

Treatment of pain in juvenile arthritis occurs secondary to the treatment of inflammation. ASA is the first line of treatment and the aim is to maintain blood levels of 20–30 mg% for several months (Schaller, 1984) (see chapter 4 for a discussion of ASA). ASA, at this level, usually provides adequate analgesia. Because of its relative lack of anti-inflammatory action acetaminophen is rarely used in the juvenile arthritis. For children who do not respond to ASA, non-steroidal anti-inflammatory drugs (NSAIDs) are sometimes helpful.

The use of the non-steroidal anti-inflammatory drugs with children is not clear. Some of the non-steroidal anti-inflammatory drugs have been recommended by authors (e.g., mefenamic acid, naproxen and ibuprofen by Huskisson (1984), naproxen and ibuprofen by Flower et al. (1985)) but only tolmetin and naproxen are recommended (in Canada) for use in children under 12. No clinical studies in children or adolescents are available. The non-steroidal anti-inflammatory drugs have also been recommended in dental pain, headache, dysmenorrhea, and musculoskeletal trauma. In the United States ibuprofen is now available as an over-the-counter medication.

Non-steroidal anti-inflammatory drugs are thought to have their action by inhibiting the synthesis of prostaglandin and also in some cases by antagonizing the effects of prostaglandins at the receptor sites (Flower et al., 1985).

3. Reflex sympathetic dystrophy

Reflex sympathetic dystrophy is a generic term used to indicate a constellation of signs and symptoms following injury to bone and soft tissue. Synonyms for the disorder include: Sudeck's atrophy, minor causalgia, mimocausalgia, shoulder-hand syndrome, post-traumatic pain syndrome, sympathalgia, chronic traumatic edema, reflex hyperemic deossification, traumatic reflex osteodystrophy, reflex trophoneurosis, acute bone atrophy, post-traumatic painful osteoporosis (Imanuel et al., 1981; Payne, 1986). We prefer to follow the International Association for the Study of Pain's nomenclature and use the term reflex sympathetic dystrophy (Merskey, 1986). The syndrome usually begins with a minor trauma that results in spontaneous pain, usually aching or burning in nature. The skin is initially warm, red and dry, changing to cold, bluish and sweating. There is local edema and increased hair and nail growth. The dystrophic stage begins 3–6 months after injury with continuing pain, cracked grooved ridged nails, decreased hair growth, decreased range of motion, muscle wasting, osteoporosis and edema (Payne, 1986). The final stage is marked by pain, decreased skin temperature, pale cyanotic skin, irreversible changes in the skin and subcutaneous structures and bony demineralization. Complications include: disuse atrophy of the involved limb, depression, drug abuse and suicide (Merskey, 1986).

The prevalence of the disorder in children and adolescents is unknown. Although some authors claim that there is a psychological predisposition to the disorder (Bernstein et al., 1978), there is no good evidence that this is so. It is our impression, however, that poor compliance with treatment may be important in treatment failure and that psychological and family factors may impinge on compliance. Treatment has not been carefully evaluated but typically aggressive physiotherapy is the first line of treatment. Physiotherapy may include exercises, movement and attempts to reverse the disuse that has developed. Transcutaneous electrical nerve stimulation has been reported in anecdotal case studies but has not been adequately evaluated (Stiltz et al., 1977; Richlin et al., 1978). Sympathetic block, sympathectomy and high-dose corticosteroids are used in advanced cases with adults.

4. Limb pains

Limb pain can be due to trauma, orthopedic conditions, rheumatic disease, infectious disease, malignancies, benign bony tumors, endocrine disorders, nutritional abnormalities, miscellaneous disorders, syndromes of unknown origin and psychogenic syndromes. Determination of causality is based on history, physical examination and some lab tests. Pain in the knee should always trigger careful examination of the hip as pain may be referred.

The three most common limb pain syndromes which, happily, are benign, are: growing pains, patellofemoral pain and Osgood-Schlatter's disease.

4.1. Growing pains

Growing pains have been known since earliest recorded medical history but relatively few references in the medical literature can be found for this relatively common problem. Oster and Nielsen (1972) defined the symptoms as consisting of intermittent and frequently quite incapacitating pain localized deeply in the arms and/or legs. The pain is not in the joints and it is not accompanied by tenderness, redness or swelling. There may be restlessness. The pain is nocturnal and there is no abnormality of gait. The pains are usually bilateral. There are no abnormal physical or laboratory findings and the pain does not affect daytime activities. Growing pains do not develop into pathologic conditions.

The prevalence of growing pains depends on the criteria, the method of ascertainment (British Medical Journal, 1972) and the population surveyed. Naish and Apley (1951) questioned children and their mothers attending school clinics for routine school examinations. They used very strict criteria of non-arthritic limb pains of at least 3 months duration and severe enough to interfere with activities. They estimated an incidence of 4.2%. At the other extreme, Hawksley (1939) estimated growing pains (undefined criteria) to occur in 33.6% of children attending hospital clinics. Oster and Nielsen (1972) found an incidence of 12.5% in boys and 18.4% in girls by questioning the children alone.

The cause of growing pains is unknown. With advancing knowledge of rheumatic fever and rheumatoid arthritis, rheumatic causes have now been discredited. Similarly, growth per se has been discounted as a cause. Children with growing pains do not grow differently from those who do not have growing pains and these pains do not occur during periods of maximum growth. Three theories of causation are current. They are that growing pains are caused by psychosocial problems, orthopedic abnormalities or fatigue.

Naish and Apley (1951), Apley (1970), Oster and Nielsen (1972) endorsed a psychogenic model. No studies using standardized measurement and appropriate design have been done investigating the psychogenic model. Rarely are the minimally acceptable criteria for psychogenic pain (chapter 14) met in children with growing pain.

Orthopedic abnormalities, in particular, flat foot, knock knee, or poor posture have been suggested by Hawksley (1939) as causative of growing pain. Again, no properly controlled studies have been published supporting this viewpoint.

Finally, fatigue has been suggested by Naish and Apley (1951) but their data suggested that pain following exertion was prevalent particularly with children who had predominantly diurnal pain. The authors suggested that exertion in combination with psychologic disturbance was causative.

Growing pains are typically managed by reassurance that the child would outgrow it or by non-specific interventions such as heat, massage and ASA or acetaminophen. The only randomized trial of treatment known to us is one recently completed by Baxter (1986). She randomly assigned 36 children between 5 and 14 years of age with growing pains to either a follow-up condition or a stretching exercise regimen. Each child had been examined for

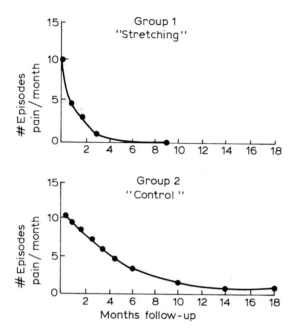

Fig. 1. Effects of stretching exercises on growing pain. (Reprinted from Baxter, 1986, with permission.)

orthopedic abnormality (hip range of motion; scoliosis, degree of SLR; degree of tibial torsion; presence of LLD; presence of foot deformities) and none were found. As can be seen in Fig. 1, the stretching group's pain quickly resolved, whereas the follow-up group did not significantly improve.

The stretching treatment was based on a fatigue model which hypothesized that fatigue in predisposed individuals caused growing pains. The exact mechanism is not known.

4.2. Patellofemoral pain

Patellofemoral pain is often called chondromalacia patellae. The term was coined by Aleman (1928) because of presumed patellar cartilage changes. However, arthroscopy has shown that changes in cartilage are not associated with the clinical symptoms (Insall, 1979). Patellofemoral pain is diagnosed by a history of usually anteromedial pain aggravated by stair climbing, cycling, or prolonged sitting with the knee flexed. There is often clicking, catching or giving way. There may be locking. Persistent effusion is not characteristic.

There is no atrophy and no systemic findings. The adolescent female athlete may be the most frequent sufferer. True chondromalacia patella with softening, fibrillation, fissuring or erosion of the cartilage (Bentley, 1970) does occur but is an infrequent cause of patellofemoral pain in children (Insall, 1979).

The rate of occurrence of the disorder is not known. However, in a recent survey of a sample of 446 adolescents aged 13–17 years, 31% reported knee pain (Fairbank et al., 1984). Boys and girls were equally represented in the pain group. Of this group, 25 adolescents (18%) had stopped sports because of the pain and 40 adolescents (29%) reported visiting a doctor because of the pain. No measures of the severity of pain were taken.

The most widely accepted hypothesis is that the problem is due to malalignment and subsequent abnormalities of patellar tracking (Insall, 1979). Mechanical causes have also been suggested. There is however little empirical support for any specific etiology. Fairbank et al. (1984) found no relationship between having pain and a series of objective measurements of joint mobility, the Q-angle, genu valgum and anteversion of the femoral neck. The only statistically significant finding was that 55% of the pain group reported engaging in sports as much as possible whereas only 40% of the pain-free group said they did sports as often as possible. Although statistically significant, the clinical meaning of this difference is not clear. No actual measure of participation was taken. The authors concluded that chronic overloading rather than faulty mechanics cause pattelofemoral pain.

Treatments that have been suggested include surgery, bracing, and stretching and strengthening exercises. There is no clear evidence for the efficacy of any of these interventions and no controlled studies have been done.

The natural history of the disorder is benign. Sandow and Goodfellow (1985) found that almost all of 54 female adolescents presenting with patellofemoral knee pain still experienced some pain when followed 2–8 years after initial presentation but many (46%) reported reduced severity and few (13%) reported worsening of symptoms. Only 17% of patients had restricted their sports activity due to pain. None had developed significant knee pathology.

4.3. Osgood-Schlatter's disease

Osgood-Schlatter's disease is marked by pain, swelling and tenderness in the tibial tuberosity. There is often a limp. Pressure on the tibial tuberosity reproducing the pain is virtually diagnostic. Radiograph will usually show an abnormal tibial tuberosity but a radiograph is unnecessary in the typical case (Feldman et al., 1987).

The prevalence of the disorder is unknown but a recent survey of 446 pupils found six boys with what was thought to be mild Osgood-Schlatter's disease (Fairbank et al., 1984).

Osgood-Schlatter's disease is treated by avoidance of activities that cause pain, or by taking analgesics prior to exercise. There is no evidence that children who continue activity in the face of pain do themselves any harm.

5. Other orthopedic pain

5.1. Hip pain

Transient synovitis of the hip is the most common cause of painful hips in children and has been suggested as a precursor to Legg-Calvé-Perthes disease (Jacobs, 1971). Legg-Calvé-Perthes disease is aseptic necrosis of the femoral head. It is found primarily in children under 10 years of age. Diagnosis is by X-ray. Treatment is by bracing or traction while revascularization occurs (Bowyer and Hollister, 1984). The exact prevalence and causation of these disorders is unknown.

5.2. Back pain

Back pain is exceedingly common in adults (Spitzer, 1986). However, it is rare in children and when it occurs, back pain is frequently of pathological origin (King, 1984). Bunnell (1982) has suggested four categories of pediatric back pain: mechanical problems, developmental abnormalities, inflammatory processes and neoplastic processes.

King (1984) has warned of the danger of lightly diagnosing psychological causation:

> Children, like adults, are affected by stress and their environment. However, children rarely respond to stress with physical complaints that have no evidence of organic pathology. For this reason, a child's complaint should not be attributed to hysteria and/or malingering *(King, 1984, p. 1094)*.

No studies have been done on the quality of back pain in children or the correlates of back pain in children.

There have been proposals to teach children 'back hygiene' consisting of proper posture and back exercises in order to prevent back pain in adulthood (Fine, 1982). Such a program may be helpful in preventing back pain. On the other hand, it may be useless or harmful (McGrath and Manion, 1987). No evaluation of such programs has been done.

5.3. Rickets

Rickets are not infrequent in Asian immigrants and can occur in any child. The main factors causing rickets in Asian immigrants have been suggested as: lack of exposure to sunlight, sometimes due to covering for modesty; vegetarian diets; use of unfortified cow's milk for infant feeding; maternal deficiency of vitamin D during pregnancy (Black, 1984). Rickets is a painful disease and may present in infancy to adolescence. Pain is experienced in the back and legs and may be severe enough to delay walking or induce a previously walking toddler to stop walking. In adolescence, deformities are unlikely but limb pain or backache are common presenting problems (Black, 1984).

5.4. Fibrositis, fibromyalgia or myofibritis

This disorder of unknown etiology is characterized by aches, pains and stiffness at multiple sites. The condition is exacerbated by fatigue, stress, inactivity and cold, damp weather. Victims also suffer from sleep disturbances, headaches, irritable bowel syndrome, feelings of numbness and subjective feelings of swelling (Bowyer and Hollister, 1984). Laboratory investigations are normal except for a deficiency of stages 3 and 4 non-REM sleep. Although psychological causes have been suggested, the best evidence is that psychological factors are not causative (Campbell et al., 1983). The prevalence of this disorder in children is unknown.

Treatment usually involves non-steroidal anti-inflammatory drugs, warmth and suggestions for increasing exercise and increasing opportunities for sleep.

6. *Clinical guidelines*

In general, musculoskeletal pain in children and adolescents should not be regarded as of psychogenic origin unless there is clear evidence of psychogenicity. Conservative management is less invasive and has less potential for possible harm to the child.

7. Future directions

(1) Incidence and prevalence studies of childhood arthritic diseases, of specific subtypes of arthritic disease and of reflex sympathetic dystrophy are necessary.
(2) Evaluation of conservative management of growing pains, patellofemoral pain, and Osgood-Schlatter's disease are vital.
(3) Examination of the pharmacokinetics, safety and efficacy of the non-steroidal anti-inflammatory drugs in children is required.
(4) Evaluation of treatments of reflex sympathetic dystrophy in children is needed.

References

Aleman, O. (1928) Chondromalacia posttraumatica patellae. Acta Chir. Scand. 63, 149–190.

Apley, J. (1970) Clinical canutes: A philosophy of paediatrics. Sect. Paediatr. 63, 479–484.

Baxter, M. (1986) Growth pains and growing pains. Paper presented at Clinical Review Day Children's Hospital of Eastern Ontario.

Beales, J.G., Keen, J.H. and Lennox Holt, P.J. (1983) The child's perception of the disease and experience of pain in juvenile chronic arthritis. J. Rheumatol. 10, 61–65.

Bentley, G. (1970) Chondromalacia patellae. J. Bone Jt. Surg. Ser. A 52, 221–232.

Bernstein, B.H., Singsen, B.H., Kent, J.T., Kornreich, H., King, K., Hicks, R. and Hanson, V. (1978) Reflex neurovascular dystrophy in childhood. J. Pediatr. 93, 211–215.

Black, J. (1984) The New Paediatrics: Child Health in Ethnic Minorities (British Medical Journal Press, London) pp. 23–24.

Bowyer, S.L. and Hollister, J.R. (1984) Limb pain in childhood. Pediatr. Clin. North Am. 31, 1053–1081.

British Medical Journal (1972) Growing pains, 5823, 365–366.

Bunnell, W.P. (1982) Back pain in children. Orthop. Clin. North Am. 13, 587–604.

Campbell, S.M., Clark, S., Tindall, E.A., Forehand, M.E. and Bennett, R.M. (1983) Clinical characteristics of fibrositis. I. A blinded controlled study of symptoms and tender points. Arthritis Rheum. 26, 817–824.

Fairbank, J.C.T., Pynsent, P.B., Van Poortvliet, J.A. and Philips, H. (1984) Mechanical factors in the incidence of knee pain in adolescents and young adults. J. Bone Jt. Surg. Ser. B 66, 685–693.

Feldman, W., Rosser, W. and McGrath, P.J. (1987) Primary Medical Care of Children and Adolescents (Oxford University Press, New York), pp. 202–204.

Fine, J. (1982) Spinal Column. Back to Back 2, 1–4.

Flower, R.J., Moncada, S. and Vane, J.R. (1985) Analgesic-Antipyretics and Anti-Inflammatory Agents; Drugs Employed in the Treatment of Gout. In: A.G. Gilman, L.S. Goodman, T.W. Rall and F. Murad (Eds.), Goodman and Gilman's the Pharmacological Basis of Therapeutics, 7th edn. (Macmillan, New York) pp. 674–715.

Hawksley, J.C. (1939) The nature of growing pains and their relation to rheumatism in children and adolescents. Br. Med. J. 1, 155–157.

Huskisson, E.C. (1984) Non-narcotic analgesics. In: P.D. Wall and R. Melzack (Eds.), Textbook of Pain (Churchill Livingstone, Edinburgh) pp. 505–513.

Imanuel, H.M., Levy, F.L. and Geldwert, J.J. (1981) Sudeck's atrophy: A review of the literature. J. Foot Surg. 20, 243–246.

Insall, J. (1979) Chondromalacia patellae: Patellar malalignment syndrome. Orthop. Clin. North Am. 10, 117–127.

Jacobs, B.W. (1971) Synovitis of the hip in children and its significance. Pediatrics 47, 558–566.

King, H.A. (1984) Back pain in children. Pediatr. Clin. North Am. 31, 1083–1095.

Laaksonen, A.L. and Laine, V. (1961) A comparative study of joint pain in adult and juvenile rheumatoid arthritis. Ann. Rheum. Dis. 20, 386–387.

McGrath, P.J. and Manion, I.G. (1987) Prevention of pain problems. In: K.D. Craig and S. Weiss (Eds.), Prevention and Early Intervention: Biobehavioral Perspectives (Springer, New York), in press.

Merskey, H. (Ed.) (1986) Classification of chronic pain: description of chronic pain syndromes and definition of pain terms. Pain suppl. 3, S29–S30.

Naish, J.M. and Apley, J. (1951) 'Growing pains': A clinical study of non-arthritic limb pains in children. Arch. Dis. Child. 26, 134–140.

Oster, J. and Nielsen, A. (1972) Growing pains: A clinical investigation of a school population. Acta Paediatr. Scand. 61, 329–334.

Passo, M.H. (1982) Aches and limb pain. Pediatr. Clin. North Am. 29, 209–219.

Payne, R. (1986) Neuropathic pain syndromes, with special reference to causalgia and reflex sympathetic dystrophy. Clin. J. Pain 2, 59–73.

Richlin, D.M., Carron, H., Rowlingson, J.C., Sussman, M.D., Baugher, W.H. and Goldner, R.D. (1978) Reflex sympathetic dystrophy: successful treatment by transcutaneous nerve stimulation. J. Pediatr. 93, 84–86.

Ross, D.M. and Ross, S.A. (1984) Childhood pain: the school-aged child's viewpoint. Pain 20, 179–191.

Sandow, M.J. and Goodfellow, J.W. (1985) The natural history of anterior knee pain in adolescents. J. Bone Jt. Surg. 67, 36–38.

Schaller, J.G. (1984) Chronic childhood arthritis and the spondylarthropathies. In: A. Calin (Ed.), Spondylarthropathies (Grune and Stratton, New York) pp. 187–208.

Scott, P.J., Ansell, B.M. and Huskisson, E.C. (1977) Measurement of pain in juvenile chronic polyarthritis. Ann. Rheum. Dis. 36, 186–187.

Spitzer, W. (1986) Rapport du Groupe de Travail Quebequois sur les Aspects Cliniques des Affections Vertebrales chez les Travailleurs (Task Force on Spinal Disorders, Quebec Workers' Health and Safety Commission, Quebec).

Still, G.F. (1897) On a form of chronic joint disease in children. Med. Chir. Trans. 80, 47–59.

Stiltz, R.J., Carron, H. and Sanders, D.B. (1977) Reflex sympathetic dystrophy in a 6-year-old: Successful treatment by transcutaneous nerve stimulation. Anesth. Analg. 56, 438–443.

Thompson, K.L., Varni, J.W. and Hanson, V. (1987) Comprehensive assessment of pain in juvenile rheumatoid arthritis: An empirical model. J. Pediatr. Psychol., in press.

Varni, J.W., Thompson, K.L. and Hanson, V. (1987) The Varni/Thompson Pediatric Pain Questionnaire: I. Chronic musculoskeletal pain in juvenile rheumatoid arthritis. Pain 28, 27–38.

CHAPTER 10

Cancer pain

1. Introduction

In the layman's mind, cancer and pain are almost synonymous. A recent survey (Levin et al., 1985) found that cancer was perceived to be an extremely painful disease relevant to other medical conditions. Cancer pain has been identified by the World Health Organization as an important global health issue (Stjernsward, 1985). The clinical management of pain for young cancer victims has long concerned parents and clinicians but, because almost no research has been done, little is known about pediatric cancer pain.

In this chapter, we will discuss the prevalence of pain from cancer and the management of cancer pain which may be due to the disease itself and/or to its treatment. We will also consider several special issues of pediatric cancer pain, that is, the meaning of pain to the child, reactions of significant people to the child, disruption of school and social life, and the Damocles syndrome. Finally, we will propose guidelines for clinical practice and future directions for pediatric cancer pain research.

2. Prevalence

There is ample evidence that a large number of adult cancer patients endure a great deal of pain. In his extensive review of prevalence studies of pain in cancer, Bonica (1985) tabulated the results of 47 reports on cancer pain. He concluded that 68% of far advanced cancer patients and 50% of other cancer patients had serious pain problems.

Foley (1985) has suggested that patients with cancer pain can be classified into five groups: (1) patients with acute cancer-related pain associated either with the diagnosis or treatment of the cancer; (2) patients with chronic, cancer-related pain associated with cancer progression or cancer therapy; (3) patients with pre-existing chronic pain and cancer-related pain; (4) patients with a history of drug addiction and cancer-related pain; (5) dying patients with cancer-related pain. An alternative, which may be more appropriate for children, is to classify the pain as: (1) due to the disease itself; (2) due to the diagnostic procedures involved; or (3) due to the treatment (chemotherapy or irradiation). The usefulness of each of these classifications has not been demonstrated. However, both Bonica (1985) and Foley (1985) note that pain is often from more than one site or source.

Studies of the prevalence of cancer pain suffer from several deficiencies. The vast majority of these studies derive their data from medical records rather than from direct measurement of pain reported by the patients themselves. Such data are from multiple sources whose reliability and validity are unknown. Most of the studies are based on undescribed samples of patients. Therefore, the studies often do not detail the extent or nature of cancer pain from the different types of disease and the various treatments and procedures. Finally, none of the studies have considered the pain experienced by children.

Writers such as Beales (1979) have noted that severe intractable pain is frequent in adult cancer victims but less frequent in children. For many children, however, pain is an important and distressing feature of their disease. Pain has been described as an important component in the most common solid tumors.

> Pain is a constant, even if not always early sign of systemic or disseminated neoplasms (leukaemia, Ewing's tumor, Hodgkin or non-Hodgkin lymphoma, primary or secondary bone tumor) *(Ottolenghi and Marradi, 1984, p. 391)*.

Ventafridda et al. (1984) reported that an analysis of 135 cases from 1 to 18 years of age revealed that the prevalence of physical pain appears in decreasing order for Ewing sarcoma, leukemia, lymphoma, embryonal rhabdomyosarcoma, neuroblastoma, malignant hemangioma and in cancer of the ovaries in puberty. However, no data were presented upon which to base these conclusions.

P.A. McGrath et al. (1985) very briefly reported on the intensity of pain experienced by children undergoing procedures for treatment of their cancer. The procedures were rated on a 150 mm visual analogue scale. The ratings were: finger prick, 6.3; intravenous, 13.4; lumbar puncture, 31.7. Unfortunately, the sample is not described in any detail and even the number of subjects or their recruitment is not clear. There is no description of pain due to the disease itself. As well, there appear to be a number of contradictions in the data. For example, children with lumbar punctures under sedation were reported to experience more pain than children undergoing lumbar punctures without sedation. This may be due to the pain caused by the use of intramuscular injection to produce sedation, because patients who were more likely to be distressed were sedated, or because the sedation itself increased pain.

The need for better data on the prevalence of cancer pain in children led us (McGrath et al., 1986) to undertake a survey of all the children in the Oncology Clinic at the Children's Hospital of Eastern Ontario. Each child over 7 years and the parents were asked to rate the intensity of pain from various procedures, from treatment and from their disease. For children under 7 years only the parents were surveyed. The study is in progress but preliminary results indicate that a high percentage of children report considerably more pain both from disease and from what are considered minor procedures such as venipuncture, than has been previously reported.

3. Management of pain from treatment

Several studies have focussed on measurement of pain due to procedures. Measurement studies were discussed in chapter 3. The most extensive literature in pediatric cancer pain has been on the management of pain due to procedures. The major focus of these studies has been pain due to diagnostic lumbar punctures and bone marrow aspirations. Little consideration has been given to pain as a side effect of treatment. For example, chemotherapy and radiation treatments may result in painful mucositis. Surgery used to treat the cancer may cause considerable pain during recovery.

Anxiety is of major importance in cancer pain. With children, the anticipation of pain from aversive procedures frequently increases with each negative experience so that each subsequent procedure becomes more painful (Katz et al., 1980). Theoretically, the impact of anxiety on pain should be on the affective aspect of the pain rather than on the sensory aspect (Melzack, 1983). However, the differential measurement of these aspects have not been validated in children. Of course, pain is no less real if its intensity is enhanced by anxiety.

Poor technique resulting in botched attempts to get samples may be important if inexperienced staff are expected to do testing without training. As in the neonatal intensive care unit, sophisticated teaching modules with computer-assisted models to learn how to do these procedures may be helpful.

3.1. Psychological methods

The majority of research in this area has focussed on the use of hypnosis. In one of the first reports of management of pain due to cancer treatment, Hilgard and Morgan (1976) described a clinical series in which 24 consecutive patients aged 4–19 years were referred for pain relief. Three patients had continuous pain from their disease, five reported problems with intravenous injections and changing bandages and 16 patients had problems dealing with lumbar punctures and bone marrow aspirations. Hypnosis was not successful with the children with disease-related pain. Four of the five children with pain from short procedures obtained substantial to excellent pain relief with hypnosis. Only one of the ten 4–6-year-olds who were referred for pain from lumbar punctures and bone marrow aspirations were helped by hypnotic procedures. Four of the six older children (7–19-year-olds) were substantially helped. Olness (1981) reported that 21 of a clinical series of 25 patients agreed to use hypnotic techniques, and 19 of these patients demonstrated substantial symptom relief. She emphasized that hypnosis was most effective when it was first used near the time of the child's initial diagnosis of cancer, so that few negative experiences with procedures were allowed to occur. Unfortunately, no control groups were used and measurement consisted of the unstandardized judgement of the authors in these clinical series.

Several non-controlled studies of hypnotic pain relief have used standardized measurement. Hilgard and LeBaron (1982) obtained baseline measures on 63 children and adolescents with cancer who were undergoing lumbar punctures and bone marrow aspirations. Twenty-four children and adolescents accepted the invitation to participate in a hypnotic pain control program. Nineteen of the 24 children were highly hypnotizable. Ten of these participants reduced self-reported pain substantially by the first hypnotic treatment and five more reduced self-reported pain by the second treatment. None of the four less hypnotizable subjects were successful. The results of this project are described in detail in Hypnotherapy of Pain in Children with Cancer (Hilgard and LeBaron, 1984). This volume also contains a great deal of clinical detail that will be of interest to the clinician or researcher.

In another, non-controlled hypnosis study, Kellerman et al. (1983) treated 18 adolescents. Nine of them had problems with bone marrow aspirations. Two adolescents had difficulty with lumbar punctures and seven reported that injections were the problem. Two patients rejected hypnosis and the remaining 16 adolescents participated in the hypnosis treatment. Patients were given an explanation of hypnosis that emphasized self-help. Initial induction using eye fixation or hand levitation was followed by suggestions for progressive relaxation, slow rhythmic breathing, increased feelings of well being, and visualization of a pleasant scene or event. Patients practised the hypnosis before the procedure and were prompted at the time of the lumbar puncture, bone marrow aspiration or venipuncture. The results were most encouraging with statistically significant group differences and 16 of 18 patients reporting significant pain reduction. Pain was measured by a 0–10 rating by two independent judges and also by self-report on the same scale. Decreases in situational anxiety and trait anxiety were also found.

In a recent paper, P.A. McGrath and De Veber (1986) described an integrated approach using hypnosis, relaxation training, visual imagery, distraction and desensitization to reduce pain and anxiety in children undergoing lumbar punctures. In their prospective series of 14 children, they found that children above 5 years of age were able to use these methods to reduce pain, as measured by reports of a parent and a nurse on visual analogue scales and a behavioral checklist.

Case studies and clinical series such as have been described up to this point are helpful in generating ideas but, because they do not have appropriate experimental controls, they provide only very weak evidence for the effectiveness of the treatment methods used.

Using a single subject experimental design, Jay et al. (1985) demonstrated the efficacy of psychological intervention for five subjects undergoing bone marrow aspiration between 3.5 and 7 years of age. The design was a multiple baseline design across subjects with a staggered baseline. The psychological intervention consisted of: reinforcement for coping; breathing exercises; imagery; role playing; behavioral rehearsal; and filmed modelling by a 'coping' model. The child was accompanied by his or her parent and the psychologist who coached the child in the use of these procedures. The results demonstrated a uniformly effective reduction of distress as measured by the observational scale of behavioral distress (Jay et al., 1983). Single subject designs such as that used by Jay et al. (1985) do provide experimental control but the results are less generalizable to other children than are randomized controlled trials.

In a randomized controlled trial, Zeltzer and LeBaron (1982) compared hypnotic and non-hypnotic techniques in helping 27 children and adolescents with bone marrow aspiration and 22 children and adolescents during lumbar puncture. Non-hypnotic techniques included a combination of deep breathing, distraction and practice sessions. Hypnotic techniques focussed on imagery. During bone marrow aspiration, pain was reduced to a large extent by hypnosis and to a smaller but significant extent by non-hypnotic techniques. Only hypnosis was effective in reducing anxiety. Although, in general, this was an excellent study, one thing might have been confounded. The children in the hypnosis group were given more information as to the exact timing of each element of the procedures than were the children in the non-hypnotic group. It may be that this ability to predict each part of the procedure may have been important in the success of treatment. Moreover, objective observational measures were not used. Ratings by observers, which were used in this study, have the disadvantage that the behaviors on which the raters based their estimations of pain and distress are not identified.

In a recent randomized trial, Katz et al. (1987) studied 36 children between the ages of 6 and 11 years of age with acute lymphoblastic leukemia who had experienced distress when undergoing bone marrow aspiration. The design included hypnosis and non-directed play as the two treatment conditions, with dependent measures taken during baseline and intervention bone marrow aspirations. In order to ensure blindness of the nurses and raters, hypnosis was not done during the actual procedures but post-hypnotic suggestion with a covert cue was used. The psychologist accompanied children in both groups into the treatment room and provided encouragement to all children. Children in both the hypnosis and the non-directed play groups showed significant decreases in self-reported fear and pain during bone marrow aspirations. Behavioral distress as measured by the procedures behavior rating scale (revised) (Katz et al., 1982) did not decline in either group. Rapport between the therapist and the child showed moderate correlation with self-report measures of pain for two of three of the post-treatment bone marrow aspirations. There were no ethnic differences. Girls tended to exhibit more distress behavior than boys.

The Katz et al. (1987) study is an example of the difficulty in conducting well designed clinical research. In order to ensure that the raters and the nurses involved in the procedures were not biased, the hypnosis was not done during sessions. The failure to find significant differences between the two groups may have been because of attenuation of the power of the hypnosis because of this methodologically correct maneuver. Unfortunately, there are no easy solutions to this type of problem.

Kuttner et al. (1985) used a randomized controlled trial to compare hypnotic techniques with distraction and standard medical treatment in helping 48 children between 3 and 10 years of age cope with bone marrow aspiration. Standard medical treatment consisted of providing information of what was about to happen and friendly warm conversation. The hypnotic technique and a wide range of distraction and breathing techniques used with the younger children have been described in detail (Kuttner, 1984) and is demonstrated in a commercially available videotape: No Fears...No Tears (Kuttner, 1986). Basically, the technique involved asking the children to relate their favorite story and then the therapist interweaves this story with the actual events occurring during the bone marrow aspiration. Treatment was carried out during the procedures so that raters could not be blinded. Measurement was self-report, raters' judgements and an objective scale (the procedures behavior rating scale, revised (Katz et al., 1982)). They found that hypnosis was most effective for the younger (3–6-year-olds) group. The older group (7–10-year-olds) did well with both experimental strategies but there was a trend to do somewhat better using distraction strategies. All groups at both age levels did well on the second post-treatment procedure. This may have been due to contamination of the control groups as the clinical staff became aware of the success of the treatments. Hypnosis tended to work in an all or none fashion. However, the distraction strategies worked in a graded pattern suggesting that a skill was being learned. The availability of a technique to help young cancer patients undergoing aversive medical procedures is particularly important since leukemia is most frequent in this age group.

A prominent debate in the hypnosis literature focusses on the nature of hypnosis and, indeed, whether hypnosis should be regarded as a distinct state or simply as a situation of enhanced suggestibility in which the person who is hypnotized engages in role playing and goal directed behavior. The opposite sides of the debate have been clearly argued by Hilgard (1977) who maintains that hypnosis is an altered state and by Spanos (1986) who believes that hypnosis is best conceptualized in terms of relaxation, imagery and suggestion. Fortunately, for the clinician interested in alleviating children's pain, the debate is academic. If the procedures described as hypnosis are detailed sufficiently to allow reproducibility, it does not matter whether they are due to hypnotic trance or due to other mechanisms.

3.2. Pharmacological methods

Pharmacological methods for helping children deal with the pain from treatments are widely used but have not been systematically researched. Typically, children who are undergoing lumbar punctures and bone marrow aspirations are infiltrated subcutaneously with a local anesthetic prior to needle injection. This reduces the surface puncture pain.

The use of sedation during lumbar puncture and bone marrow aspiration is not uncommon, especially in younger children. Many children report that they do not like the feeling of sedation and would rather not be sedated in these procedures (Ross and Ross, 1982). Diazepam is most commonly used. Alternatively, a cocktail is used to sedate children for a variety of procedures. Bray (1969) suggested a mixture of 25 mg of meperidine, 6.25 mg of promethazine and 6.25 mg of chlorpromazine per 1 ml of solution given i.m. 45 min before the procedure. The recommended dose is 0.1 ml/kg with a maximum dose of 2 ml. Recently, at our hospital, the above mixture has been used in conjunction with oral chloral hydrate (50 mg/kg) with excellent results. Unfortunately, the mixture must be given intramuscularly and the pain of the needle may be very frightening to the child. General anesthetics are not commonly used in North America ostensibly because of cost and medical risk. The practice in most North American Centers to use general anesthetic only with very resistive children who present a safety hazard when they are not anesthetized. However, general anesthetic is routine in British and European centers. Ketamine, for example, is used extensively with little risk and little additional cost.

In a randomized, double-blind crossover, placebo-controlled study, Clarke and Radford (1986) evaluated the use of a topical anesthetic cream (EMLA) in the reduction of pain due to venipuncture in children undergoing repeated venipuncture for chemotherapy. The cream is a combination of equal parts of lignocaine and prilocaine in an emulsion. Pain was measured using visual analogue scales and a four category, author-developed scale which asked the child to relate the amount of pain to the typical venipuncture. Fourteen of 15 children completed the study. Results clearly favored the active treatment. The authors suggested the use of anesthetic cream with children who require regular venipuncture.

Similar results were reported by Wahlstedt et al. (1984) who also found that technicians rated EMLA-assisted venipuncture as easier than placebo-assisted venipuncture.

Mucositis (inflammation of the lining of the mouth) is a painful and irritating side effect of chemotherapy and local radiation treatment. Systemic analgesics (both opioid and non-opioid) are sometimes helpful. Topical anesthetics, in the form of a mouth wash, have been used but cause numbness of the mouth which is unpleasant for many and may lead to accidental injury. ASA gum may provide brief relief. Recently, a non-steroidal anti-inflammatory agent in topical form, benzydamine, has been developed and tested. Used as a mouth wash, benzydamine has been shown superior to placebo for treatment of mucositis in a number of randomized trials with adults (Mahon and De Gregorio, 1985). No trials have been done for this indication with children. It should be as effective as with adults for any child old enough to gargle and willing to comply.

3.3. Surgical and other methods

In children with serious problems in coping with the pain, especially from intravenous procedures, and who have poor peripheral venous access, the use of a Hickman-type catheter (Hickman et al., 1979) is sometimes advisable. The procedure involves surgical implantation of an external catheter. Unfortunately, external catheters carry high risk of infection, may limit activities such as swimming and are often seen as disfiguring by children and adolescents. Newer, totally implantable systems, such as the Port-a-Cath, have the advantages of substantially less care in terms of dressing changes and heparin flushes, reduced risk of infectious complications (Lokich et al., 1985) and unobtrusiveness. McDowell et al. (1986) have established the practice of implanting a Port-a-Cath in all children under 4 who were to receive prolonged chemotherapy as well as in older children when indicated.

4. Management of pain from the disease

4.1. Pharmacological methods

The literature on pharmacological pain control in pediatric cancer has virtually ignored the control of common cancer pain and has focussed on the terminal or very seriously distressed patient.

Routine pharmacological management of pain in pediatric cancer should follow the general strategies that have been developed for adults. There is no doubt that adequate pain control exists for almost everyone, no matter how severe the pain is (Angell, 1982). Simple stepwise programs of cancer pain therapy such as that recommended by the Canadian Expert Advisory Committee (Scott, 1984), if implemented, would control almost all severe cancer pain. Fig. 1 details the four-step program progressing from non-opioids (ASA or acetaminophen) for mild pain to strong opioids, such as morphine, for severe pain. Emphasis is placed on prevention of pain by use of

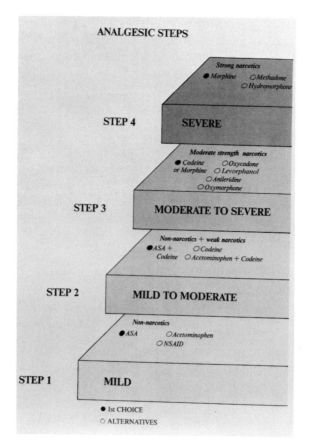

Fig. 1. Stepwise analgesic program. (Reprinted from Scott, 1984, and used with permission of the author and Health and Welfare, Canada.)

scheduled medication and on the use of simple regimens well known to the prescribing physician.

The average pediatric cancer patient will probably be helped by judicious medications on the first steps of the ladder in Fig. 1 by use of acetaminophen, or ASA. The second step may include peripherally acting analgesics in combination with centrally acting analgesics such as ASA or acetaminophen + codeine.

With infants and young children, specific problems arise. These problems are similar to those that arise with post-operative pain (see chapter 4). Lack of knowledge and familiarity in using opioids with children and the difficulty in measuring pain in children complicate adequate provision of pain relief.

Undermedication may result from a fear of addiction. Respiratory depression can be a serious difficulty if not monitored carefully.

Miser and her colleagues have published clinical series outlining their work with opioid analgesics with pediatric oncology patients. Miser et al. (1980) described their experience with eight children in the terminal stages of malignancy whose pain could not be controlled by oral or intermittent parenteral opioids. These children were treated with morphine sulfate administered as a continuous intravenous infusion using a constant infusion pump. Infusions lasted from 1 day to 16 days and pain relief was deemed adequate in three cases and complete in five cases. The dosage range that was needed for complete pain relief ranged from 0.025 to 2.6 mg/kg per h and the median dose was 0.04–0.07 mg/kg per h. The investigators found that the intravenous infusion provided uniform pain relief, avoided the marked fluctuations common with intermittent parenteral administration and resulted in only mild and easily controlled side effects.

In another clinical series, Miser et al. (1983) examined the use of subcutaneous infusion of morphine in 17 children with severe cancer pain. A constant infusion syringe pump connected to a 25 or 27 gauge needle by means of a line as long as 107 cm was used. The needle was inserted subcutaneously into the front of the thigh and the site was rotated every 24–48 h. Freedom from pain more than 95% of the time was accomplished for every case. Dosage was similar (range 0.025–1.79 mg/kg per h; median dosage 0.06 mg/kg per h) to those used for intravenous infusion. Drowsiness occurred in nine of the 12 patients but did not interfere with the child's interaction with family, friends and staff. In five out of 15 patients, mild respiratory depression to a rate of 10–15 breaths/min developed. Constipation was not an important problem in any patient. A notable feature of the subcutaneous route was that three of the patients were able to be treated at home.

Oral methadone, with a starting dose of 0.1 mg/kg given every 4 h or the equivalent daily dose given less frequently, was studied in a series by Miser and Miser (1986). They found that of the 22 courses given to 19 children, who were not controlled on other oral medication, 21 courses gave adequate pain control.

Rafart et al. (1984) briefly reported on success using a syrup similar to Brompton's cocktail with 18 children with advanced cancer. The syrup containing morphine, cocaine, orange syrup, gin, chlorpromazine and water was given every 4 h.

The routine use of oral sustained release morphine tablets in children with cancer pain has been pioneered by Goldman and Bowman (1987) at the

Hospital for Sick Children at Great Ormond Street, London, England. They reported on a series of 46 children with an age range of 1–18 years (median 6 years). Their practice has evolved with experience but they now have a general starting dose of 1 mg/kg per dose, with short acting opioids for breakthrough pain. Constipation and initial drowsiness were frequent side effects. Bad dreams and hallucinations were reported by two patients, and intolerable itching by two patients. Nausea was transient and uncommon; vomiting was rare. Respiratory depression was noted in one patient given an inappropriate initial dose. The authors concluded that oral sustained release morphine tablets are effective, convenient and acceptable in treating pain in the home care of the terminally ill child with cancer.

Clinicians should be aware that children may need pain control more at night when outside stimuli are minimal and they may feel lonely and isolated. Many children with cancer fear going to bed because of the fear of pain and distress once the lights are out.

4.2. Psychological methods

Although no systematic research has been done, it is evident from clinical practice that combining psychological methods and medication may provide optimum relief. Hilgard and LeBaron (1984) described six types of activities that they have noted to improve cancer pain control. These are: personal contact, fantasy activities, story telling and story reading, appropriate television stories, games, and filling unfilled time. Skills such as relaxation, meditative breathing and self-hypnosis can be used to augment pharmacologic pain relief. As Beales (1979) emphasized, everyone involved in the care of the child with cancer has a role to play in psychological pain management. Parents can play a major role in providing reassurance during painful procedures and they can help reduce the unpleasant associations that children have about the disease. Parents can also cue pain control strategies in their children. An important role that should not be underestimated is that of advocacy if appropriate pain relief is not being provided. Finally, parents can minimize the impact of the disease and reduce pain by helping the child live a full life.

4.3. Surgical and other methods

Surgical methods for pain relief in cancer are of four types: (1) to reduce compression on nerves or structures; (2) to ablate 'pain pathways'; (3) to destroy 'pain centers'; or (4) to orthopedically reconstruct damage due to disease or previous surgery.

Transcutaneous electrical nerve stimulation (TENS) has been described by Pichard et al. (1985) as particularly effective in deafferentation pain.

Regional blocks may be of use in specific cases (Pichard et al., 1985) but have not been extensively described for pediatric cancer pain.

5. Special issues

Since pain is not simply a sensory event, the entire context of the individual must be considered. Only a holistic approach will enable the problems of the child or adolescent with cancer to be understood.

5.1. The meaning of the pain to the child

As we discussed in chapter 2, Gaffney and Dunne (1987) have shown that many children believe that pain is a punishment for their transgressions. Moreover, children tend to believe that illness is due to misbehavior (Peters, 1978). In effect, children with pain and cancer are in double jeopardy for blaming themselves for their condition. Self-blame by children with cancer pain will increase their suffering and may make treatment more difficult. Children who blame themselves may not report pain and may not co-operate with pain treatment because they may feel that they deserve to suffer.

5.2. Reaction of significant others

Most laymen believe that childhood cancer is a sentence of death and indeed, until recently, most children who were victims of cancer did die. However, the survival rate for childhood cancer has now dramatically improved. Blotcky et al. (1985), in a study of 32 pediatric cancer patients 3 months postdiagnosis, found that parental coping behavior and their subjective distress were good predictors of the childrens' feelings of hopelessness. Parents, who were able to foster family integration and to maintain their own stability, had children who were more optimistic about their disease. Although this was not tested in this study, it is reasonable to believe that optimism about one's disease would tend to decrease the pain and distress from procedures, treatment and from the disease.

Children with cancer arouse strong emotions in parents, teachers and other adults. In many cases, these feelings include pity and a strong desire to protect the child from any possible harm. Pity may lead to lower levels of expectation and fewer maturity demands. Similarly, excessive concern over possible harm may result in overprotection (Parker, 1983). Finally, medical staff working with pediatric cancer patients must guard against a tendency to become inappropriately attached in a way that discourages independent coping. These styles of interaction can rob the child of a sense of self-worth or power and decrease ability to cope with pain. Koocher and O'Malley (1981) have detailed what they call the Damocles syndrome that affects families whose children are in remission from cancer. They noted that the child in remission and the family are under constant threat of possible reoccurrence of disease. This long-term uncertainty can lead to serious psychological problems if they cannot learn to ignore the uncertainty and adopt a positive, optimistic, hopeful attitude.

Parental discord and divorce in the face of childhood cancer (even if not in any way caused by the disease) will be an added burden on the afflicted child and the other children in the family.

Siblings of cancer patients may be deprived of much of their parents' attention and may resent their ill sibling. Cairns et al. (1979) found that siblings of pediatric cancer patients were more at risk for psychological problems than were the patients themselves. Siblings may also exhibit school problems because of their personal difficulties and reduction in supervision by over-extended parents.

The routine availability of a mental health specialist in the clinic will allow patients and their families to seek help without labelling themselves as 'crazy'. For many families, a therapist, who is familiar with and sensitive to the issues involved in childhood cancer, will be invaluable in assisting the family to cope with the stress involved in having cancer. A child and family, who are coping well with the illness, will be better able to cope with and participate in treatment for pain. However, all members of the team must have the responsibility of promoting the psychological well being of the patient and the family.

5.3. Disruption of school and social life

Disruption of school and family life due to cancer does not directly cause pain but may trigger depression and reduce the ability of the patient to cope with the pain. Absence from school because of disease or because of medical appointments can be a serious impediment to school success (Schlieper,

1985). Moreover, there is good evidence that treatment by central nervous system irradiation and perhaps intrathecal methotrexate may cause learning problems (Lansky et al., 1984; Copeland et al., 1985).

Ross and Ross (1984) have reported that, for children with leukemia, the worst thing about having the disease is being teased upon return to school. Children are teased because of baldness (from chemotherapy), obesity (from steroids), or being gaunt and pale (from the disease). They describe a training program which helps the child with cancer fight back against teasing. Their program consisted of discussion, behavioral rehearsal and feedback. Their experience suggests that the program is very effective but no properly controlled studies are available.

6. Clinical guidelines

(1) Pain from procedures and from disease should be routinely evaluated. Unless children are asked, they are unlikely to report pain. All procedures should be considered. Venipunctures, which may be regarded as painless by the professional, may be quite aversive to the child.
(2) Pain should be treated aggressively. At this point there is no clear indication that psychological strategies are more or less effective than pharmacologic strategies. Use of both, together, may be most effective.
(3) The meaning of the disease and the pain should be explored with the child and the family on a regular basis.
(4) Pediatric cancer centers should consider the approach used by the Hospital for Sick Children at Great Ormond Street in London, England. A special team consisting of a pediatric oncologist and two nurses is dedicated to providing symptom relief, support and liaison throughout active treatment and remission as well as assisting with terminal care and bereavement (Goldman et al., 1987).

7. Future directions

(1) More research is needed on the extent and treatment of all aspects of pediatric cancer pain.
(2) Methods of disseminating hypnotic techniques should be developed and evaluated.
(3) Research is needed to develop and evaluate ways of reducing the

aversiveness of diagnostic procedures, such as lumbar punctures, bone marrow aspirations and venipunctures, used in management of pediatric cancer.

(4) Evaluation of the need for the current frequency of aversive procedures and research designed to reduce the frequency of aversive procedures is needed.

(5) Further development and implementation of programs aimed at helping children undergoing cancer treatment cope with teasing would be invaluable.

References

Angell, M. (1982) The quality of mercy. New Engl. J. Med. 306, 98–99.

Beales, J.G. (1979) Pain in children with cancer. In: J.J. Bonica and V. Ventafridda (Eds.), Advances in Pain Research and Therapy, Vol. 2 (Raven, New York) pp. 89–98.

Blotcky, A.D., Raczynski, J.M., Gurwitch, R. and Smith, K. (1985) Family influences on hopelessness among children early in the cancer experience. J. Pediatr. Psychol. 10, 479–493.

Bonica, J.J. (1985) Treatment of cancer pain: Current status and future needs. In: H.L. Fields, R. Dubner and F. Cervero (Eds.), Advances in Pain Research and Therapy, Vol. 9 (Raven, New York) pp. 589–616.

Bray, P.F. (1969) Neurology in Pediatrics (Year Book Medical, Chicago, IL) p. 487.

Cairns, N.U., Clark, G.M., Smith, S.D. and Lansky, S.B. (1979) Adaptation of siblings to childhood malignancy. J. Pediatr. 95, 484–487.

Clarke, S. and Radford, M. (1986) Topical anaesthesia for venepuncture. Arch. Dis. Child. 61, 1132–1134.

Copeland, D.R., Fletcher, J.M., Pfefferbaum-Levine, B., Jaffe, N., Reid, H. and Maor, M. (1985) Neuropsychological sequelae of childhood cancer in long-term survivors. Pediatrics 75, 745–753.

Foley, K.M. (1985) The treatment of cancer pain. New Engl. J. Med. 313, 84–95.

Gaffney, A. and Dunne, E.A. (1987) Children's understanding of the causality of pain. Pain 29, 91–104.

Goldman, A. and Bowman, A. (1987) Oral sustained release morphine tablets (MST) for analgesia in children with malignant disease. Paper to be presented at the 1987 Meeting of Children's Hospice International.

Goldman, A., Beardsmore, S. and Hunt, J. (1987) A 'hospice' approach to care of children with malignant disease throughout the course of their illness. Paper to be presented at the 1987 Meeting of Children's Hospice International.

Hickman, R.O., Buckner, C.D., Clift, R.A., et al. (1979) A modified right atrial catheter for access to the venous system in marrow transplant recipients. Surg. Gynecol. Obstet. 148, 871–875.

Hilgard, E.R. (1977) Divided Consciousness (Wiley, New York).

Hilgard, J.R. and LeBaron, S. (1982) Relief of anxiety and pain in children and adolescents with cancer: Quantitative measures and clinical observations. Int. J. Clin. Exp. Hypn. 30, 417–442.

Hilgard, J.R. and LeBaron, S. (1984) Hypnotherapy of Pain in Children with Cancer (Kaufmann, Los Altos, CA).

Hilgard, J.R. and Morgan, A.H. (1976) Treatment of anxiety and pain in childhood cancer through hypnosis. In: F.H. Franbel (Ed.), Hypnosis at Its Bicentennial (Plenum Press, New York) pp. 281–287.

Jay, S.M., Ozolins, M., Elliott, C.H. and Caldwell, S. (1983) Assessment of children's distress during painful medical procedures. Health Psychol. 2, 133–147.

Jay, S.M., Elliott, C.H., Ozolins, M., Olson, R.A. and Pruitt, S.D. (1985) Behavioral management of children's distress during painful medical procedures. Behav. Res. Ther. 23, 513–520.

Katz, E.R., Kellerman, J. and Siegel, S.E. (1980) Distress behavior in children with cancer undergoing medical procedures: developmental considerations. J. Consult. Clin. Psychol. 48, 356–365.

Katz, E.R., Sharp, B., Kellerman, J., Marsten, A., Hirschman, J. and Siegel, S.E.(1982) β-Endorphin immunoreactivity and acute behavioral distress in children with leukemia. J. Nerv. Ment. Dis. 170, 72–77.

Katz, E.R., Kellerman, J. and Ellenberg, L. (1987) Hypnosis in the reduction of acute pain and distress in children with cancer. J. Pediatr. Psychol., in press.

Kellerman, J., Zeltzer, L., Ellenberg, L. and Dash, J. (1983) Adolescents with cancer: Hypnosis for the reduction of the acute pain and anxiety associated with medical procedures. J. Adolesc. Health Care 4, 85–90.

Koocher, G.P. and O'Malley, J.E. (1981) The Damocles Syndrome: Psychosocial consequences of surviving childhood cancer (McGraw-Hill, New York).

Kuttner, L. (1984) Favourite stories: A hypnotic pain reduction technique for children in acute pain. Paper presented at the American Society for Clinical Hypnosis, San Francisco, CA, November.

Kuttner, L. (1986) No Fears...No Tears (Canadian Cancer Society, BC and Yukon Division, 955 West Broadway, Vancouver, BC V5Z 3X8, Canada).

Kuttner, L., Bowman, M. and Teasdale, M.J. (1985) Psychological treatment of distress, pain and anxiety for young children with cancer. Unpublished manuscript, Vancouver Children's Hospital.

Lansky, S.B., Cairns, G.F., Cairns, N.U., Stephenson, L., Lansky, L.L. and Garin, G. (1984) Central nervous system prophylaxis. Am. J. Pediatr. Hematol. 6, 183–190.

Levin, D.N., Cleeland, C.S. and Dar, R. (1985) Public attitudes toward cancer pain. Cancer 56, 2337–2339.

Lokich, J.J., Bothe, A., Benotti, P. and Moore, C. (1985) Complications and management of implanted venous access catheters. J. Clin. Oncol. 3, 710–718.

McDowell, H.P., Hart, C.A. and Martin, J. (1986) Implantable subcutaneous venous catheters. Arch. Dis. Child. 61, 1037–1038.

McGrath, P.A. and De Veber, L.L. (1986) The management of acute pain evoked by medical procedures in children with cancer. J. Pain Symp. Man. 1, 145–150.

McGrath, P.A., De Veber, L.L. and Hearn, M.T. (1985) Multidimensional pain assessment in children. In: H.L. Fields, R. Dubner and F. Cervero (Eds.), Advances in Pain Research and Therapy, Vol. 9 (Raven, New York) pp. 387–393.

McGrath, P.J., Hsu, E., Luke, B., Goodman, J.T. and Dunn-Geier, B.J. (1986) Pain in Pediatric Oncology: A Survey. Children's Hospital of Eastern Ontario, Research Protocol.

Mahon, W.A. and DeGregorio, M. (1985) Benzydamine: A critical review of clinical data. Int. J. Tissue React. 7, 229–235.

Melzack, R. (1983) Concepts in pain measurement. In: R. Melzack (Ed.), Pain Measurement and Assessment (Raven, New York) pp. 1–6.

Miser, A.W. and Miser, J.S. (1986) The use of oral methadone to control moderate and severe pain in children and young adults with malignancy. Clin. J. Pain 1, 243–248.

Miser, A.W., Miser, J.S. and Clark, B.S. (1980) Continuous intravenous infusion of morphine sulphate for control of severe pain in children with terminal malignancy. J. Pediatr. 96, 930–932.

Miser, A.W., Davis, D.M., Hughes, C.S., Mulne, A.F. and Miser, J.S. (1983) Continuous subcutaneous infusion of morphine in children with cancer. Am. J. Dis. Child. 137, 383–385.

Olness, K. (1981) Imagery (self-hypnosis) as adjunct therapy in childhood cancer – Clinical experience with 25 patients. Am. J. Pediatr. Hematol. Oncol. 3, 313–321.

Ottolenghi, A. and Marradi, P. (1984) Diagnostic and therapeutic problems in neoplastic pain of childhood. In: R. Rizzi and M. Visentin (Eds.), Pain: Proceedings of Joint Meeting of the European Chapters of the International Association for the Study of Pain (Piccin/Butterworths, Padua) pp. 391–396.

Parker, G. (1983) Parental Overprotection: A Risk Factor in Psychosocial Development (Grune and Stratton, New York).

Peters, B.M. (1978) School aged children's beliefs about causality of illness: A review of the literature. Matern. Child Nurs. J. 7, 143–154.

Pichard, E., Gauvain-Piquard, A., Poulain, P. and Montagne, F. (1985) La douleur de l'enfant cancéreux et son traitement: diagnostic, évaluation, conduite pratique (Institute Gustave-Roussy, Villejuif).

Rafart, A., Espinosa, W., Illa, J., Fabregas, C. and Borrego, A. (1984) Different kinds of analgesia in pediatric oncology: Oral medication. In: R. Rizzi and M. Visentin (Eds.), Pain: Proceedings of Joint Meeting of the European Chapters of the International Association for the Study of Pain (Piccin/Butterworths, Padua) pp. 401–403.

Ross, D.M. and Ross, S.A. (1982) A Study of the Pain Experience of Leukemic Children. Final report submitted to the David and Lucille Packard Foundation.

Ross, D.M. and Ross, S.A. (1984) Teaching the child with leukemia to cope with teasing. Issues Compr. Pediatr. Nurs. 7, 59–66.

Schlieper, A. (1985) Chronic illness and school achievement. Dev. Med. Child Neurol. 27, 75–79.

Scott, J.F. (1984) Cancer Pain: A Monograph on the Management of Cancer Pain (Government of Canada, Supply and Services, Ottawa).

Spanos, N. (1986) Hypnotic behavior: A social psychological interpretation of amnesia, analgesia and 'trance logic'. Behav. Brain Sci. 9, 449–502.

Stjernsward, J. (1985) Cancer pain relief: An important global public health issue. In: H.L. Fields, R. Dubner and F. Cervero (Eds.), Advances in Pain Research and Therapy, Vol. 9 (Raven, New York) pp. 555–558.

Ventafridda, V., Rogers, A. and Valera, L. (1984) Pain in the child with cancer. In: R. Rizzi and M. Visentin (Eds.), Pain: Proceedings of Joint Meeting of the European Chapters of the International Association for the Study of Pain (Piccin/Butterworths, Padua) pp. 377–382.

Wahlstedt, C., Kohlberg, H., Moller, C. and Uppfeldt, A. (1984) Lignocaine-prilocaine cream reduces venepuncture pain. Lancet ii, 106.

Zeltzer, L. and LeBaron, S. (1982) Hypnotic and non-hypnotic techniques for the reduction of pain and anxiety during painful procedures in children and adolescents with cancer. J. Pediatr. 101, 1032–1035.

CHAPTER 11

Other medical pain

1. Introduction

This chapter will discuss a variety of medical pains including ear pain, eye pain, phantom limb pain, genito-urinary pain, rectal pain, and oral pain. Finally, we will discuss pain from blood disorders.

2. Ear pain

> It (ear ache) felt like something inside your ear like a sticker from a rose bush poking deep inside your ear, like way harder than just pricking *(boy, aged 9 years, quoted in Ross and Ross, 1984, p. 184)*.

We will discuss three types of ear pain: pain from air pressure change, pain from otitis media and ear pain from other causes.

2.1. Pain from air pressure change

Infants travelling in aircraft frequently suffer ear pain during descent. Byers (1986) observed 37 mother-infant pairs during aircraft descent in commercial aircraft and subsequently interviewed the mothers. She found that generally infants cried during descent and were not consoled by the comforting strategies that had been previously effective. Seventy-eight percent of the non-feeding infants cried, compared with 29% of the bottle feeding babies. All infants with colds cried, whether they were feeding or not. Crying typically occurred more than 9 min after adults perceived a need to clear their ears. Only four of the mothers with crying infants attributed the crying to ear pain.

Byers (1986) attributed the crying to ear pain from air pressure due to inadequate ventilation of the middle ear. She suggested the use of bottle feeding during descent with infants who are flying. Because of the potential for middle ear damage, she suggested that infants who have colds should not fly. If they must fly, medication such as pseudoephedrine hydrochloride can be used to reduce congestion and allow clearing of ears during descent.

Given the apparent incidence of pain in infants flying, feeding during descent, if proven effective in further research, could be a simple, appealing, and inexpensive intervention.

2.2. Otitis media

Otitis media is probably the most frequent infection in children with the cumulative incidence of otitis during the first 6 years of life among children in the United States being above 90% (McInerny et al., 1978). More than two-thirds of children will have at least one attack in the first 3 years of life (Bluestone, 1982).

Pain is the most frequent way that parents become aware of otitis media in their children. However, pain is not always present in otitis. Hayden and Schwartz (1985), in a prospective study of 335 consecutive episodes of acute otitis media with effusion diagnosed in a suburban American pediatric practice, found that 83% of the episodes resulted in pain. Pain was graded as not present if there was no evidence on direct questioning of parents and child of pain, fussiness or sleep problems. Mild pain was diagnosed if the child was slightly fussy or querulous. Moderate pain was said to exist if the child was extremely fussy. Severe pain occurred if the child was crying. Pain was mild in 19% of the cases, moderate in 21% and severe in 42% of children. Pain was more frequent in older (more than 2 years of age) than in younger children.

There are two different aspects to the treatment of ear pain: non-specific treatment of the pain and specific treatment of the cause of the pain. Pain should be treated with acetaminophen or acetylsalicylic acid. Topical analgesics in the form of drops are not effective (Feldman et al., 1987). Antimicrobial agents are recommended. Antihistamines and decongestants are not effective in the treatment of otitis. Surgical treatment (myringotomy) for simple repeated otitis is controversial (Feldman et al., 1987).

2.3. Other ear pain

Other ear pain is most commonly due to otitis externa or the occurrence of a boil in the ear canal. Otitis externa often occurs in children who swim frequently, in children with seborrhea or in children who scratch or poke their ear canals. The ear canal is swollen, there is pus and the child experiences pain when the ear is moved. Topical antibiotics are used in otitis externa. Warm water in the ear canal, systemic antibiotics and surgical drainage are used to treat boils in the ear.

3. Eye pain

Pain in the eye is most commonly from bacterial or viral infection, from a foreign body in the eye, from a blow, from a chemical burn or (in the case of a neonate) from medical treatment. Most North American infants start life with mild eye pain because of silver-nitrate induced conjunctivitis. Silver nitrate is routinely infused into the eyes of the newborn to prevent the serious sequelae of gonococcal infection. Although there is no clear evidence that reaction to silver nitrate produces significant problems, chloramphenicol or erythromycin can be substituted (Feldman et al., 1987).

Eye pain should be treated according to its cause. Immediate copious flushing of the eye is important for chemical burns. Hot soaks are all that are of use in viral infections. Antibiotics and hot soaks are helpful in bacterial infection. Topical analgesics may be useful in conjunctival or corneal tears from foreign body or an injury. Eye patch or surgery may be required in eye pain from foreign body or injuries. Proper eye protection is needed by children participating in sports such as hockey, racket sports and baseball to prevent injuries.

4. Phantom limb pain

Fortunately, amputation is rare in childhood. Phantom limb sensation of any sort is rarely found in congenital amputees or in children who have been amputated before about 6 years of age (Riese and Bruck, 1950). However, older children and adolescents may experience phantom limb pain. Pain can be either stump pain, preamputation pain or actual phantom pain. The incidence of phantom limb pain in adults ranges from 2% to nearly 100% (Jensen and Rasmussen, 1984). The incidence of phantom limb pain in children may well be lower than in adults. Treatment of phantom limb pain can be medical, using analgesics, antidepressants, anticonvulsive drugs, or beta-blockers. Alternatively, electrical stimulation or surgery of the stump are sometimes effective.

5. Genito-urinary pain

5.1. Urinary tract infections

Urinary tract infections are much more common in girls than in boys and may or may not be symptomatic. The best evidence is that asymptomatic infections occur in about 1% of girls and symptomatic infections occur even less often (Kunin, 1971).

Flank pain and burning pain on urination are typical of symptomatic urinary tract infection, but abdominal pain with fever may be a more common presentation in adolescence (Barr, 1983). Young children frequently cannot describe their symptoms and parents often cannot discern the relationship between pain and urination. Consequently, children under 2 years of age who look sick but who have fever without any discernible reason should be investigated for urinary tract infection (Feldman et al., 1987). Treatment is with antimicrobial drugs but reoccurrence is common.

5.2. Pelvic pain

Pelvic pain may be due to salpingitis or pelvic inflammatory disease, endometriosis, postoperative adhesions, congenital abnormalities of the uterus, chronic hemoperitoneum, functional ovarian cysts and uterine serositis (Goldstein et al., 1979; Shafer et al., 1982; Barr, 1983). Only one estimate of the prevalence of various causes of pelvic pain has been published. Goldstein et al. (1979) reported on a clinical series of 109 adolescent women between the age of 10.5–19 years seen at the Gynecology Service at Children's Hospital Medical Center, Boston. On laparoscopy they found that 45% had endometriosis, 16% had postoperative adhesions and 9% had each of congenital abnormalities of the uterus, pelvic inflammatory disease and no pathology. The prevalence of endometriosis, in this series, is surprisingly high and the rate of pelvic inflammatory disease and no pathology, surprisingly low. These findings may be due to a referral filter bias to this tertiary care gynecology service and probably does not represent the causes of pelvic pain in the general population.

5.3. Other genito-urinary pain

Dysmenorrhea is a common complaint in the adolescent female. There is little evidence for psychological causation but psychological factors may be important in coping with the pain. For example, an adolescent with dysmenorrhea and poor coping skills may avoid many social and academic activities, while another adolescent with good coping skills might alter activities but participate in less demanding activities. Dysmenorrhea appears to be related to changes in myometrial activity, secretion of prostaglandins, and increased sensitivity of pain receptors to prostaglandins and/or uterine ischemia (Barr, 1983).

Treatment should be in a stepped fashion. Initially ASA or acetaminophen (which both inhibit prostaglandins) may be tried. Non-steroidal anti-inflammatories have been demonstrated as effective in more severe cases. Finally, ovulation can be prevented with resulting inhibition of production and release of prostaglandins, using standard oral contraceptives.

Testicular pain can be momentary or continuing. Acute testicular pain that is more than momentary, should always be taken seriously and investigated urgently to rule out testicular torsion. Bennett et al. (1987) studied 83 boys between 3 months to 16 years who were admitted to hospital with acute testicular pain or swelling. Seventy cases had exploratory surgery. In 55% of the 27 cases of torsion, the testicle was lost. Delay in seeking treatment was an important factor and no testis was saved in which torsion was present for more than 18 h. The major reason for the poor results was that the patient or his parents delayed seeking treatment. Extrapolating from their data, the authors suggested that about 400 boys per year in the U.K. lose a testicle from torsion and concluded that education of potential patients and their parents is needed to prevent this unnecessary morbidity.

6. Chest pain

> It (irregular painful heartbeat) felt like a rock was bouncing round in my chest hitting the sides hard *(boy, aged 6 years, quoted in Ross and Ross, 1984, p. 184)*.

For most people, chest pain is perceived as an indicator of an impending heart attack. Fortunately in children and adolescents with no previously known pathology, this is virtually never the case (Feldman et al., 1987).

Chest pain has become a major cause for referral to pediatric cardiology clinics in the United States (Brenner et al., 1984) and it accounts for 650 000 patient visits annually in patients aged 10–21 years (Ezzati, 1978). Its prevalence among a sample of 562 urban black youth was 12.8% but only 32% of those with pain saw a doctor (Brunswick et al., 1979).

Distinguishing common benign chest pain from the rare pathological chest pain is done by means of history and physical examination (Feldman et al., 1987). Laboratory procedures including chest X-ray and ECG have virtually no yield, unless specifically indicated and have the danger of increasing anxiety, i.e., the physician tells the patient that there is no serious problem but he is worried enough to do tests.

Understanding the benign nature of recurrent chest pain in children will help to prevent the transformation of an occasional pain into a chronic pain problem with attendant school absence and other restriction of activities (Coleman, 1984).

Table 1 outlines the key elements in distinguishing benign chest pain from chest pain that requires medical action. The causes of chest pain in children have been exhaustively described by Perry (1985).

TABLE 1
Narrowing down on chest pain.
(Reprinted from Feldman et al., 1987.)

Finding	Narrowing down	Management
Normal physical examination; pain not anginal; no palpitations or dyspnea	Hyperventilation; normal breasts; psychogenic; GI	Explanation and reassurance; treat disability
Pain elicited by palpation	Costochondritis; chest wall syndrome; breast problems	Explanation and reassurance; treat disability
Acute pain elicited by respiration	Chest X-ray to diagnose pneumonia, pneumothorax	Treat as indicated
Chronic pain elicited by respiration	Chest X-ray to diagnose allergic, cold or exercise bronchospasm	Treat as indicated
Angina, syncope, dyspnea, palpitations or fever, cough and friction rub	Myocardial disease; pericarditis EKG; chest X-ray	Referral to consultant

Pain which is anginal in nature, accompanied by dyspnea, syncope or palpitations should arouse suspicion of cardiac disease. Fortunately, this is rare.

Pantell and Goodman (1983) evaluated 100 consecutive patients who had presented at an adolescent primary care clinic with chest pain. They diagnosed the cases as follows: musculoskeletal problems (31%); costochondritis (14%); chest wall syndrome (13%); skeletal trauma (2%); ribcage anomalies (2%); hyperventilation (20%); breast-related problems (5%); idiopathic (39%) (Pantell and Goodman, 1983, p. 883). Thirty-one percent of the patients had a significant negative life event prior to coming to the clinic. Unfortunately, the lack of a control group precludes any firm conclusions about the relationship of chest pain and life events.

A related study involved the same patients with chest pain and one control group of adolescents with abdominal pain and another control group of pain-free adolescents (Goodman and Pantell, 1984). There were no differences among the three groups on age, race, family constellation, school failure, incidences of headaches, anorexia, insomnia, feelings of uselessness, loss of pleasure, and use of medications, street drugs or cigarettes. Girls were over-represented in the abdominal pain group. Adolescents with pain were more likely to have more clinic visits, to limit their activities, to worry, to reproach themselves, to see their health as problematic, and to see their health as interfering with school. Thirty-two percent of the chest pain patients and 37% of the abdominal pain group reported they missed 3 or more days a month from school compared to 16% of the pain-free group. Using DSM III criteria, there were no differences between the groups (7% of subjects) on incidence of depression.

Driscoll et al. (1976) examined 43 pediatric patients whose main complaint was chest pain. The diagnoses were: idiopathic (45%); costochondritis (22.5%); coughing and bronchitis (12.5%); miscellaneous (10%); muscle strain (5%); trauma (5%). They found that although most children were concerned about their pain, there was no evidence of psychiatric causation of pain. There was no standardized measurement of psychological functioning and no control group in this study.

In a retrospective study, Selbst (1985) reviewed the charts of 267 pediatric patients presenting with chest pain to a pediatric emergency room. The diagnoses were: idiopathic (28%); functional anxiety (17%); musculoskeletal (15%); costochondritis (10%); gastrointestinal (7%); cough or URI (6%); asthma (4%); trauma (4%); arrhythmia (3%); pneumonia (2%); and other (4%). Selbst (1985) noted that pain due to cardiorespiratory problems (cough, asthma, pneumonia, pleuritis and arrhythmia) were more common in younger children and functional pain was more common in adolescents. No standardized measurement of psychological functioning was used.

Thirty-six children with psychogenic chest pain were studied by Asnes et al. (1981) who concluded that specific stressful situations related to onset of pain could be identified in most patients. They also found that 55% of children had other recurrent somatic complaints and 30% of children had sleep disturbances. The study is suspect because no criteria for psychogenicity were detailed; no control group was used; and no standardized measures were utilized.

In a study of 100 children attending a cardiology clinic, Kashani et al. (1982) identified four children with benign chest pain. All four were diagnosed as having clinical depression as measured by DSM III criteria. Contrary to the authors, we feel this small sample of four children is much too small on which to base any conclusions.

The studies on chest pain in children are generally poorly designed and as a result their conclusions are suspect. However, there are some consistent findings: children with chest pain generally feel that they have a serious disease either heart disease or cancer and their chest pain puts them at higher risk for reducing activities at school (cardiac non-disease) (Bergman and Stamm, 1967). The adult literature on chest pain in patients with no coronary disease, also supports the notion that continuing chest pain is associated with an exaggerated preoccupation with health and a subjective perception that one is vulnerable to heart disease (Weilgosz and Earp, 1986).

7. Rectal pain

7.1. Proctalgia fugax

Proctalgia fugax is a condition characterized by infrequent recurrent attacks of very severe, deep, non-radiating rectal pain. The pain occurs day or night and resolves without residue in less than 10–20 min (Thompson, 1979). The disorder occurs in over 10% of the population (Thompson, 1979) and although usually beginning after 16 years of age, cases of children have been recorded (Hayden and Grossman, 1959). No treatment has been evaluated but some patients report pressure and heat are helpful.

7.2. Constipation

Rappaport and Levine (1986) have described a self-perpetuating cycle which begins with mild constipation from any number of sources, including:

changes in food, toilet training, fear of bathroom, anal fissure, illness, and avoidance of school bathroom. The mild constipation causes some pain upon defecation. This leads the child to retain feces which results in subsequent hardening of the stool and more pain. The pain-retention-pain cycle then maintains itself resulting in more severe constipation and pain. The prevalence of this problem is unknown. Rappaport and Levine (1986) suggested that a combined program of education, increased dietary fiber, and stool softeners will be effective. No evaluation of this type of strategy for the reduction of pain has been completed. However, numerous studies have demonstrated the effectiveness of such an approach with encopretic and constipated children (e.g., Levine and Bakow, 1976) and in children with recurrent abdominal pain (see chapter 6).

8. Oral pain

8.1. Temporomandibular pain and dysfunction syndrome

There has been much consideration given to the study of aching in the temporomandibular joint and the muscles involved in chewing. The disorder goes by a large number of names the most popular of which are myofascial pain dysfunction syndrome and temporomandibular joint pain. The International Association for the Study of Pain has labelled the syndrome 'temporomandibular pain and dysfunction syndrome' (Merskey, 1986) and defined it as: aching in the muscles of mastication plus, in some cases, an occasional brief severe pain on chewing, possibly leading to restricted jaw movement (Merskey, 1986). The pain is usually felt as a dull, continuous, poorly localized ache. Typically, the pain is unilateral but on occasion it is bilateral (Sharav, 1984). There are often no evident radiological changes. Problems due to some known disorder such as arthritis or trauma are not considered to be temporomandibular pain and dysfunction syndrome. Although hundreds of papers have been written on the syndrome, the research is generally poor, the results confusing and contradictory (Eversole and Machado, 1985). Although not specifically focussed on children, the recent review by Eversole and Machado (1985) is a model of clarity both for its organization and because of the critical appraisal of the quality of evidence in each study.

The prevalence of the syndrome in children and adolescents has been documented in a number of studies in Europe. Egermark-Eriksson et al. (1981) found that 39% of 7-year-olds, 67% of 11-year-olds and 74% of 15-

year-olds reported symptoms occasionally. More frequent symptoms and multiple symptoms were reported by 4%, 7% and 11% of 7-, 11- and 15-year-old children, respectively. Similarly, Nilner (1981) and Nilner and Lassing (1981) found that 36% of 7–14-year-old children had at least one symptom of the syndrome whereas 41% of the 15–18-year-old adolescents exhibited one or more symptoms.

The etiology of the disorder is unknown. Etiological theories have focussed on psychogenic causation and occlusal disturbances. Psychogenic hypotheses suggest that emotional factors are paramount. The argument is that tense individuals, when under stress or in response to depression, grind or clench their teeth, creating heightened muscle tension and resultant pain. The hypothesis of occlusal disturbance is that occlusal imbalances predispose to parafunctional habits, muscle incoordination, myospasm and pain. Both types of hypotheses consider muscle tension as the major etiologic factor but posit different causes for the muscle tension.

Studies investigating etiology of temporomandibular pain and dysfunction syndrome have suffered from numerous problems. It is difficult to separate cause and effect. Children may develop temporomandibular pain and dysfunction syndrome because they are psychologically disturbed or they may be psychologically disturbed because of the pain and limitations from the disorder. Similarly, occlusal abnormalities might cause or be caused by temporomandibular pain and dysfunction syndrome. Consequently, the finding of a higher rate of psychological disturbance or occlusal problems in children with temporomandibular pain and dysfunction syndrome compared to controls does not tell us anything about the cause of the disorder. However, it should be noted that the opposite is not quite true. In spite of the difficulties in interpreting failure to find a difference, the failure to find higher rates of psychological disturbance in temporomandibular pain and dysfunction syndrome patients would tend to discount that theory of causation.

Other problems in the research include a failure to account for referral bias. For example, it is more likely that children referred to a psychologist for temporomandibular pain and dysfunction syndrome would have psychological problems than would a population sample of all such patients. Further, most studies use measurements of unproven reliability and validity. Finally, the assumption is made that temporomandibular pain and dysfunction syndrome is one disorder with a unitary cause in all cases. This is unlikely to be the case.

Relatively few studies have been done on children. Belfer and Kaban (1982) found that 35% of their pediatric patients with temporomandibular pain and dysfunction syndrome were suffering from reactive depression. They suggested that treatment consist of psychotherapy, soft diet, heat therapy, and anti-inflammatory analgesics and muscle relaxants. Unfortunately, the measurement of depression was not described, nor was the treatment formally evaluated. Moreover, the referral bias of the tertiary care center may have led to an unusual sample of children with temporomandibular pain and dysfunction syndrome.

In the same vein, no convincing studies implicating occlusal problems as the cause of temporomandibular pain and dysfunction syndrome in children and adolescents have been published.

No properly designed treatment studies have been published on children and adolescents. In practice, many children will not be treated at all, most children who are, will be treated dentally with rest, soft diet, dental splints and appliances, correction of bite and, as a last resort, by surgery. Some children will be treated medically with muscle relaxants and a few will be treated psychologically with psychotherapy, biofeedback or stress management.

Recently Pillemer et al. (1987) have suggested a strategy of classifying children with temporomandibular pain and dysfunction syndrome. They suggested three categories. Group I consists of patients with a true somatic disorder where organic or anatomic pathology is responsible for the pain. There may be anxiety, depression, insomnia or anger but these resolve with treatment of the organic or anatomic pathology. Group II are referred to as having a psychosomatic disorder in which psychological and organic factors are intertwined. In these patients, there is thought to be a physiological vulnerability such as malocclusion plus psychosocial dysfunction. Children in this category will often express psychological tension via myofascial activity. Finally, group III patients are seen to have pseudosomatic disorders in which there are no objective signs of organic or anatomic joint dysfunction. In their clinical series of 53 children and adolescents, Pillemer et al. reported that 9% were in group I (true somatic disorder); 66% were in group II (psychosomatic disorder); and 25% were in group III (pseudosomatic disorder). Group III patients are similar to what we would describe as chronic intractable pain patients (chapter 13). The authors mentioned the problem with referral bias but noted that a similar referral pattern in adult patients did not result in nearly as many patients in group III. The authors suggested that medical treatment including anti-inflammatory drugs, medical counselling, muscle relaxants, occlusal splints, orthodontics and surgery are appropriate for group I patients. Behavioral treatment, muscle relaxants and occlusal splints were recommended for group II patients. Psychotherapy, psychopharmacologic drugs were suggested for group III patients. The reliability of this classification system and its utility has not been evaluated. However, it does provide a first step in approaching pediatric temporomandibular pain and dysfunction syndrome.

8.2. Dental pain

> As soon as I get in the chair I pretend he's the enemy and I'm a secret agent and he's torturing me to get secrets and if I make one sound I'm telling him secret information and I never do. I'm going to be a secret agent when I grow up so this is good practice *(boy, aged 10, at the dentist, quoted in Ross and Ross, 1984, p. 186)*.

Dental pain in children and adolescents can arise from dental disease (tooth decay and peridontal disease) or from treatment of dental problems.

Prevalence of dental pain has not been well-documented in itself but cavities affect nearly everyone. By age six, the average American child has three decayed or filled primary teeth and by age 14, six permanent teeth have decayed (Leske et al., 1980). Peridontal disease is one of the most widespread diseases of mankind affecting approximately half of the child population and almost the entire adult population (World Health Organization, 1961). Pain from dental procedures, including restorations and orthodontic procedures is of unknown prevalence.

8.2.1. Pain from disease
Unlike most pain in children and adolescents, there are well validated methods of preventing dental pain.

The most effective single primary prevention method for dental cavities and resulting pain is fluoridation of community water supplies to approximately one part per million (Leske et al., 1980). Water fluoridation reduces caries and resultant dental pain by about 50%. Additional effective methods of delivering fluoride include fluoridation of school water supplies, fluoride added to food, supplementary fluoride, or topical fluoride. These methods are more expensive and less universal than fluoridation of communal water.

A second type of primary prevention for dental pain problems involves changing dietary habits. Specifically, reducing the frequent consumption of sugars, particularly sticky sugars or sugars that remain in the mouth for extended periods (such as bottles of juice or milk given to babies as they fall asleep or chewy candy given to children) may well reduce the incidence of nursing dental caries and childhood caries. Changes in dietary practice are particularly difficult to implement and the impact of efforts to change dietary practice to reduce tooth decay have not been evaluated.

A third method for the primary prevention of dental pain involves the teaching of appropriate dental skills by behavioral methodology. Both flossing skills and brushing skills have been effectively taught and maintained in both children and adults (Iwata and Becksfort, 1981; Dahlquist et al., 1985). Although it is clear that flossing and brushing are effective deterrents to peridontal disease (but not cavities), large-scale long-term prevention programs based on oral hygiene methods have not demonstrated reduction in dental disease (Leske et al., 1980). Behavioral methods of promoting generalization across settings and time (durability) may be particularly worth exploring in large scale studies.

8.2.2. Pain from procedures

8.2.2.1. Restorations   Advances in the past 15 years in dental analgesia have dramatically decreased the amount of pain experienced by children during restorations (Spiro, 1981). There are, however, no controlled trials with children.

Although, there have been a number of well-designed studies examining cognitive/behavioral procedures in children undergoing restorations, the focus of the measurement has been on distress or anxiety and cooperative behavior rather than pain per se.

In a series of well-controlled studies, Melamed and her colleagues (Melamed et al., 1975a,b, 1977; Melamed, 1979) demonstrated that filmed modelling effectively reduced children's fear and distress behavior in the dental operatory.

Siegel and Peterson (1980, 1981) demonstrated that teaching specific coping skills and/or providing information about the sensory aspects of the dental experience were effective in reducing children's ratings of anxiety and discomfort, as well as in lowering physiological arousal. The coping skills used included muscle relaxation, pleasant imagery, and calming self-instruction.

Finally, Nocella and Kaplan (1982) in a randomized controlled trial studied 30 children between 5- and 13-years-of-age who had prior dental experience. They found that children, who were taught cognitive coping strategies, evidenced fewer disruptive behaviors than did children in the attention control or the no treatment group. Cognitive training consisted of 15 min of instruction on breathing exercise, muscle relaxation, and positive coping statements.

Studies focussing specifically on pain from restorative procedures have not been done.

8.2.2.2. Orthodontic procedures

> When he's doing it (orthodontic session) it's like one big dagger after another right into my teeth *(girl, aged 11, quoted in Ross and Ross, 1984, p. 186).*

Many children undergo orthodontic banding to straighten their teeth. The procedure is painful. Mischel et al. (1986) randomly assigned 25 children between 8 and 15 years of age to one of three groups: distraction training, reframing training and irrelevant training control. Assessment of pain included heart rate, self-ratings and ratings by the orthodontist and his assistants. Distraction training consisted of diverting attention from painful procedures by engaging in mental activities such as counting backwards by sevens, remembering lists or imagining pleasant events. Reframing training involved creating alternative contexts or frameworks for the pain such as being an injured tennis star. Both cognitive strategies were superior to the control condition in the first half of the banding. All groups of children experienced reduced distress in the second half of the procedure.

8.3. Teething

Although teething is a universal phenomenon and an apparent cause of pain in many babies, little research has examined the occurrence of distress or the effectiveness of treatments. In a British longitudinal survey of 4480 episodes of primary tooth eruption, local medication was applied by parents to the gums of 52% of the infants for primary central and lateral incisor tooth eruption (Seward, 1969). During eruption of the canine and primary molar teeth, local medication was used for 62% of the babies.

In a subsequent randomized double-blind placebo-controlled trial, Seward (1969) evaluated a teething solution applied to the gums of infants aged 5 months to 31 months for relief of pain and discomfort. One hundred and fifty-five infants were in the experimental group and 136 infants were in the control group. The teething solution consisted of active ingredients: lignocaine (0.30%), benzyl alcohol (0.30%) and tincture of myrrh (0.80%) in a sweetened aqueous base. The placebo solution was identical except for the active ingredients. The solution was effective in reducing pain. There was a tendency for the solution to be more effective for male infants and for infants over 1 year of age. There was no difference between applying the solution before or after the tooth had erupted. The teething solution was equally effective during the day, at naps, or at night. Most of the mothers (82%) found it easy to apply and 90% of the infants were reported to like the solution.

Alternative interventions include systemic analgesics such as acetaminophen, teething rings, cold or massage of the gums. None has been systematically evaluated.

9. Blood disorders

Both hemophilia and sickle cell disease are genetic blood disorders that cause considerable pain.

9.1. Hemophilia

Hemophilia is a disorder of blood coagulation which is marked by recurrent internal bleeding episodes. Acute bleeds can be quite painful requiring opioid analgesics. As well, repeated bleeds into joints can cause a type of painful osteoarthritis. Pain is typically controlled by a combination of opioid and non-opioid analgesics. No studies have been reported documenting the extent of the pain of hemophilia or the efficacy of long-term analgesic usage.

Varni and his associates have demonstrated the use of biobehavioral methods in helping children and adults with pain in hemophilia. For example, Varni et al. (1981) in a case study, taught a 9-year-old boy with classic hemophilia, progressive muscle relaxation, meditative breathing and guided imagery. Table 2 summarizes the change from 1 year prior to treatment to the year following treatment. There was marked reduction in pain, analgesic use, hospitalizations and days missed from school. There were substantial improvements in the child's ability to walk up stairs.

A second case report (LeBaron and Zeltzer, 1985) demonstrated reduction in codeine usage by an 18-year-old severe hemophiliac by hypnotherapy. The patient had been using an average of 49.5 grains of codeine a month. Hypnotherapy allowed a steady decline in use of codeine and reported control of hemorrhaging by hypnosis. The authors cautioned that there was a return to heavy codeine use after treatment was terminated and that there was no objective evidence of control of bleeds by hypnosis. They also noted that the patient reported accidentally triggering a bleed by hypnosis.

Although there was no experimental control in either of these case studies, they provide tantalizing hope of possible help for these children in coping with the pain of their disease.

TABLE 2

Parameters associated with pain intensity.
(Reprinted from Varni et al., 1981, p. 124, with permission.)

Parameters	1 year pre self-regulation training	1 year post self-regulation training
Pain intensity (1 = mild; 10 = severe)	7[a]	2[b]
Meperidine	74 tablets (50 mg/ea.)	0 tablets
Acetaminophen/codeine elixir	438 doses (24 mg codeine/dose)	78 doses (24 mg codeine/dose)
Physical therapy measures		
Range of motion	Normal r. knee 0°–150° Arthritic l. knee 15°–105°	R. knee 0°–150° L. knee 0°–140°
Quadriceps strength (0–5 scale)	Normal r. knee 4 − Arthritic l. knee 3 +	R. knee 4 + L. knee 4
Girth (knee joint circumference)	Not available	R. knee 26 cm L. knee 25.8 cm
Ambulation on stairs	2–3 maximum	No limitation
School days missed	33	6
Hospitalizations		
Total days	11	0
Number admissions	3	0

[a] 2.5-week pre assessment during pain just prior to self-regulation training.
[b] 1 year average rating during pain episodes when using self-regulation techniques.

9.2. Sickle cell disease

In sickle cell disease, there is an abnormality of the hemoglobin which causes the red blood cells to form a sickle shape when exposed to low oxygen tension. Sickle cells aggregate in the microcirculation causing infarction. The sickle cell gene is widely distributed throughout mid-Africa and the descendants of the people of Africa who were dispersed by the slave trade. The gene also occurs in the indigenous population of the north coast of the Mediterranean, Saudi Arabia and in some parts of India (Black, 1985). The gene is carried by about one in ten and the disease affects approximately one in 400 of the affected groups (Black, 1985). The pain from sickling crises can be mild but it is frequently moderate or severe. In a sample of 50 sickle cell disease patients, there was an average of 2.3 hospitalizations per year before age 5 years, dropping to 1.2 in the 12–16 year age range. Similarly, emergency room visits dropped from an average of 3 to 1.5 in the same age range. Crises with mild to moderate pain occurred once every 2 weeks to once a month across the age ranges (Hurtig and White, 1986).

Parfrey et al. (1984) have suggested that the pain crisis itself may be a significant cause of death. They found that 45% of sickle cell patients dying during crisis had no other cause of death whereas only 7.8% of patients dying outside of a pain crisis had unexplained cause of death. The mechanism of death is unknown but may be related to intravascular sickling.

Painful episodes of sickle cell disease are treated with ASA and acetaminophen on a routine basis. Morphine is the preferred opioid. Opioids generally are reserved for hospital use (Black, 1985) because of concern with possible abuse. Schechter (1985) has challenged the concern with abuse and pointed out that there are no studies on the problem of addiction in individuals with sickle cell disease. He argued that the prevalence of abuse is likely close to the rate of abuse in cancer patients who have been on high doses of opioids for long periods of time. It is widely agreed that addiction is not a major problem in cancer patients. He concluded that fear of addiction should not prevent the adequate treatment of pain in patients with sickle cell.

A retrospective clinical series reported by Cole et al. (1986) describes their 5 year experience with intravenous opioid therapy during sickle cell crisis used with 38 patients during 98 crises. The standard protocol which was used in 78% of the crises called for a bolus intravenous injection of 0.15 mg/kg of morphine sulfate or 1.0 mg/kg of meperidine followed by a morphine sulfate infusion at a dose rate of 0.07–0.10 mg/kg per h or a meperidine hydrochloride infusion at a dose rate of 0.5–0.7 mg/kg per h. If needed the dose was titrated upwards by increments of approximately 25% every 3–4 h until sufficient analgesia was obtained. The authors believed their strategy to be superior to the more common use of intramuscular injection of opioids. The intravenous route is usually established anyway to provide hydration; rapid and sustained serum opioid levels are obtained, titration is easy and there is no pain from repeated injections. Side effects were common but not usually serious. Chest syndrome was a frequent complication and respiratory depression occurred in three patients. The role of the opioid infusion in these complications was not clear. There was no evidence of addiction.

In a case report, Zeltzer et al. (1979) discussed two young adults with sickle cell disease who were taught to use self-hypnosis with suggestions of vasodilation to help them cope with sickling crises. The results were impressive with reductions in emergency room visits from 54 for the 12 months prior to hypnosis to 3 in the 12 months after hypnosis. Days hospitalized dropped from 95 to zero.

Unfortunately, no further studies have been published using these strategies with sickle cell disease patients.

Children and adolescents with sickle cell disease are almost always black and are frequently from poor families. Although no research has investigated the issue, it is possible that race and class biases may be barriers to adequate analgesic management. Poor black adolescents may be viewed by health care providers as more likely to be exaggerating their pain and more likely to abuse opioid analgesics.

10. *Clinical guidelines*

(1) Parents travelling by plane with infants should be advised of the possible efficacy of feeding during descent to prevent ear pain.
(2) Adolescents with benign chest pain and their parents should be counselled regarding the benign nature of the disorder and cautioned to be careful to prevent the development of chronic illness behavior (cardiac non-disease).
(3) Simple behavioral methods, such as distraction and relaxation, should be used to help children cope with dental treatment.
(4) Adequate analgesics should be provided for children with sickle cell disease. Aggressive analgesic therapy may reduce manipulative behavior on the part of these patients.

11. *Future directions*

(1) Studies using adequate control groups and standardized measures are needed in adolescent chest pain to determine the psychological correlates of chest pain and to determine if cardiac non-disease is a problem.
(2) Interdisciplinary studies of temporomandibular pain and dysfunction syndrome are needed using standardized measures and proper controls. Both case control and intervention studies are required.
(3) Studies investigating pain relief (both pharmacological and psychological) in sickle cell disease and hemophilia are required. The issue of opioid use in outpatient treatment of sickle cell disease needs careful examination.

References

Asnes, R.S., Santulli, R. and Bemporad, J.R. (1981) Psychogenic chest pain in children. Clin. Pediatr. 20, 788–791.

Barr, R.G. (1983) Abdominal pain in the female adolescent. Pediatr. Rev. 4, 281–289.

Belfer, M.L. and Kaban, L.B. (1982) Temporomandibular joint dysfunction with facial pain in children. Pediatrics 69, 564–567.

Bennett, S., Nicholson, M.S. and Little, T.M. (1987) Torsion of the testis: why is the prognosis so poor? Br. Med. J. 294, 824.

Bergman, A.B. and Stamm, S.J. (1967) The morbidity of cardiac non-disease in schoolchildren. New Eng. J. Med. 276, 1008–1013.

Black, J. (1985) The New Paediatrics: Child Health in Ethnic Minorities (British Medical Journal, London) pp. 21–32, 51–64.

Bluestone, C.D. (1982) Otitis media in children: To treat or not to treat. New Engl. J. Med. 306, 1399–1404.

Brenner, J.I., Engel, R.E. and Berman, M.A. (1984) Cardiologic perspectives of chest pain in childhood: A referral problem? To whom? Pediatr. Clin. North Am. 31, 1241–1258.

Brunswick, A.F., Boyle, J.M. and Tarica, C. (1979) Who sees the doctor? A study of urban black adolescents. Soc. Sci. Med. 13A, 45–56.

Byers, P.H. (1986) Infant crying during aircraft descent. Nurs. Res. 35, 260–262.

Cole, T.B., Sprinkle, R.H., Smith, S.J. and Buchanan, G.R. (1986) Intravenous narcotic therapy for children with severe sickle cell pain crisis. Am. J. Dis. Child. 140, 1255–1259.

Coleman, W.L. (1984) Recurrent chest pain in children. Pediatr. Clin. North Am. 31, 1007–1026.

Dahlquist, L. M., Gil, K.M., Hodges, J., Kalfus, G.R., Ginsberg, A. and Holborn, S.W. (1985) The effects of behavioral intervention on dental flossing skills in children. J. Pediatr. Psychol. 10, 403–412.

Driscoll, D.J., Glicklich, L.B. and Gallen, W.J. (1976) Chest pain in children: A prospective study. Pediatrics 57, 648–651.

Egermark-Eriksson, I., Ingervall, B. and Carlsson, G.E. (1981) Prevalence of mandibular dysfunction and orofacial parafunction in 7-, 11- and 15-year-old Swedish children. Eur. J. Orthod. 3, 163–172.

Eversole, L.R. and Machado, L. (1985) Temporomandibular joint internal derangements and associated neuromuscular disorders. J. Am. Dent. Assoc. 110, 69–79.

Ezzati, T. (1978) Ambulatory Care Utilization Patterns of Children and Young Adults: Vital and health statistics, Series 13, no. 39 (United States Department of Health, Education and Welfare Publication no. PHS, 78–1790).

Feldman, W., Rosser, W. and McGrath, P. (1987) Primary Medical Care for Children and Adolescents (Oxford University Press, New York) pp. 18–19, 72–76, 80–83, 105–110.

Goldstein, D.P., DeCholnoky, C., Leventhal, J.M. and Emans, S.J. (1979) New insights into the old problem of chronic pelvic pain. J. Pediatr. Surg. 14, 675–679.

Goodman, B.W. and Pantell, R.H. (1984) Chest pain in adolescents: Functional consequences. West. J. Med. 141, 342–346.

Hayden, R. and Grossman, M. (1959) Rectal, ocular and submaxillary pain. Am. J. Dis. Child. 97, 479–482.

Hayden, G.F. and Schwartz, R.H. (1985) Characteristics of earache among children with acute otitis media. Am. J. Dis. Child. 139, 721–723.

Hurtig, A.L. and White, L.S. (1986) Psychosocial adjustment in children and adolescents with sickle cell disease. J. Pediatr. Psychol. 11, 411–427.

Iwata, B.A. and Becksfort, C.M. (1981) Behavioral research in preventive dentistry: Educational and contingency management approaches to the problem of patient compliance. J. Appl. Behav. Anal. 14, 111–120.

Jensen, T.S. and Rasmussen, P. (1984) Amputation. In: P.D. Wall and R. Melzack (Eds.), Textbook of Pain (Churchill-Livingstone, Edinburgh) pp. 402–412.

Kashani, J.H., Labidi, Z. and Jones, R.S. (1982) Depression in children and adolescents with cardiovascular symptomatology: The significance of chest pain. J. Am. Acad. Child Psychiatr. 21, 187–189.

Kunin, C.M. (1971) Epidemiology and natural history of urinary tract infection in school age children. Pediatr. Clin. North Am. 18, 509–528.

LeBaron, S. and Zeltzer, L. (1985) Hypnosis for hemophiliacs: Methodologic problems and risks. Am. J. Pediatr. Hematol. Oncol. 7, 316–319.

Leske, G.S., Ripa, L.W. and Leske, M.C. (1980) Dental public health. In: J.M. Last (Ed.), Public Health and Preventive Medicine, 11th edn. (Appleton Century Crofts, New York) pp. 1473–1513.

Levine, M.D. and Bakow, H. (1976). Children with encopresis: A study of treatment outcome. Pediatrics 58, 845–852.

McInerny, T.K., Roghmann, K.J. and Sutherland, S.A. (1978) Primary pediatric care in one community. Pediatrics 61, 389–397.

Melamed, B.G. (1979) Behavioral approaches to fear in dental settings. In: M. Hersen, P. Eisler and P. Miller (Eds.), Progress in Behavior Modification, Vol. 7 (Academic Press, New York) pp. 171–203.

Melamed, B.G., Weinstein, D., Hawes, R. and Borland, M. (1975a) Reduction of fear related dental management problems using filmed modelling. J. Am. Dent. Assoc. 90, 822–826.

Melamed, B.G., Hawes, R., Heiby, E. and Gluck, J. (1975b) The use of filmed modelling to reduce unco-operative behavior of children during dental treatment. J. Dent. Res. 54, 797–801.

Melamed, B.G., Hawes, R., Hutcherson, S., and Fleece, L. (1977) Fear level, previous experience and the effects of filmed modelling in dentistry. J. Dent. Res. 56, 431.

Merskey, H. (Ed.) (1986) Classification of chronic pain: Descriptions of chronic pain syndromes and definitions of pain terms. Pain suppl. 3, pp. S27–S30, S59–S60, S65, S40–S43, S140.

Mischel, H.N., Fuhr, R. and McDonald, M.A. (1986) Children's dental pain: The effects of cognitive coping training in a clinical setting. Clin. J. Pain 1, 235–242.

Nilner, M. (1981) Prevalence of functional disturbances and diseases of the stomatognathic system in 15–18 year olds. Swed. Dent. J. 5, 173–187.

Nilner, M. and Lassing, S. (1981) Prevalence of functional disturbances and diseases of stomatognathic system in 7–14 year olds. Swed. Dent. J. 5, 173–187.

Nocella, J. and Kaplan, R.M. (1982) Training children to cope with dental treatment. J. Pediatr. Psychol. 7, 175–178.

Pantell, R.H. and Goodman, B.W. (1983) Adolescent chest pain: A prospective study. Pediatrics 71, 881–887.

Parfrey, N.A., Moore, W. and Hutchins, G.M. (1984) Is pain crisis a cause of death in sickle cell disease? Am. J. Clin. Pathol. 84, 209–212.

Perry, L.W. (1985) Pinpointing the cause of pediatric chest pain. Contemp. Pediatr., Nov./Dec. issue, 27–42.

Pillemer, F.G., Masek, B.J. and Kaban, L.B. (1987) Temporomandibular joint dysfunction and facial pain in children: An approach to diagnosis and treatment. Pediatrics, in press.

Rappaport, L.A. and Levine, M.D. (1986) The prevention of constipation and encopresis: A developmental model and approach, Pediatr. Clin. North Am. 33, 859–869.

Riese, W. and Bruck, G. (1950) Le membre fantôme chez l'enfant. Revue Neurol. (Paris) 83, 221–222.

Ross, D.M. and Ross, S.A. (1984) Childhood pain: The school-aged child's viewpoint. Pain 20, 179–191.

Schechter, N.L. (1985) Pain and pain control in children. Curr. Probl. Pediatr. 15, 54.

Selbst, S.M. (1985) Chest pain in children. Pediatrics 75, 1068–1070.

Seward, M.H. (1969) The effectiveness of a teething solution in infants: A clinical study. Br. Dent. J. 127, 457–461.

Shafer, M.A., Irwin, C.E. and Sweet, R.L. (1982) Acute salpingitis in the adolescent female. J. Pediatr. 100, 339–350.

Sharav, Y. (1984) Orofacial pain. In: P.D. Wall and R. Melzack (Eds.), Textbook of Pain (Churchill-Livingstone, Edinburgh) pp. 338–349.

Siegel, L.J. and Peterson, L. (1980) Stress reduction in young dental patients through coping skills and sensory information. J. Consult. Clin. Psychol. 48, 785–787.

Spiro, S.R. (1981) Pain and Anxiety Control in Dentistry (Jack K. Burgess, Englewood, NJ)

Thompson, W.G. (1979) The Irritable Gut: Functional Disorders of the Alimentary Canal (University Park Press, Baltimore MD) pp. 125–130.

Varni, J.W., Gilbert and Dietrich, S.L. (1981) Behavioral medicine in pain and analgesia management for the hemophilic child with Factor VIII inhibitor. Pain 11, 121–126.

Weilgosz, A.T. and Earp, J. (1986) Perceived vulnerability to serious heart disease and persistent pain in patients with minimal or no coronary disease. Psychosom. Med. 48, 118–124.

World Health Organization (1961) Peridontal disease. Technical Report Series no. 207. Report of an Expert Committee on Dental Health (WHO, Geneva).

Zeltzer, L., Dash, J. and Holland, J.P. (1979) Hypnotically induced pain in sickle cell anemia. Pediatrics 64, 533–536.

CHAPTER 12

Injuries

I told myself to go soft all over and start rolling in deep snow *(boy, aged 8, about burn treatment, quoted in Ross and Ross, 1984, p. 186)*.

1. Introduction

Injuries frequently cause pain. This chapter will briefly review the literature on accidental injuries, intentional injuries and sports injuries. Particular emphasis will be placed on the prevention of injuries and the resulting pain.

2. Accidental injuries

Accidental injuries are an important cause of morbidity and mortality in children. In the United States, it has been estimated that 22 000 children die each year from injuries and for every child who dies approximately 1270 are treated in a medical facility for injuries (Feldman et al., 1987).

The cause of serious injuries vary with the age of the child but the major causes are: choking, motor vehicle accidents, pedestrian motor vehicle accidents, burns, drowning, falls and poisoning. Most injuries cause pain.

2.1. Prevention

The prevention of injuries is the most effective method of curtailing the pain and resultant suffering. Unfortunately, there are only a few methods of prevention that have been shown to be effective. We will not review the many suggestions that have been made to reduce accidents for which there is no evidence of their validity.

2.1.1. Motor vehicle accidents

Child car restraints can substantially reduce morbidity and mortality. Legislation requiring child restraint has resulted in increased compliance

(Williams and Wells, 1981). Raising the driving age could also reduce injuries in the 15–19-year-old group of adolescents (Hingson et al., 1985). Simple engineering improvements such as reducing curves and hills in roads and reducing or protecting rigid structures such as bridge abutments could reduce highway injuries (Feldman et al., 1987).

2.1.2. Pedestrian motor vehicle accidents

Pedestrian motor vehicle accidents can be reduced by designing roadways in residential areas so as to reduce and slow traffic and to keep pedestrians separate from automobiles (OECD, 1983). Crosswalks, cross guards, and school safety programs have all been used to reduce pedestrian motor vehicle accidents but their effectiveness is unknown.

2.1.3. Burns

Burns result from fires, scalds, electrical sources and chemical contact. Legislation requiring smoke detectors may be effective in reducing mortality from house fires (U.S. Fire Administration, 1983). Scalds from hot tap water could be substantially eliminated if legislation setting hot water tank thermostats at 50°C was enacted (Rosser et al., 1987). Alteration in design of a coffee maker reduced scalds from this source in children in Denmark (Sorenson, 1976).

2.1.4. Falls

The Canadian Medical Association (1987) has recommended that infant walkers be banned because they are hazardous to children. They estimate that 40% of children that use walkers will eventually suffer accidents. The most serious of these accidents usually involve falling down stairs.

Falls from playground equipment can be significantly reduced by a comprehensive program of inspection and monitoring (Warner, 1982).

2.2. Pain control during treatment

Not only can injuries cause pain but the treatment of injuries may cause pain. Two types of common treatment of injuries in childhood will be considered in this section: treatment of burns, and suturing of cuts.

2.2.1. Burns

Severely burned children are subjected to excruciating pain both from the injury and from the treatment. As well as causing suffering, the pain itself and the children's reaction to it may interfere with treatment (Beales, 1982;

McGrath and Vair, 1983) and may influence postrecovery adaptation (Long and Cope, 1961).

A survey of burn units in the United States (Perry and Heidrich, 1982) yielded responses from 93 burn facilities. The survey collected some demographic information about each facility; information about common analgesic practice and pain assessment using a vignette of a 'typical' adult and child patient; information about general pain issues in burn units.

The vignette to assess medication for debridement (tanking) for the child patient was:

> The patient is a 3-year-old, 14 kg boy who has suffered 28% second and third degree burns to his lower extremities. He has been on the unit for 2 weeks, is physiologically stable and has no respiratory compromise. What would be a typical medication order for tanking *(Perry and Heidrich, 1982, p. 268)?*

The adult vignette was the same except for the age and weight of the patient. Twenty-four respondents did not recommend opioid analgesics for child debridement whereas in adult debridement only four respondents thought opioids were unnecessary. Among those respondents suggesting opioid analgesics, the average recommended dosage of opioids on a mg/kg basis was higher for children than for adults. Psychotropic drugs in conjunction with opioids were used less than with adults (24% versus 52%). The mean assessment of pain for children and adults was very similar (2.9 and 3.0 on a 5 point scale) indicating moderate pain. There were no differences in perceived pain level depending on the use of analgesics. The authors estimated that the respondents had experience with over 10 000 patients and not one case of iatrogenic opioid addiction could be recalled.

There is good evidence that even with opioid analgesics, children suffer a great deal of pain during burn dressing changes. Szyfelbein et al. (1985) had 15 children age 8–17 years rate their pain during the components of burn dressing changes, and measured plasma levels of β-endorphin immunoactivity before and after the procedure. For 28 of the 33 burn dressing changes, children were given Percocet, a proprietary mixture of 5 mg oxycodone and 325 mg of acetaminophen. Children rated their pain on a large vertical thermometer with numbers from 0 to 10 with 0 representing 'no pain' and 10 representing 'pain as bad as it could be'. As can be seen in Table 1, in spite of the use of analgesics children rated their pain as quite severe. The ratings of pain were consistent with their behaviors at the time of the ratings (Table 1) and with the measures of β-endorphin.

No studies could be found which evaluated the use of analgesics in controlling the pain of children's burn treatment.

TABLE 1
Pain scores associated with various procedures and behaviors.
Procedures and behaviors during BDC documented in the observer's records are presented with the mean pain scores occurring at the time of these events (Reprinted from Szylfelbein et al., 1985, p. 178, with permission.)

	Pain score (±SD)	no. of observations
Procedure		
Removal of outer layer of bandage	1.5±1.31	25
Removal of innermost layer of bandage	8.6±1.78	28
Debridement	6.9±2.81	111
Silver nitrate poured on wound or bandage	4.1±3.93	16
Salve applied to burn injury	3.2±3.16	27
Behavior		
Sleepy	1.1±1.46	7
Eating or drinking	1.4±1.65	10
Talking (conversation)	3.5±2.16	11
'It hurts'	7.3±2.25	15
Shouting, yelling	8.3±2.45	26
Moaning or crying	8.3±1.53	36
Expletives	9.1±1.64	8
Screaming	10.0±0	14

The use of psychological interventions in controlling pain during burn treatment has been investigated in both uncontrolled and controlled studies. Some studies focussed on global well-being and others have focussed specifically on pain.

One of the first reports was that of Bernstein (1963) who described the use of hypnosis with three children (two aged 8 years and one aged 11 years) who were having considerable difficulty coping with burn treatment. All three were successfully treated with hypnosis although in no case was hypnotic analgesia induced. The major changes in the behavior of the children was increased cooperation, decreased anxiety and improved mood. No measurement was used and there was no experimental design.

In a similar anecdotal report, Le Bau (1973) studied 23 severely burned children and reported major improvements in eating and a reduction in soiling and wetting through the use of hypnosis.

Shorkey and Taylor (1973), in a case study, discussed the use of signalling a child when an aversive procedure was to be done. This signalling allowed the child to let down her guard and relax at other times.

Case studies with hypnosis have also been reported by Weinstein (1976), and Stoddard (1982). In no case was there appropriate measurement or experimental design.

Varni et al. (1980) studied a 3-year-old girl who was showing significant pain behavior in using knee extension splints required in treatment of fixed muscle contraction from second and third degree burns. A design which combined multiple baseline across settings and a reversal was used to demonstrate effectiveness of treatment. Using an operant model, coping, non-pain behavior was reinforced socially and with tangible rewards, while ignoring was used to extinguish pain behavior. The child's pain behavior declined dramatically when the contingencies were imposed. As well, the child's behavior during splinting changed from resistive to helpful.

Kelley et al. (1984) used a single subject reversal design to evaluate the effects of cartoon viewing and a star feedback chart on the pain behavior of two children aged 4 and 6 years of age who were undergoing open treatment for second and third degree burns. The combination of an operant and a respondent component appeared to be effective in reducing the motoric and verbal pain behavior of both children. The ratings of pain and cooperativeness by the mother and the therapist were positively correlated with the pain behavior. However, the children's ratings of pain were not correlated with the ratings of the mother or therapist or the pain behavior.

Elliott and Olson (1983) used a combined multiple baseline and reversal design to examine the efficacy of a therapist-mediated, stress reduction, and cognitive coping skills program to reduce behavioral distress in four children undergoing hydrotherapy and debridement. The treatment was moderately effective for three of the four children. The treatment did not generalize to situations where the therapist was not actively coaching the children in the use of the techniques.

Tarnowski et al. (1987) in a single subject reversal design compared self-mediated debridement to therapist-mediated debridement with a 10-year-old boy. In the self-mediated debridement, the child controlled his own debridement and removed devitalized surface tissue. During therapist-mediated treatment, the therapist debrided the tissue. Pain behavior or distress was measured by means of the same objective scale used in the Kelley et al. (1984) study. Pain behavior was markedly reduced in the self-mediated treatment. However, because of the location of the burns some treatment had to be done by the therapist. During therapist controlled debridement immediately following self-debridement, pain behaviors were exacerbated.

Controlled group studies have been done by Wakeman and Kaplan (1978) and by Kavanagh (1983). Wakeman and Kaplan (1978) conducted two studies, one with patients suffering less than 30% burns and the second was with patients with burns from 30 to 60% of their bodies. Patients were assigned to either a hypnosis condition or a non-hypnosis condition. It does not appear that patient assignment was random. Patients in the hypnosis group were trained in hypnotic techniques of hypnoanalgesia, hypnoanesthesia, or dissociation and reduction of anxiety and fear. Initially therapist-mediated hypnosis was used but autohypnosis was then instituted. Patients in the non-hypnosis condition were given an equivalent amount of therapist attention. Subjects in the hypnosis group requested less analgesic medication than did the subjects in the non-hypnotic group. In both groups, patients between 7 and 18 years did better than the adult subjects. There were no other measures taken. The study although suggestive was seriously lacking. Subject assignment was apparently not random; no measures of pain were taken; only the hypnosis group gave informed consent; and there was no control for staff or patient expectancies.

Kavanagh (1983) studied nine children between the age of 2 and 11.5 years who had second and third degree burns. Two different procedures were used. The first was 'super standard care' in which the staff controlled the treatment and the child had little input into the procedure. The second treatment maximized the predictability and control of the child over the burn dressing changes. Children were not randomly assigned to treatments although they were roughly equivalent. As well, the reliability and validity of the nursing reports and the behavior inventories used was not assessed. However, there were important advantages to the group that received the experimental treatment in which there was more predictability and in which the children had more control of the burn dressing changes. The control group was more depressed at discharge and demonstrated more maladaptive behavior during the first 2 weeks of hospitalization.

Although the studies have serious methodological problems, taken together they indicate the promise of treatments that teach children relaxation, imagery and cognitive skills to control pain during debridement and give the children as much control over their treatment as possible. This type of treatment should be evaluated by careful experimental studies.

2.2.2. Suturing

Pain from suturing of cuts and other wounds has not been extensively researched. Alcock et al. (1985) evaluated the effects of a child life intervention in the emergency department suturing of 372 children. Self-report of pain was measured using a visual analogue scale, while pain behavior was measured with the procedures behavior rating scale (Katz et al., 1980). Four- to 6-year-old children reported feeling the most pain and displayed the most pain behavior. Older children (11–14 years of age) reported and displayed the least pain. Facial injuries resulted in greater pain than bodily injuries independent of the extent of the injury.

Child life intervention did not appear to have effects on pain but did impact on perceived satisfaction of parents' and on children's anxiety in some subgroups.

3. Sports and school injuries

3.1. Prevalence

The prevalence of sports injuries is not clear. However, in a recent survey of 729 adolescents, Feldman et al. (1986) found that 20% of adolescents were concerned about sports injuries.

Similarly, Hodgson et al. (1984) found that with routine reporting, there was an annual incidence rate of 5.4 per 100 children for both serious and non-serious injuries. Using more intensive reporting strategies, Hodgson et al. (1984) found that the true rate was approximately five times that rate. Serious injuries, those involving fractures, loss of consciousness, dislocations, sprains, torn ligaments or cartilage, chipped or broken teeth and internal injuries, accounted for 29% of all injuries. Organized sports were the major cause of injuries (35.3% of all injuries and 53.7% of serious injuries). The next most important causes were falls and body contact during playing/fighting.

Specific sports may produce specific injuries. For example tackle football may produce severe knee injuries (Andrish, 1985); elbow pain is common in baseball players (Pappas, 1982); sprains and strains to ankles and knees occur in soccer players (Ekstrand et al., 1983).

The most sensible ways of reducing pain due to sports injuries are prevention and appropriate management.

3.2. Prevention

There has been little well done research in the prevention of sports injuries. An exception to this is the exemplary randomized trial conducted by Ekstrand et al. (1983). This study examined the effectiveness of a prophylactic program in reducing the rate of a variety of soccer-related injuries incurred over a 6 month period in young adults. Their comprehensive prevention program included changes in training techniques, provision of adequate equipment, ankle taping, controlled rehabilitation, exclusion of players with grave knee instability, information on the importance of disciplined play and the danger of injuries during training, and correction and supervision by physiotherapists and doctors. Each component of their program was directed against a different type of injury. Results indicated 75% fewer injuries in test teams compared to controls.

Ekstrand et al. (1983) emphasized the need to develop prevention programs. Such programs must be based on careful study of the incidence, type, and localization of specific injuries associating a given sport with the mechanisms behind the injuries. A concern is the cost of their program. The professional supervision that they proposed represents a major expense. It would be important to evaluate the effectiveness of such a program without this component, particularly with reference to compliance to program recommendations. As the effectiveness of a variety of preventive measures in the area of sports injury is established, the problem of compliance with such measures remains. However, the Ekstrand et al. (1983) study stands out as a model for pain prevention research.

A poorly designed study has shown that a comprehensive approach to prevention and management does increase appropriate care and prevention behavior (Rice et al., 1985) in high school athletics.

3.3. Management

Management of sports injuries may reduce pain by reducing the immediate pain or by reducing long-term complications. There is ample evidence to believe that the management of sports injuries is woefully lacking. For example, Hodgson et al. (1984) in their school study found that only half of the fractures that occurred in their study were immediately referred to a hospital or doctor. Adults trained in first aid were present during a minority of physical education classes and intramural and interscholastic sports.

4. Intentional pain

4.1. Discipline

Pain has been a means of disciplining children throughout history (see chapter 1). Indeed the words pain and punishment derive from the same Latin root 'poena'. The prevalence of the use of pain in disciplining children is unknown but is probably very high in North American society. Most commentators do not currently encourage the use of pain in discipline. Spock (Spock and Rothenberg, 1985) decried the 'American tradition' of spanking and suggested that the widespread use of spanking may contribute to violence in society. Others, even in academic pediatric circles, do suggest spanking. Christopherson (1982, p. 286) for example, in a protocol for bedtime problems suggested the use of spanking:

> When your child gets up, give him one spank, and put him back to bed. Make this as matter-of-fact as possible.

Legislation or case law protects parents in many jurisdictions from criminal liability for 'reasonable' use of force in disciplining their children. For example, the Criminal Code of Canada states:

> Every schoolteacher, parent or person standing in the place of a parent is justified in using force by way of correction toward a pupil or child, as the case may be, who is under his care, if the force does not exceed what is reasonable under the circumstances.

This type of provision, either in statute or in case law, is the norm. However, there are exceptions. In 1979, Sweden inserted a clause in their legislated Code on Parenthood and Guardianship (Foraldrabalken) which states:

> A child may not be subjected to physical punishment or other injurious or humiliating treatment *(chapter 6, paragraph 3, section 2)*.

The impact of advice of experts or legislation on the extent of pain inflicted on children in the course of discipline is unknown. For example, we do not know if the extent of children being spanked has changed because of the introduction of the 'anti-spanking law' in Sweden.

4.2. Child abuse

Child abuse is a major social problem whose extent is not entirely known. However, nearly one million cases of child abuse and neglect are reported to child protection agencies in the United States each year (American Humane Association, 1984). The many strategies for prevention of child abuse including: teaching parenting skills to high risk families (Wolfe et al., 1987); teaching teachers about abuse and neglect (McGrath et al., 1987); altering community support systems; increasing awareness; and improving social agency, judicial and police response to domestic violence, although promising, have yet to be shown effective.

5. Clinical guidelines

(1) Automobile child restraints and seat belts should be used at all times.
(2) Decrease the extreme pain associated with debridement, hydrotherapy, and splinting for burn patients by self-mediated treatment and appropriate use of analgesics.
(3) The purchase of infant walkers should be discouraged.
(4) Implementation of sports prevention programs especially at the high school level should be encouraged.

6. Future directions

(1) Evaluation of the use of analgesics in relieving pain from debridement is needed.
(2) Implementation and evaluation of the prevention of injuries in and from automobiles, as well as from burns and sports injuries is required.
(3) Research of the effectiveness of programs to prevent child abuse are vital.
(4) New techniques of delivery of analgesics such as nebulizers (Masters, 1986) or percutaneous 'band-aid analgesia' for injured children who are in pain and shock should be developed. These children frequently do not readily absorb intramuscular injections and intravenous delivery may be difficult.

References

Alcock, D.S., Feldman, W., Goodman, J.T., McGrath, P.J. and Park, M. (1985) Evaluation of child life intervention in emergency department suturing. Pediatr. Emerg. Care 1, 111–115.

American Humane Association (1984) Trends in Child Abuse and Neglect: A National Perspective (AHA, Denver, CO).

Andrish, J.T. (1985) Knee injuries in gymnastics. Clin. Sports Med. 4, 111–121.

Beales, J.G. (1982) Factors influencing the expectation of pain among patients in a children's burns unit. Burns Incl. Therm. Inj. 9, 187–192.

Bernstein, N.R. (1963) Management of burned children with the aid of hypnosis. J. Child Psychol. 4, 93–98.

Canadian Medical Association (1987) Ban sale of baby walkers, CMA urges. Can. Med. Assoc. J. 136, 57.

Christopherson, E.R. (1982) Incorporating behavioral pediatrics into primary care. In: E.R. Christopherson (Ed.), The Pediatric Clinics of North America, Vol. 29, no. 2, Symposium on Behavioral Pediatrics (W.B. Saunders, Toronto) pp. 261–313.

Criminal Code of Canada (Queen's Printer, Ottawa) chapter 51, section 43.

Ekstrand, J., Gillquist, J. and Liljedahl, S. (1983) Prevention of soccer injuries. Am. J. Sports Med. 11, 116–120.

Elliott, C.H. and Olson, R.A. (1983) The management of children's distress in response to painful medical treatment for burn injuries. Behav. Res. Ther. 21, 675–683.

Feldman, W., Hodgson, C., Corber, S. and Quinn, A. (1986) Health concerns and health-related behaviours of adolescents. C. Med. Assoc. J. 134, 489–493.

Feldman, W., Rosser, W. and McGrath, P. (1987) Primary medical care of children and adolescents (Oxford University Press, New York).

Hingson, R., Morrigan, D. and Heeron, T. (1985) Effects of Massachusetts raising its legal drinking age from 18 to 20 on deaths from teenage homicide, suicide and non-traffic accidents. Pediatr. Clin. North Am. 32, 221–232.

Hodgson, C., Woodward, C.A. and Feldman, W. (1984) A descriptive study of school injuries in a Canadian region. Pediatr. Nurs., May/June issue, 215–220.

Katz, E.R., Kellerman, J. and Siegel, S. (1980) Behavioral distress in children with cancer undergoing medical procedures: Developmental considerations. J. Consult. Clin. Psychol. 48, 356–365.

Kavanagh, C. (1983) Psychological intervention with the severely burned child: Report of an experimental comparison of two approaches and their effects on psychological sequelae. J. Am. Acad. Child Psychiatr. 22, 145–156.

Kelley, M.L., Jarvie, G.J., Middlebrook, J.L., McNeer, M.F. and Drabman, R.S. (1984) Decreasing burned children's pain behavior: Impacting the trauma of hydrotherapy. J. Appl. Behav. Anal. 17, 147–158.

Le Bau, W.L. (1973) Adjunctive trance therapy with severely burned children. Int. J. Child Psychother. 2, 80–92.

Long, R.T. and Cope, O.C. (1961) Emotional problems of burned children. New Engl. J. Med. 264, 1121–1127.

McGrath, P.J. and Vair, C. (1983) Psychological aspects of pain management of the burned child. Child. Health Care 13, 15–19.

McGrath, P.J., Wiseman, D., Allan, B., Khalil, N. and Cappelli, M. (1987) Teacher awareness program on child abuse: A randomized controlled trial. Child Abuse Neglect 11, 125–132.

Masters, N. (1986) Nebulised pain relief for children. Arch. Dis. Child. 61, 1142.

Organization for Economic Cooperation and Development (1983) Traffic Safety of Children. Report of a scientific expert group, Paris.

Pappas, A.M. (1982) Elbow problems associated with baseball during childhood and adolescence. Clin. Orthop. Relat. Res. 164, 30–41.

Perry, S. and Heidrich, G. (1982) Management of pain during debridement: a survey of U.S. burn units. Pain 13, 267–280.

Rice, S.G., Schlolfield, J.D. and Foley, W.E. (1985) The Athletic Healthcare and Training Program: A comprehensive approach to the prevention and management of athletic injuries in high school. West. J. Med. 142, 352–357.

Ross, D.M. and Ross, S.A. (1984) Childhood pain: the school-aged child's viewpoint. Pain 20, 179–191.

Rosser, W., Feldman, W. and McGrath, P. (1987) A critical look at the family physician's role in preventing childhood injuries. Can. Fam. Phys. 33, 733–740.

Shorkey, C.T. and Taylor, J.E. (1973) Management of maladaptive behavior of a severely burned child. Child Welfare 52, 543–547.

Sorenson, B. (1976) Prevention of burns and scalds in a developed country. J. Trauma 16, 249–258.

Spock, B. and Rothenberg, M.B. (1985) Baby and Child Care (Pocket Books, New York) pp. 398–409.

Stoddard, F. (1982) Coping with pain: A developmental approach to treatment of burned children. Am. J. Psychiatr. 139, 736–742.

Szyfelbein, S.K., Osgood, P.F. and Carr, D.B. (1985) The assessment of pain and plasma β-endorphin immunoactivity in burned children. Pain 22, 173–182.

Tarnowski, K.J., McGrath, M.L., Calhoun, M.B. and Drabman, R.S. (1987) Pediatric thermal injury: Self- versus therapist-mediated debridement. J. Appl. Behav. Anal., in press.

Varni, J.W., Bessman, C.A., Russo, D.C. and Cataldo, M.F. (1980) Behavioral management of chronic pain in children: Case study. Arch. Phys. Med. Rehabil. 61, 375–379.

Wakeman, R.J. and Kaplan, J.Z. (1978) An experimental study of hypnosis in painful burns. Am. J. Clin. Hypn. 21, 3–12.

Warner, P. (1982) Playground injuries and voluntary product standards for home and public playgrounds. Pediatrics 69, 18–20.

Weinstein, D.J. (1976) Imagery and relaxation with a burned patient. Behav. Res. Ther. 14, 481.

Williams, A. and Wells, J. (1981) Evaluation of the Rhode Island child restraint law. Am. J. Public Health 71, 742–743.

Wolfe, D.A., Edwards, B., Manion, I. and Koverola, C. (1987) An evaluation of parent training and family support approaches to child abuse and neglect early intervention. J. Consult. Clin. Psychol., in press.

U.S. Fire Administration (1983) An Ounce of Prevention (Federal Emergency Management Agency, Washington, DC).

CHAPTER 13

Chronic intractable pain

1. Introduction

In this chapter, we will first delineate a syndrome that we call chronic intractable pain and subsequently discuss the factors that may be related to the causation of the syndrome. Finally, we will focus on the management of the syndrome and its impact on the individual and the family.

2. Definition of chronic intractable pain

A difficulty arises when defining chronic pain. If chronic pain simply refers to any pain that lasts longer than some predetermined length of time, say 3 or 6 months, then all of the recurrent pains of childhood (headache, recurrent abdominal pain and growing pains) or pain from arthritis and many pains from cancer should be considered chronic pain and those suffering such pain are chronic pain patients. However, we prefer to consider chronic pain in terms of the psychosocial impact of the pain rather than its duration. Crue (1985) distinguishes four types of long-term pain: recurrent acute, ongoing acute, chronic benign and chronic benign intractable pain syndrome.

Recurrent acute pain refers to pain from underlying recurrent or continued nociceptive input. Examples are migraine or arthritis. Ongoing acute pain refers to pain from malignant disease. Chronic benign pain, according to Crue (1985) refers to ongoing pain with no known nociceptive input but with adequate coping. Chronic benign intractable pain syndrome refers to chronic pain with poor patient coping. Since we agree with Bonica (1985) that no long-term pain is benign, we have chosen to label the syndrome of poor coping with long-term pain which is not accounted for by known nociceptive input, chronic intractable pain. We consider pain to be chronic intractable pain if it is long lasting and interferes, in a major way, with the child's life. Any of the types of pain can become chronic intractable pain problems. In our opinion, it is not the type or frequency of the pain which defines chronic intractable pain. Rather it is the ability of the child to cope with the pain and the degree to which the pain interferes with daily activities that makes long term pain into a chronic problem. Unfortunately, the pain literature has ignored what we believe to be the majority of people who have long-term pain but who cope. Pain sufferers who are coping seldom attend pain clinics and are unlikely to be subjects of chronic pain studies.

It is quite clear that most children who have chronic or recurrent types of pain cope quite well. However, there is a small group of children who do not cope. Very little is known about factors which may differentiate between those children who are coping well with their pain and those who are not.

The definition of what constitutes significant disruption of a child's life or failure to cope is difficult. In practice, a clinical judgement can be made considering social, academic and family life. For research purposes, we (Dunn-Geier et al., 1986) have used school absence as the criterion for non-coping.

The prevalence of chronic intractable pain in children is unknown but we do know it is quite rare. Chronic intractable pain can be of unknown cause. For example, in the case of children disabled by abdominal pain there is usually no discernible cause. On the other hand, there may be a cause for pain but the child's pain far exceeds the known cause. The child may remain disabled long after the cause should be operative. An example of this latter case would be the child who has a minor sprain and gives up social activities for several months. Pain that is due to specific causes such as arthritis, sickle cell disease or cancer is discussed in specific chapters. Pain that is psychologically caused, psychogenic pain, is discussed in chapter 14.

3. Factors influencing chronic intractable pain

Six factors have been described as important in the etiology of coping with chronic pain: family functioning, modelling, depression, stress, reinforcement and somatization disorder.

3.1. Family functioning

Family overinvolvement or enmeshment of parents in the lives of their children has been cited as a cause of chronic pain by clinicians (Stone and Barbero, 1970; Apley, 1975; Hughes and Zimin, 1978). Each has noted that children suffering from chronic benign pain frequently have parents who are overinvolved in their children's lives and that the children encourage or permit this level of involvement. The classic work of Engel (1959), which involved adults recalling their childhood, emphasized that aggression, suffering and pain during childhood (often imposed by a punitive or abusive parent) played an important role in chronic intractable pain. Engel (1959) also felt that chronic pain problems might be the heritage of cold or distant parents.

Minuchin and his colleagues (Minuchin et al., 1975) have most extensively developed a model of family functioning in coping with chronic pain. The model was originally developed in relationship to diabetics and anorexics but has been widely applied to families with chronic pain. They suggested that three factors are necessary for the development of severe 'psychosomatic' illness in children. First, the family must be physiologically vulnerable. Second, the family must possess the following characteristics: enmeshment, overprotectiveness, rigidity and lack of conflict resolution. Finally, the child must play an important role in the family's pattern of conflict avoidance and this role must be important in the reinforcement of the child's symptoms.

Clinically, in our practice we have found that the overinvolvement appears to include elements of excessive parental caregiving but, more importantly, excessive control (Parker, 1983). This pattern of behavior is often evident even in the initial clinical interview when questions addressed to the child are repeatedly answered by the parent. Our clinical impression is that a number of elements come together to produce the overinvolvement of the family of the pediatric chronic intractable pain patient. The first is long-term pain of any type. The second is at least one parent who is overinvolved. Often this takes the form of a very sympathetic and domineering parent. Third, the other parent must be collaborating in the overinvolvement or be absent physically or emotionally. Finally, the child or adolescent must be unassertive in dealing with the pain and his/her parents. We have not found any avoidance of conflict in these families. The typical situation is that of a teenage girl who has headaches, an overinvolved mother and an absent father. We have seen, however, all possible combinations. It should be noted that we have no objective data to support this model in toto and we regard this model as too simplistic to reflect the complexity of individual families.

In order to examine some of these issues in a more rigorous way we (Dunn-Geier et al., 1986) compared adolescents, who were not coping with long-term benign pain, and their mothers with a matched group of adolescents, who were coping, and their mothers. We struggled with a definition of coping and finally decided to use school attendance as a measure of coping. School attendance was chosen because it is the best single indicator of the extent to which an adolescent is fulfilling his/her principal developmental demand. Children in our coping group had missed an average of 0.4 days in the preceding 2 months and the non-coping children had missed 14.7 days. Mother-child interaction was videotaped during two, 15 min sessions in which the mother supervised a series of exercises (arm-curls, sit-ups and step-ups) which were designed to simulate naturally occurring situations that would trigger pain. Videotapes were blindly scored at 10 s intervals using a variant of Mash and Terdal's (1981) response class matrix. A pain diary was kept for 1 week and questionnaires were given to the subjects. The two groups did not significantly differ on the amount of pain they reported on a 1 week pain diary or on the duration of their pain problem. The personality and family questionnaires did not yield differences. However, the behavioral interaction was very telling (Table 1). Non-coping adolescents engaged in significantly more negative behavior. The mothers of non-copers were more intrusive in the tasks both in encouraging and discouraging coping and non-coping. Discriminant analysis with one variable, mother discouraging coping, correctly classified 100% of copers and 70% of non-copers. Although, it is clear that the mothers in our sample of non-copers were more intrusive and encouraged more pain behavior it is not clear if this parental behavior is a

TABLE 1

Means, SDs and *t* values of the frequency of child antecedent and parent behaviors. (Reprinted from Dunn-Geier et al., 1986, with permission of the author and Elsevier.)

Variable	Copers		Non-copers		
	M	SD	M	SD	*t*
Child behaviors					
Pain expression	1.60	1.26	7.00	7.07	2.38
On-task	173.40	9.05	151.40	28.50	2.33
Off-task	3.90	8.76	13.70	21.69	1.32
Negative	1.10	1.37	7.90	6.30	3.34*
Parent behaviors					
Encourage coping	1.30	1.34	3.80	3.55	2.08
Discourage coping	1.50	1.35	8.50	5.30	4.05*

*$P < 0.05$.

$n = 10$ per group.

cause or a result of having a child who is not coping with pain. It may be that having to deal with a child who is not coping with pain generates the type of behavior that we observed in these parents.

3.2. Modelling

The notion that children learn how to cope or not cope with their pain from their parents is intuitively appealing. A number of researchers have noted a family aggregation of chronic intractable pain. For example, Apley (1975) reported that abdominal pain was six times more likely to occur in siblings of and parents of abdominal pain patients than in controls. Although a number of authors have suggested that children with chronic intractable pain come from 'pain-prone' families, the evidence is weak since no standardized way of determining pain prone has been used and usually no control groups are used. For example, as noted in chapter 6, Christensen and Mortensen (1975) followed up 34 children who had been hospitalized for recurrent abdominal pain approximately 30 years earlier. They found that the children of these patients were no more likely than controls to be experiencing pain. However, children whose parents were currently experiencing pain were more likely to have pain themselves. This suggested that the children were modelling the pain behavior of their parents. No measure of severity of pain or coping with the pain was used. We have not found increased pain in the families of children who have recurrent abdominal pain (McGrath et al., 1983). We have not examined the family aggregation of pain in chronic intractable pain.

Edwards et al. (1985) found that college students who reported that they had more relatives with long lasting pain were more likely to report more pain. Similarly, Sternbach (1986) reported a generational effect in that individuals with pain had parents with pain problems.

Experimental studies of modelling of pain behavior with adults provide strong support for the potential power that modelling may play in pain perception and reaction to pain (Craig, 1978, 1983; Prkachin and Craig, 1985).

3.3. Depression

The role of depression in chronic intractable pain can be conceptualized in two ways. The first is to see depression as the result of having a long-standing pain disorder. The second is to see chronic pain as a symptom of depression.

It is likely that both are important in specific cases. The primacy of depression as a reaction to chronic pain versus depression as a cause of chronic pain in any sample of children may well depend on the selection or referral bias of the group studied. Samples of children selected because they have pain may have somewhat elevated depression scores depending on the severity of their pain but will not typically have scores in the clinically depressed range (Cunningham et al., 1987). On the other hand, depressed adolescents and children will likely have a greater incidence of various aches and pains. Studies of specific types of pain have tended to find a somewhat higher incidence of depressive feelings in children with pain but not a high rate of clinical depression. Each of these has been discussed in the specific chapter on that type of pain. No surveys of pain experienced by depressed children have been reported.

3.4. Stress

As we have described in chapters on specific pains, stress is frequently seen as a precipitant of recurrent abdominal pain and headache for which there are no clear organic causes. The evidence is not strong, particularly because of the difficulty of gathering data that is not hopelessly confounded. No research on stress in chronic intractable pain in children has been reported. Children who are not coping well with pain may not only experience more stressful situations but they are likely to precipitate more stressful events in their lives.

3.5. Reinforcement

Reinforcement of pain behavior has been shown to be an important determinant of not coping with pain in adults (Fordyce, 1976). Although it is a popular belief that reinforcement is a common cause of chronic intractable pain in children, little research has been done. In our lab, in one study, we demonstrated that children with chronic pain are reinforced for their pain behavior. Dunn-Geier et al. (1986) did show that mothers of children not coping with pain did reinforce their children for pain behavior more than did mothers of children with pain who were coping.

Single case treatment studies have also demonstrated the role of operant factors in specific children who were not coping well with abdominal pain (Sank and Biglan, 1974; Miller and Kratchowill, 1979) and headache (Ramsden et al., 1983).

3.6. Somatization disorder

Routh and Ernst (1984) found that children who have recurrent abdominal pain for which no organic cause can be determined had more symptoms of somatization disorder than children with an organic abdominal pain disorder. Somatization disorder refers to a psychiatric disorder in which the patient reports multiple physical symptoms (at least 14 in women or 12 in men) which have interfered with everyday life and for which no organic cause can be found (American Psychiatric Association, 1980). As well, children, who were attending the clinic and who had experienced pain for several years, had more symptoms of somatization disorder than children with recurrent abdominal pain of a more recent onset. Relatives of these children were also found to have a higher incidence of somatization disorder (Ernst et al., 1984). These data can best be interpreted as evidence that a subgroup of children (approximately 17%), who have recurrent abdominal pain for more than 1 year, may develop into adult patients with somatization disorder. Children who have numerous widespread or changing pain symptoms without specific physical findings, who are missing school and whose parents have similar types of problems are clearly at risk for developing a chronic pain disorder.

4. Management of chronic intractable pain

Although the principles of treatment for children for whom a cause of their pain is known and those for whom no cause is known are the same, it may be easier to treat children with a definite medical diagnosis (McGrath et al., 1986). Children with no diagnosis are usually defensive about the pain being 'all in their heads' or the suspicion that they may be malingering. We will review the management of these children focussing on the same factors as mentioned in etiology of poor coping. Studies focussing on specific diseases are reviewed in their respective chapters.

4.1. Family functioning

No studies have evaluated interventions focussing on family functioning. However, it is our judgement as well as the consensus of the literature that the family (Minuchin et al., 1975) must be involved in any treatment program. Our own bias is to use a behavioral model of family therapy but other approaches may be equally effective.

4.2. Modelling

Modelling of coping responses by parents could provide a powerful tool for children who are not coping. However, in those families with parents with chronic intractable pain we have found changing parental pain behavior to be difficult. However, in some cases, parents become motivated to improve their own coping to help their children.

4.3. Depression

Treatment of depression can be medical or psychological. Medical treatment involves antidepressant medication in particular the tricyclics. The efficacy of using tricyclics is well-established in adult depression and appears effective with children and adolescents but no controlled studies have been done. Psychological treatment can be in the form of psychotherapy or cognitive behavioral strategies. Again, these strategies have been evaluated with adults but not with children but are likely to be helpful with adolescents.

4.4. Stress

Reduction of the effects of stress can be done by reducing stressors or by teaching better coping skills such as relaxation or cognitive restructuring. Randomized trials on the treatment of specific pains have shown effectiveness of these treatments (e.g., Richter et al., 1986, with migraine) but no studies have been done with children with chronic intractable pain. It is our clinical experience that stress management is necessary but not sufficient treatment for children with chronic intractable pain.

4.5. Reinforcement

Masek et al. (1984) have outlined a series of suggestions for parents to help children cope with pain. These guidelines focus on encouraging normal activity and discouraging pain behavior. Suggestions for encouraging normal behavior revolve around frequent approval for normal activity patterns and strong advocacy for school attendance as the norm. Discouraging pain behavior is accomplished by ignoring verbal and non-verbal pain complaints, preventing escape or avoidance of responsibilities, dispensing any pain medication on a schedule rather than in response to complaints, and not asking questions about the pain. No evaluation of these suggestions has been done. Our experience is that, if implemented, these suggestions are extremely helpful to children with chronic intractable pain. However, we have found that obtaining parental compliance is frequently difficult.

4.6. Somatization disorder

No evaluation of treatment of somatization disorder in children has been published. Treatment of somatization disorder in adults is usually very difficult and unrewarding. No controlled trials have been published.

5. Effects on the child of chronic intractable pain

The child with chronic pain, who is not coping with a long-term pain problem, is at serious risk for major psychosocial problems. First of all, from studies of children with a long-standing pain problem (Andrasik et al., 1987; Cunningham et al., 1987) we know that they are at increased risk for psychosocial problems. Similarly, children with chronic illness are at higher risk for psychosocial problems (Satterwhite, 1978; Pless, 1983) and those with reduced mobility may be at greatest risk (Cadman et al., 1987). Children with chronic pain are burdened with social isolation and high risk for academic failure which prevent the child from learning age-appropriate skills. Finally, children with chronic pain may well grow up into adults with chronic pain.

6. Effects on the family of long-term pain

No studies have examined the impact on the family of having a child who is not coping with a long-term pain problem. The literature on the impact on the family of having a chronic disease and our clinical impressions are all we have to draw on. Our own clinical impression is that these families are consumed by the search for a cure for their child's pain. Although the child's problem may provide a focus for the family and a sense of meaning and purpose (Minuchin et al., 1975), the cost is high.

7. Pharmacological treatment

The analgesic treatment of specific disorders, such as cancer, headache and arthritis, has been discussed in relevant chapters. Since chronic intractable pain has two components, pain and failure to cope, analgesic pharmaco-therapy must be accompanied by more comprehensive psychological inter-vention. The use of pharmacotherapy as a sole treatment in chronic intractable pain is contraindicated. Although experience with children is limited, there is extensive evidence from the adult literature that analgesic therapy alone in chronic intractable pain may lead to problems of doctor-shopping, poly-drug abuse and deterioration of the ability to function (Aronoff and Evans, 1985).

ASA and acetaminophen are the most widely used and the best analgesics for children with pain (see chapter 4). Non-steroidal anti-inflammatory drugs are also of some use in some children (see chapter 9 for a discussion of these drugs).

In sharp contrast to postoperative pain and cancer pain, the use of opioid analgesics may be problematic in children with chronic intractable pain as it frequently is in adults with chronic intractable pain (Aronoff and Evans, 1985). The tendency is for chronic intractable pain patients to expect analgesics to eliminate their problems. When this does not happen, a search for a more effective drug often begins. Long-term use of opioid analgesics will result in tolerance and need for larger doses. Increasing doses also lead to more side effects and dependence. Drug abuse is a possibility with children and adolescents with chronic intractable pain.

Tricyclic antidepressants are prescribed for depression, and also may have some use in chronic intractable pain in adolescents. The analgesic action of tricyclics in chronic pain is in debate with some arguing that the effect is essentially secondary to the antidepressive effect with others maintaining that the effect is independent (Walsh, 1983; Feinmann, 1985).

The major tranquillizers, especially the phenothiazines have been suggested for their ability to potentiate opioids (Lacouture et al., 1984) but their use in chronic intractable pain has not been evaluated. Their use in children for pain has not been well documented.

The minor tranquillizers, especially the benzodiazepines, are useful in the short-term treatment of anxiety, do have sedative-type effects (Lacouture et al., 1984) but have not been shown useful in chronic intractable pain.

As Lacouture et al. (1984) have noted, anticonvulsants would seem to have no role in the management of pain. However, they have been recommended for migraine (see chapter 8), deafferentation pain, and for lancinating pain in the face.

8. Clinical guidelines

Fortunately, although many suffer pain, only a very small group of children and adolescents are chronic pain patients. Most child health specialists have little experience with these patients and their families. As well, there is little or no guidance in standard pediatric or pain texts for the clinician who is not experienced in this area. Consequently, we (McGrath et al., 1986) have developed a series of guidelines to assist the clinician in dealing with these most difficult patients and their families.

(1) Begin psychosocial assessment as soon as non-coping occurs. Psychosocial assessment should be an intrinsic part of all cases when the child is not coping. Children who are not attending school regularly or who are curtailing their social activities because of pain are not coping. Assessment consists mostly of interviewing, record keeping and observation of the child and the family. Standardized psychological tests have not been shown to be of use in assessing childhood chronic intractable pain. Early assessment may reduce the probability of the development of chronic problems of school absence and social withdrawal. Patients and their families are more likely to accept a psychological referral and not feel abandoned if it is presented as a routine procedure in all cases of long-term pain causing disruption of normal activities.

(2) Unless the cause of the pain is clearly evident, avoid the organic/psychogenic dichotomy. Most chronic intractable pain of childhood cannot be diagnosed as either organic or psychogenic and is of unknown origin (Barr and Feuerstein, 1983). Consequently, much time and effort may be expended with little yield. The failure to find an organic cause of the pain does not mean that it is psychogenic. Psychogenic and organic causes of pain can coexist, and as a result, a finding of psychological causation cannot rule out organic factors.

(3) Emphasize coping rather than curing. The alternative to focussing on the organic/psychogenic dichotomy is to focus on coping with the pain. Children should be encouraged to engage in as many activities as they can that do not result in physical harm or debilitating levels of pain. There should be an expectation that pain will continue but will not dominate the life of the child or the family. Parents should be encouraged to ignore minor complaints and to pay attention to coping behavior. Appropriate use of analgesics will often be helpful in coping but will rarely eradicate the pain experienced by these patients.

(4) Focus on family strengths. Although we do not advocate a slavish

adherence to any one model or school of therapy we are absolutely convinced that in all cases the families must be included in treatment. Individual sessions, family sessions and sessions with the parents may be required. It is far too easy to locate and explore only the pathological aspects of a family. Successful management will, however, be based on strengths not on weaknesses. The strengths of each family will vary. In one family, enmeshment can be reframed into closeness. In another family, strong identification with a parent can be used to model coping behavior or rebellion can be constructively channelled.

(5) Investigate the school situation. A major part of a child's life is spent at school. A child, who is not coping with chronic intractable pain, may have a number of school-related stresses that could be triggering avoidance behavior and non-coping pain behavior. On the other hand, a child may be succeeding in school but have an overwhelming fear of failure. Telephone calls to the child's teacher may reveal serious stresses. Private discussions with the child may uncover hidden problems. The clinician should also be aware of the possibility that the stress of a learning problem and consequent repeated failure may encourage non-coping behavior. Direct intervention to correct a social problem such as an intolerable schoolbus ride or instituting a more rewarding educational program by identifying and remediating a learning problem can quickly enhance coping.

(6) Teach coping skills. Teaching specific cognitive and behavioral coping skills such as relaxation and cognitive restructuring will give parents and families a sense of control over the situation as well as reducing pain and its effects.

(7) Listen to the patient. As in any clinical situation, it is crucial to carefully listen to the concerns of the patient and family. It is rarely if ever helpful to try to convince a family or a patient that the pain they are experiencing is psychological, not physical or that the patient is malingering. Never doubt a patient's statement that he is in pain. First of all, since pain is a phenomenological event only the person in pain can say how much pain he is feeling. Furthermore, challenging a patient that he is not in pain is only likely to cause an increase in pain behavior to prove the validity of the pain.

It is helpful to know the patient's view or theory of what is causing the pain (Beales, 1982). Not only will patient defensiveness be reduced if they feel they are understood, but also errors in information can be corrected. A diary of pain intensity and mitigating factors that is read and queried by the therapist can provide excellent information from which discussion can begin. As well, the diary can enhance the adolescent's feelings that he is being taken seriously. At the same time, having a child keep a pain diary can reduce unproductive complaining by ensuring he will be heard.

Chronic pain sufferers, who are not coping, are difficult to get into therapy and difficult to keep in therapy. The trust in the therapist may often be the most powerful incentive to continue.

Part of listening to one's patients is being open to second opinions. If you do not appear open to another evaluation, you may force doctor-shopping on your patient.

(8) Do not blame the patient or family. Chronic intractable pain patients and their families frequently provoke strong, hostile reactions in health professionals and it is easy to attribute blame. Blaming the patient may be a response to our own frustration and inability to help. Some chronic intractable pain patients may be skilled in triggering such responses. Patients and families easily discern if they are being blamed. Blaming is not functional nor is it valid. It is no more the patients' fault if they are unable to cope with pain than it is their fault if their immune system is deficient. To successfully help a patient cope one must form an alliance with the family against the pain and carefully avoid all reference to blame. The patient, family and doctor must be a team not adversaries.

Patients may turn the issue of blame around and be hostile in accusing doctors of not finding what is wrong with them. Professional defensiveness, in this situation, is seldom helpful. After all, they are right – we have failed to find the cause and the cure for their pain.

(9) Educate about pain. The more the patient is educated about his pain the better able he will be to form an alliance with the doctor. Knowledge can make the family and child feel in a stronger position to discuss their situation with health professionals. In addition, education can correct misconceptions about pain and help the family understand issues such as: hurt does not always mean damage; avoidance will cause further fear; one can be productive and in pain. Knowledge about the type of symptoms that should and should not cause concern can assist the patients and their family in discriminating between variations in a symptom that are meaningful from those that are not.

(10) Understand without pitying. Although the health professional must be understanding about chronic intractable pain, they must also provide reasonable expectations that are frequently lacking in families of non-

copers. There is no place in chronic intractable pain for encouraging self-pity. Tender loving care and extra attention for pain is appropriate when the pain is acute but is destructive for the patient who is not coping with chronic pain (Sternbach, 1974). Firm expectations can provide a model for parents and a hope for the child.

Goals should be realistic given the family's current ability. Short-term goals or shaping of target behavior is often appropriate. A child who has been away from school for weeks may have to return in steps. Unrealistic goals will only encourage failure and future avoidance.

9. Future directions

(1) Education of health care professionals in the treatment of chronic intractable pain in children is needed.
(2) Research on the correlates and treatment of intractable pain is required.
(3) Pharmacotherapy in chronic intractable pain requires investigation.

References

American Psychiatric Association (1980) Diagnostic and Statistical Manual of Mental Disorders, 3 edn. (A.P.A., Washington DC).

Andrasik, F., Kabela, E., Quinn, S., Blanchard, E.B. and Rosenblum, E.L. (1987) Psychological functioning of children who have recurrent migraine, manuscript under review.

Apley, J. (1975) The Child with Abdominal Pains, 2nd edn. (Blackwell, London).

Aronoff, G.M. and Evans, W.O. (1985) Pharmacological management of chronic pain. In: G.M. Aronoff (Ed.), Evaluation and Treatment of Chronic Pain (Urban and Schwarzenberg, Baltimore, MD) pp. 435–449.

Barr, R.G. and Feuerstein, M. (1983) Recurrent abdominal pain syndrome: How appropriate are our basic clinical assumptions? In: P.J. McGrath and P. Firestone (Eds.), Pediatric and Adolescent Behavioral Medicine: Issues in Treatment (Springer, New York) pp. 13–27.

Beales, J.G. (1982) The assessment and management of pain in children. In: P. Karoly, J.J. Steffen and D.J. O'Grady (Eds.), Child Health Psychology; Concepts and Issues (Pergamon, New York) pp. 154–179.

Bonica, J.J. (1985) Importance of the problem. In: G.M. Aronoff (Ed.), Evaluation and Treatment of Chronic Pain (Urban and Schwarzenberg, Baltimore, MD) pp. xxxi–xliv.

Cadman, D., Boyle, M., Szatmari, M. and Offord, D.R. (1987) Chronic illness, disability and mental and social well-being: Findings of the Ontario Child Health Study.

Christensen, M.F. and Mortensen, O. (1975) Longterm prognosis in children with recurrent abdominal pain. Arch. Dis. Child. 50, 110–114.

Craig, K.D. (1978) Social modelling influences on pain. In: R.A. Sternbach (Ed.), The Psychology of Pain (Raven Press, New York) pp. 73–109.

Craig, K.D. (1983) Modelling and social learning factors in chronic pain. In: J.J. Bonica, U. Lindblom and A. Iggo (Eds.), Advances in Pain Research and Therapy (Raven Press, New York) pp. 813–827.

Crue, B.L. (1985) Foreword. In: G.M. Aronoff (Ed.), Evaluation and Treatment of Chronic Pain (Urban and Schwarzenberg, Baltimore, MD) pp. xv–xxi.

Cunningham, S.J., McGrath, P.J., Ferguson, H.B., Humphreys, P., D'Astous, J., Latter, J., Goodman, J.T. and Firestone, P. (1987) Personality and behavioral characteristics in pediatric migraine. Headache 27, 16–20.

Dunn-Geier, B.J., McGrath, P.J., Rourke, B.P., Latter, J. and D'Astous, J. (1986) Adolescent chronic pain: the ability to cope. Pain 26, 23–32.

Edwards, P.W., Zeichner, A., Kuczmierczyk, A.R. and Bockowski, J. (1985) Familial pain models: The relationship between family history of pain and current pain experience. Pain 21, 379–384.

Engel, G.L. (1959) 'Psychogenic' pain and the pain-prone patient. Am. J. Med. 26, 899–918

Ernst, A.R., Routh, D.K. and Harper, D.C. (1984) Abdominal pain in children and symptoms of somatization disorder. J. Pediatr. Psychol. 9, 77–86.

Feinmann, C. (1985) Pain relief by antidepressants: Possible modes of action. Pain 23, 1–8.

Fordyce, W.E. (1976) Behavioral Methods for Chronic Pain and Illness (Mosby, St. Louis, MO).

Greene, J.W., Walker, L.S., Hickson, G. and Thompson, J. (1985) Stressful life events and somatic complaints in adolescents. Pediatrics 75, 19–22.

Hughes, M.C. and Zimin, R. (1978) Children with psychogenic abdominal pain and their families: Management during hospitalization. Clin. Pediatr. 17, 569–573.

Huskisson, E.C. (1984) Non-narcotic analgesics. In: P.D. Wall and R. Melzack (Eds.), Textbook of Pain (Churchill Livingstone, Edinburgh) pp. 505–513.

Lacouture, P.G., Baudreault, P. and Lovejoy, F.H. (1984) Chronic pain of childhood: A pharmacologic approach. Pediatr. Clin. North Am. 31, 1133–1151.

McGrath, P.J., Dunn-Geier, J., Cunningham, S.J., Brunette, R., D'Astous, J., Humphreys, P., Latter, J. and Keene, D. (1986) Psychological guidelines for helping children cope with chronic benign intractable pain. Clin. J. Pain 1, 229–233.

Masek, B.J., Russo, D.C. and Varni, J.W. (1984) Behavioral approaches to the management of chronic pain in children. Pediatr. Clin. North Am. 31, 1113–1131.

Mash, E. and Terdal, L. (1981) Behavioral Assessment of Childhood Disorders (Guilford Press, New York).

Miller, A.J. and Kratchowill, T.R. (1979) Reduction of frequent stomach-ache complaints by time-out. Behav. Ther. 10, 211–218.

Minuchin, S., Baker, L., Rosman, B., Liebman, R., Milman, L. and Todd, T. (1975) A conceptual model of psychosomatic illness in children: Family organization and family therapy. Arch. Gen. Psychiatr. 32, 1031–1038.

Newburger, P.E. and Sallan, S.E. (1981) Chronic pain: Principles of management. J. Pediatr. 98, 180–189.

Parker, G. (1983) Parental Overprotection: A Risk Factor in Psychosocial Development (Grune and Stratton, New York).

Pennebaker, J. (1982) The Psychology of Physical Symptoms (Springer-Verlag, New York).

Pless, I.B. (1983) Effects of chronic illness on adjustment: Clinical implications. In:

P. Firestone, P.J. McGrath and W. Feldman (Eds.), Advances in Behavioral Medicine for Children and Adolescents (Erlbaum, Hillsdale, NJ) pp. 1–21.

Prkachin, K.M. and Craig, K.D. (1985) Influencing non-verbal expressions of pain: Signal detection analyses. Pain 21, 399–409.

Ramsden, R., Friedman, B. and Williamson, D. (1983) Treatment of childhood headache reports with contingency management procedures. J. Clin. Child Psychol. 123, 202–206.

Richter, I., McGrath, P.J., Humphreys, P., Goodman, J.T., Firestone, P. and Keene, D. (1986) Cognitive and relaxation of paediatric migraine. Pain 25, 195–203.

Routh, D.K. and Ernst, A.R. (1984) Somatization disorder in relatives of children and adolescents with functional abdominal pain. J. Pediatr. Psychol. 9, 427–437.

Sank, L.I. and Biglan, A. (1974) Operant treatment of a case of recurrent abdominal pain in a 10-year old boy. Behav. Ther. 5, 677–681.

Satterwhite, B. (1978) Impact of chronic illness on child and family: An overview based on five surveys. Int. J. Rehabil. Res. 1, 7–15.

Sternbach, R.A. (1986) Survey of pain in the United States: The Nuprin Pain Report. Clin. J. Pain 2, 49–53.

Stone, R.T. and Barbero, G.J. (1970) Recurrent abdominal pain in childhood. Pediatrics 45, 732–738.

Varni, J.W., Bessman, C.A., Russo, D.C. and Cataldo, M.F. (1980) Behavioral Management of Chronic Pain in Children: Case Study. Arch. Phys. Med. Rehabil. 61, 375–379.

Varni, J.W., Gilbert, A. and Dietrich, S.L. (1981) Behavioral medicine in pain and analgesia management for the hemophilic child with Factor VIII inhibitor. Pain 11, 121–126.

Walsh, T.D. (1983) Antidepressants in chronic pain. Clin. Neuropharmacol. 6, 271–295.

CHAPTER 14

Psychogenic pain

There has been a tendency to leap to psychological explanations when pain exhibited puzzling features which did not have a simple relation to apparent tissue damage *(Wall, 1984, p. 13)*.

1. Introduction

Psychogenic pain is pain whose cause is psychological. This chapter will review the diagnostic criteria for psychogenic pain with particular reference to the dangers of the very typical but most destructive tendency to diagnose psychogenicity on the basis of failure to find organic cause. The various etiologies of psychogenic pain will be discussed. Management of psychogenic pain will be reviewed. Finally, specific suggestions for future directions in research will be outlined.

2. Diagnostic criteria

Psychogenic pain is frequently diagnosed when children are not coping with pain and no specific organic cause can be found (Greene, 1983). Sontag (1979) noted that the tendency to ascribe psychological causation of disease has a long history. For example, it was widely believed in the 16th and 17th century that a happy man would not get the plague. Sontag (1979, p. 54) asserts:

> Theories that diseases are caused by mental states and can be cured by will power are always an index of how much is not understood about the physical terrain of a disease.

However this 'leap to the head' (Wall, 1984) is destructive and inaccurate (McGrath, 1983). First of all, children may have psychogenic pain and be coping quite well. Many children are plagued by abdominal pain when they have to speak in front of the class in elementary school. The pain is clearly psychogenic but does not interfere with performance. Secondly, a diagnosis of psychogenicity must be a positive diagnosis rather than that of exclusion. As Barr and Feuerstein (1983) have argued in the case of recurrent abdominal pain, a pain may be neither of known organic cause or of psychogenic cause. Indeed, most recurrent abdominal pain is of unknown cause. It is refreshing to note that the Diagnostic and Statistical Manual of the American Psychiatric Association (American Psychiatric Association, 1980) now explicitly states that the failure to find an organic cause is not sufficient for a diagnosis of psychogenic pain. Thirdly, psychogenic and organic disorder can coexist and the diagnosis of one cannot rule out the diagnosis of the other. A child, who is suffering from pain due to a performance anxiety, can also have a serious bowel malrotation causing pain. Moreover, as Levine and Rappaport (1984, p. 983) noted:

> Serious illnesses...may be exquisitely temperament- and stress-responsive without actually being caused by life circumstances or personality type.

Psychogenic pain may be diagnosed in an attempt to provide a sense of mastery or control over the situation by the diagnostician rather than simply admitting that the cause is not known. Finally, it is our experience that, sadly, the diagnosis of psychogenic pain is frequently used as a punishment for obnoxious patients or for failure of patients to respond to or to cooperate with treatment.

Diagnosis of psychogenic pain must be on the basis of positive evidence. The best evidence for psychogenic pain is based on time locking of pain by events. For example, pain that occurs when a child is asked to do some homework which disappears when the demand is removed or pain that regularly begins after parental arguments may well be psychogenic. A pain diary in which antecedents and consequences of the pain are recorded as illustrated in Table 1 may be useful in determining the relationship between pain and events over a period of time.

TABLE 1
Antecedent-consequence pain diary.

What happened before the pain?	Level of pain 0–10	What happened after the pain?	Comments?
Dressed for school	7	Stayed home	
Argument with sister	9	Nothing, went out	
Nothing	6	Nothing	

There are, however, circumstances in which pain may appear to be time locked by events that are triggering psychogenic pain when this is not the case. For example, a child may have abdominal pain during the school week but not on the weekend because of changes in diet and activity that correspond with the week. One of us (P.M.) once saw a child, who developed abdominal pain every Monday following a weekend with his father, who was not living with the family. Careful questioning revealed that at these times he ate 'junk' food almost exclusively. Alterations in his diet, which were arranged with his father, successfully reduced his abdominal pain.

The American Psychiatric Association (1980) also allows for the diagnosis of psychogenic pain disorder on the basis that the pain enables the individual to avoid noxious activity. No criteria are provided but, in our practice, we insist on clear evidence for avoidance. For example, simply the fact that a child does not like school does not warrant diagnosis of psychogenic pain disorder if no organic cause can be found for a specific pain.

The final criterion for psychogenic pain disorder proposed by the American Psychiatric Association (1980) is that the pain enables the individual to get support from the environment that otherwise might not be forthcoming. The problem with this criterion is, of course, that almost any pain can and should enable the child to get support from the environment.

Our practice is to try to demonstrate not only that the pain allows avoidance or garners support but also that the pain ceases to be a problem when the avoidance is blocked or the support is withdrawn before we diagnose psychogenic pain.

Our belief is that psychogenic pain is overdiagnosed in children and adolescents.

3. Etiology

The etiology of psychogenic pain varies from case to case. Psychogenic pain may be due to anxiety, avoidance, direct reward of pain behavior, or secondary to depression or psychosis (see Table 2).

3.1. Anxiety

Anxiety-based pain occurs when a traumatic event or a series of traumatic events triggers pain. The exact mechanism is unknown but it may be autonomically mediated muscle tension, changes in gut motility, or vascular

TABLE 2
Types of psychogenic pain.

Cause	Presumed mechanism	Treatment
Anxiety	Classical conditioning	Expose to feared stimuli; teach behavioral and cognitive skills
Avoidance/escape	Negative reinforcement	Prevent avoidance or escape
Reward	Positive reinforcement of pain	Extinguish pain behavior; differentially reinforce other behavior
Depression	Physiological changes Symptom over-reporting Request for help	Treat depression
Psychosis	Hallucination or physical changes	Treat psychosis

changes. Subsequently, similar events trigger pain. The traumatic events may be as dramatic as sexual abuse (Caldirola et al., 1984; Haber and Roos, 1985; Pillemer et al., 1987) or as subtle as a perception that an unreasonable demand is being made by a teacher.

3.1.1. School phobia
School phobia is often accompanied by complaints of pain. Classically, school phobia is a separation anxiety in which the child fears leaving the perceived safety of home and parents. School phobia begins when a child starts day care or kindergarten and often recurs following a time at home because of vacation or illness. Pain does not always accompany school phobia but it is common. Headaches and abdominal pain are the most frequent pains accompanying school phobia.

Kennedy (1965) has delineated two types of school phobia. Type 1, or simple school phobia, is characterized by sudden onset in a young child, usually following a legitimate absence from school because of illness or vacation. In these cases, the family is not pathological and the parents cooperate with each other in child management. Type 2, or complex school phobia occurs in older children with disturbed family relationships and a more chronic history of increasing school absence. Pain may accompany either type of school phobia.

3.1.2. Social anxiety

Levine and Rappaport (1984) have highlighted the potential role of anguish due to social failure and the stress due to name-calling, scapegoating and exclusion in the genesis of pain. Even specific inquiry into these areas by a sympathetic adult will often not result in disclosure by the child. Children with psychogenic pain often feel attacked by questions from adults. They perceive that their pain is being seen as 'all in their head' and not genuine. Only if the child feels they are not being set up will they let down their defences. Moreover, it appears that many children are actually unaware of the social stresses to which they are subjected.

3.1.3. Performance anxiety

Pain from performance anxiety is most frequently from excessive academic demands. In the clinic, we have seen a number of children who have serious undetected learning disabilities who are doing poorly in school. Thorough evaluation by a specialist in learning disabilities is the first step in therapy.

3.1.4. Sexual abuse

Sexual abuse is a very traumatic event. Two studies (Caldirola et al., 1984; Haber and Roos, 1985) have described long term pain problems as a sequela of sexual abuse. The exact mechanism and the extent of the relationship remain to be uncovered.

3.2. Avoidance or escape

> Whenever I don't want to go to swimming practice I grab my stomach and moan and make a face like eating a lemon and I say, 'Gee, Mom, I hope I don't have to miss swimming ...' *(girl, age 8, quoted in Ross and Ross, 1984, p. 188)*.

The escape or avoidance type of psychogenic pain occurs when a child learns that they can avoid or escape from an unpleasant event by reporting pain. For example, a child who is to speak in public reports a stomachache, is relieved from the obligation, and then develops tummyaches whenever asked to speak in class, can be said to have an avoidance/escape type of psychogenic pain.

3.3. Reward of pain

Reward of pain occurs when a child is given attention or special privileges for reporting pain.

3.4. Depression

Depressed children frequently report pain (Ling et al., 1970; Hughes, 1984). The mechanism may be direct physiological changes, over-reporting of symptoms or a call for help.

3.4.1. Direct physiological changes
Abdominal pain could result from depression-triggered changes in gut motility and consequent constipation. The changes could be due to changes in diet or activity or more directly due to depression. Headache can be due to sleep deprivation or perhaps even muscle tension resulting from depression.

3.4.2. Over-reporting of symptoms
Psychogenic pain in depression may be caused by a heightened awareness of normal physiological functioning and a misinterpretation of normal sensation as pain. Beck (1967) has described how a negative set is a primary hallmark of depression. Anderson and Pennebaker (1980) have demonstrated that identical physical stimulation can be perceived as either painful or pleasurable depending on the set that one has. Internal physiological stimuli that might be interpreted as neutral or not attended to at all, might provoke a pain interpretation during depression.

3.4.3. Call for help
Pain may be a calling card, a socially acceptable way for a depressed youngster to seek the help they need. Youngsters who use pain as a calling card will respond to specific questions about how their life is going with stories of widespread unhappiness.

3.5. Psychosis

Pain due to psychosis is an uncommon form of psychogenic pain but may be due to hallucination or, as in depression, may be due to changes in diet or activity.

3.6. Conversion disorder and malingering

The essential characteristic of conversion disorder is a clinical picture in which the loss or alteration of physical functioning appears to be a physical disorder but is due to psychological causes. Conversion reactions in which pain is the only symptom should not be considered conversion disorders but psychogenic pain (American Psychiatric Association, 1980).

Malingering which is prolonged deliberate lying about pain for some gain or to avoid an unpleasant situation is, in our experience, a rare form of psychogenic pain. It is extraordinarily difficult to prove malingering and in the effort to prove the case, an adversarial relationship is very likely to develop between the therapist and the patient. We prefer to treat it in the same way as chronic intractable pain (see chapter 15).

3.7. Multiple causation

The most common situation that we have seen in the clinic is a combination of the first three causes: anxiety, direct reward of pain behavior and avoidance or escape.

> *Case example*
> Ira, a 9-year-old boy was referred to the Department of Psychology by his pediatrician because of abdominal pain that was queried as being psychogenic. The initial interview revealed that Ira was the third and last child in an upper-middle-class family. He developed abdominal pain following the family's move to Ottawa 6 months previously and his change to a new school in the middle of his Grade 2 year. He typically missed 1 or 2 days of school each week. Ira presented as a bright personable child. He was reported to be above average in intelligence and well liked by his peers. Careful questioning of Ira revealed that he did not like his new teacher because she yelled a lot. He could report no positive interactions with his new teacher. A detailed description of what happened when Ira had pain showed that he was allowed to stay in his parents' bed, watch TV and was given his favorite foods. Ira's mother felt guilty for having transferred him from his former school in the middle of the year. She reported she liked spoiling him and enjoyed his company when he stayed at home. Ira's father reported that he was very busy at work and that his wife took care of things with Ira's school and doctors.
> A tentative analysis of anxiety-based pain which had been negatively reinforced by avoidance of school and positively reinforced by special attention at home was presented to the family.

4. Treatment

There have been few studies examining the treatment of psychogenic pain. Common sense would suggest that treatment should depend on a thorough and careful analysis of the cause of the pain. In all cases, care must be taken to insure that the patient and family realize that the existence of the pain is not being questioned. Psychogenic pain is real!

4.1. Anxiety

Treatment of anxiety-based psychogenic pain will depend on the type of anxiety problem.

4.1.1. School phobia

School phobia presenting as pain should be treated differently on the basis of the type.

Kennedy (1965) described a treatment program for type 1 school phobia that involved the following aspects. (1) Intervention should begin as quickly after the problem is noticed as possible. (2) A de-emphasis of pain and an insistence that the child go to school in spite of pain. (3) Resolution of realistic aspects of the school avoidance such as protection from bullies. (4) Decisive insistence on attendance at school even if physical strength is required to insure compliance. (5) Close liaison with the parents to insure that the parents take a non-emotional but firm approach. (6) Positive feedback by the parents, teachers and therapist for school attendance. (7) Follow-up to promote consolidation of gains over fear.

Kennedy (1965) reported that 100% of 50 children with type 1 school phobia were successfully returned to school and kept in school using this procedure. No randomized trials have been reported testing this method.

Gittleman-Klein and Klein (1973) studied 35 children aged 6–14 years of mixed school phobia and demonstrated that imipramine, a tricyclic antidepressant (1–3 mg/kg per 24 h) was more effective in combination with a concerted effort to return a child to school than the concerted efforts with placebo medication. Treatment of complex school phobia (type 2) has not been well evaluated but will likely require intensive therapy with the child and family.

Psychogenic pain from school phobia usually gradually remits as the school phobia is successfully treated. Interestingly, Gittleman-Klein and Klein (1973) found in their study that the children on imipramine, who were attending school, differed from children on placebo, who had returned to school, in that they felt more comfortable.

4.1.2. Social anxiety

Psychogenic pain due to social anxiety can be treated with therapy focussing on the social anxiety. There are no studies of treatment of pain from social anxiety in children.

4.1.3. Performance anxiety

Although no studies exist, our clinical experience is that children, who have undetected learning disabilities causing performance anxiety and pain, have gradual remission of pain once the appropriate educational interventions are undertaken. Other forms of performance anxiety may be treated by teaching skills or by helping the child alter unrealistic performance standards.

4.1.4. Sexual abuse

The best treatment for psychogenic pain resulting from sexual abuse would be prevention. However, in spite of the popularity of teaching children about sexual abuse, there is, as yet, no evidence that such approaches are effective. As well, although group and family treatment of the victims of child abuse is common, no well-controlled evaluations are available. The impact of such treatments on pain problems, which are hypothesized to occur years later, is unknown.

4.2. Avoidance or escape

Treatment of psychogenic pain based on avoidance or escape consists of blocking the avoidance or escape. Blocking of avoidance or escape may lead to an initial exacerbation of the pain complaints. For example, a child who is avoiding visiting a separated parent by developing pain is likely to have excruciating pain when visiting is insisted upon. If the child subsequently escapes by increased pain, the problem will be even more difficult to eradicate. Moreover, in some situations a child's avoidance or escape may serve as a reward for a significant adult. In our example, one parent may be subtly or not so subtly encouraging the failure to visit the separated parent. In effect, the child may have psychogenic pain by proxy. Consequently, any attempt to block escape or avoidance must be carefully thought out before the plan is implemented.

4.3. Direct reward of pain behavior

Removal of direct reward for pain behavior is conceptually straightforward. However, in actual practice, several problems arise. First, when reward is eliminated, pain behavior will likely increase before it decreases making it more difficult for parents to follow through on this strategy. Secondly, a parent may feel rewarded by the child's pain. For example, a lonely or isolated parent may encourage a child to stay at home because of the company she or he may provide. Thirdly, blocking escape or avoidance places an onus on the parents to teach the child more effective ways of managing a difficult situation (such as giving a speech at school or coping with a bully) than by using pain behavior.

4.4. Depression

Treatment of pain secondary to depression should focus on the depression. Both medical treatment and psychological treatments are available. No evaluations of these treatments with children and adolescents are available.

4.5. Psychosis

Treatment of pain due to psychosis is typically by antipsychotic medication.

4.6. Somatization disorder

Treatment of somatization disorder is difficult in adults. No treatments of somatization disorder in children have been reported. Long-term child and family behavior or psychotherapy would be indicated.

4.7. Conversion disorder

Conversion disorders with accompanying pain are usually treated by a combination of individual and family therapy.

4.8. Multiple causation

As mentioned, this is the most common situation encountered in a tertiary care setting such as the Children's Hospital of Eastern Ontario. We continue our case example of Ira to illustrate the type of approach we have used.

> Our plan of action consisted of: (1) Alerting Ira's teacher to the need for more positive experience at school. (2) No special attention at home for pain by instituting the rule: 'If the pain is too bad to go to school then you must be at home in your own bed, no TV or toys, resting all day with no visitors and minimal conversation with mom. No special food.' (3) Father was to spend 10 min special time playing a game Ira wanted every day he went to school. Special treat for the whole family on Friday to celebrate Ira spending a whole week at school. (4) Mother was urged to consider what type of alternatives she should consider for her own self-development. Father was urged to support mom's attempts.

Fortunately the teacher, mom, dad and Ira cooperated. Pain resolved within 3 weeks and he had not missed any school because of pain when contacted 1 year later. Ira continued to have pain every once in a while but he went to school and it usually went away.

5. *Clinical guidelines*

(1) Do not overdiagnose psychogenic pain. Psychogenic pain must be diagnosed only in the light of positive evidence.
(2) Do not discontinue observation for organic illness because of diagnosis of psychogenic pain. They are independent.
(3) Psychogenic pain is just as painful and just as disabling as organic pain.
(4) Treat specific psychogenic cause.

6. *Future directions*

(1) More research is needed on the etiology and treatment of school phobia.
(2) Family dynamics of children with psychogenic pain should be investigated in a rigorous way.
(3) The tendency to overdiagnose psychogenic pain should itself be subjected to careful research.

References

American Psychiatric Association (1980) Diagnostic and Statistical Manual of Mental Disorders, 3rd edn. (APA, Washington, DC) pp. 241–252.

Anderson, D.B. and Pennebaker, J.W. (1980) Pain and pleasure: Alternative explanations of identical stimulation. Eur. J. Soc. Psychol. 10, 207–212.

Barr, R.B. and Feuerstein, M. (1983) Recurrent abdominal pain: How appropriate are our basic clinical assumptions? In: P.J. McGrath and P. Firestone (Eds.), Pediatric and Adolescent Behavioral Medicine: Issues in Treatment (Springer, New York) pp. 13–27.

Beck, A.T. (1967) Depression: Causes and Treatment (University of Pennsylvania Press, Philadelphia, PA).

Caldirola, D., Gemperle, M., Guzinski, G., Gross, R. and Doerr, H. (1984) Chronic pelvic pain as related to abdominal pain in childhood and to psychosocial disturbance in the family. In: R. Rizzi and M. Visentini (Eds.), Pain: Proceedings of the Joint Meeting of the European Chapters of the International Association for the Study of Pain (Piccin/Butterworths, Padua) pp. 291–297.

Gittleman-Klein, R. and Klein, D.F. (1973) School phobia: Diagnostic considerations in the light of imipramine effects. J. Nerv. Ment. Dis. 150, 199–215.

Greene, M. (1983) Sources of pain. In: M.D. Levine, W.B. Carey, A.C. Crocker and R.T. Gross (Eds.), Developmental-Behavioral Pediatrics (Saunders, Philadelphia, PA) pp. 512–518.

Haber, J.D. and Roos, C. (1985) Effects of spouse abuse and/or sexual abuse in the development and maintenance of chronic pain in women. In: H.L. Fields, R. Dubner and F. Cervero (Eds.), Advances in Pain Research and Therapy, Vol. 9 (Raven, New York) pp. 889–895.

Hughes, M.C. (1984) Recurrent abdominal pain and childhood depression: Clinical observation of 23 patients and their families. Am. J. Orthopsychiatr. 54, 146–155.

Kennedy, W.A. (1965) School phobia: Rapid treatment of fifty cases. J. Abnorm. Psychol. 70, 285–289.

Levine, M.D. and Rappaport, L.A. (1984) Recurrent abdominal pain in school children: The loneliness of the long distance physician. Pediatr. Clin. North Am. 31, 969–991.

Ling, W., Oftedal, G. and Weinberg, W. (1970) Depressive illness in childhood presenting as severe headache. Am. J. Dis. Child. 120, 122–124.

McGrath, P.J. (1983) Psychological aspects of recurrent abdominal pain. Can. Fam. Phys. 29, 1655–1659.

McGrath, P.J., Goodman, J.T., Firestone, P., Shipman, R. and Peters, S. (1983) Recurrent abdominal pain: A psychogenic disorder? Arch. Dis. Child. 58, 888–890.

Pillemer, F.G., Masek, B.J. and Kaban, L.B. (1987) Temporomandibular joint dysfunction and facial pain in children: An approach to diagnosis and treatment. Pediatrics, in press.

Ross, D.M. and Ross, S.A. (1984) Childhood pain: The school-aged child's viewpoint. Pain 20, 179–191.

Sontag, S. (1979) Illness as Metaphor (Vintage Books, New York) pp. 49–56.

Wall, P.D. (1984) Introduction. In: P.D. Wall and R. Melzack (Eds.), Textbook of Pain (Churchill Livingstone, Edinburgh) pp. 1–16.

CHAPTER 15

Ethics

Jeffrey had holes cut on both sides of his neck, another hole cut in his right chest, an incision from his breastbone around to his backbone, his ribs pried apart, and an extra artery near his heart tied off. This was topped off with another hole cut in his left side for a chest tube. The operation lasted $1\frac{1}{2}$ hours. Jeffrey was awake through it all. The anesthesiologist paralyzed him with Pavulon, a curare drug that left him unable to move, but totally conscious. When I questioned the anesthesiologist later about her use of Pavulon, she said Jeffrey was too sick to tolerate powerful anesthetics. Anyway, she said, it had never been demonstrated to her that premature babies feel pain *(Lawson, 1986, p. 125)*.

1. Introduction

Our discussion of ethics in children's pain will have two foci. The first is the ethics of clinical practice and the second is the ethics of research in children's pain. Both share some common problems such as the difficulty of measurement and the extent to which premature infants, neonates and young children feel pain, but each raises unique questions.

2. Ethics in clinical practice

One of the most pressing ethical topics in children's pain is the issue of whether or not young infants feel pain. We believe that the evidence is overwhelming that, from birth, infants feel pain. As we have detailed in chapters 2, 3, 4 and 5, pain responses have been demonstrated in neonates undergoing heel lance for routine testing (Owens and Todt, 1984; Franck, 1986; Grunau and Craig, 1987), during circumcision (e.g., Williamson and Williamson, 1983) and during surgery (Anand and Aynsley-Green, 1985). Grunau and Craig (1987) also showed that the response was dependent on the state of the infant, suggesting a complex modulated response. Although no research has shown infants' memory for pain, we believe that pain is not simply a transient phenomenon, even in infants.

Even if one contests the currently available evidence for neonatal pain perception, we agree with Owens (1986) that one should adopt the assumption of neonatal pain as a working hypothesis:

> If we wrongly assume that infants feel pain, we lose little as a society or a science. If we rightly assume that infants feel pain, then we are more motivated to address it, research it and find safe and effective ways to ameliorate it *(Owens, 1986, p. 30)*.

It has been easier for all health care professionals to deny that a child could be in pain and to attribute pain behavior to feelings of fear, anxiety, anger or sadness when unavoidable pain is inflicted by health care professionals (Abu-Saad, 1984). There are three important areas of pain relief for which clinicians must assume responsibility. These are (1) anesthesia for surgical procedures, (2) relief of postoperative pain and pain from other medical procedures, and (3) pain relief from injury or disease.

2.1. Anesthesia for surgical procedures

In chapter 1 on the history of pain in childhood, it was evident that due to both the paucity of knowledge concerning pain in children and the lack of safe anesthesia itself, many children were given little or no anesthesia for surgery. As knowledge of anesthetic agents and procedures advanced, many of the initial difficulties of anesthesia have been overcome. However corresponding advances in neonatology have given rise to an important problem. As premature infants are able to survive at an increasingly earlier age and with more severe problems, they also frequently become surgical patients. The question of when premature infants should be treated for pain is compounded by the problem of providing anesthetic agents safely in this age group.

In the past, it was generally believed that infants less than 6 months of age required a relatively higher concentration of anesthetic agents to obtain satisfactory surgical anesthesia than did older children or adults (Downes and Betts, 1977). When this was thought to be the case, the risks of anesthetic agents particularly susceptibility to myocardial depression and hypotension were also increased. However, Waugh and Johnson (1984) reported that it has now been demonstrated that infants do not require more anesthetic agents than do older children. In addition to anesthesia, muscle relaxants or neuromuscular blocking drugs to prevent movement of the infant during the surgical procedure may also be used (Downes and Betts, 1977). In fact, these drugs may, if there is any doubt about the infant's ability to perceive pain, tempt the surgical team to leave the infant in unnecessary pain:

Neuromuscular blocking drugs have a most important place in the anesthetic management of young infants since they can provide optimal operating conditions with minimal doses of anesthetic or analgesic agents *(Downes and Betts, 1977, p. 59)*.

Recently, in a series of studies (described in chapter 4), Anand et al. (1987a,b) have detailed how adequate anesthesia can prevent the stress response in term and pre-term neonates undergoing surgery. The stress response is, in part, due to pain and has been implicated in morbidity and mortality.

The ethical question of whether it is sufficient to use a neuromuscular blocking drug in a surgical procedure is not new and is illustrated in the following discussion between Webb and Ward (Ward et al., 1970, p. 772) after a paper presentation on anesthetic experiences for infants under 2500 g weight:

> *Webb*:
> 'With regard to that (referring to the necessary amount of halothane, an anesthetic agent), most of these babies do not need halothane. All they need is a little ventilatory support. They do not need much agent at all. A little bit of adhesive tape holds them down.'

> *Ward*:
> 'May I just mention that in no animal laboratory in the world could you get away with anesthetizing a puppy with adhesive tape. Some of us feel that perhaps the infant is worth at least the same amount of care as a puppy.'

A further problem in surgical procedures is the presurgical preparation required to insure adequate respiratory support during the surgical procedure. For example, an endotracheal tube must be inserted for ventilation. This procedure can be done with or without an anesthetic or sedative. Ward commented about this procedure:

> I feel that generally speaking in this group of patients awake intubations are either for showoffs or sadists, unless the patient is moribund. Even if not anesthetized, these patients should be paralyzed *(Ward et al., 1970, p. 771)*.

Waugh and Johnson (1984) emphasized that awake intubation in unparalyzed and unanesthetized infants was associated with acute arterial hypertension and increases in intracranial pressure. Even in preoxygenated neonate, awake intubation could result in apnea, obstructed breathing, hemoglobin desaturation and bradycardia (Waugh and Johnson, 1984). Waugh and Johnson (1984) recommended that inhalation induction precede intubation unless there were possible abnormalities of the upper airway or if there was doubt about the anesthetist's ability to secure intubation. Randomized trials of awake versus anesthetized intubation are now in progress.

We believe that it is incumbent to insure that all possible sources of pain for infants in presurgical preparation and during the surgical procedure must be eliminated to the extent that this is possible within the margins of safety. As Waugh and Johnson (1984) argued and Anand et al. (1987a,b) have demonstrated it is good medicine as well as a sound humanitarian principle to control perioperative pain.

2.2. Postoperative pain and pain from procedures

We have previously discussed the issues involved in postoperative pain in chapter 4 and pain from procedures in chapter 5. In summary, a number of studies have demonstrated that children are given limited postoperative pain relief and frequently receive little pharmacological pain relief or psychological assistance during painful medical procedures (Eland and Anderson, 1977; Beyer et al., 1983; Mather and Mackie, 1983; Schechter et al., 1986).

When children do receive pain relief, it may be inadequate in consideration of the procedure the child has undergone. For example, in the study by Eland and Anderson (1977) of 25 children, a 6-year-old, who had intersex abnormalities requiring 13 surgical procedures, had received only one dose of pain medication during these 13 hospitalizations. A child, who had a spinal fusion, received one dose of morphine and another child with a similar surgical procedure was given two doses of aspirin.

Clinical practice must include assessment of pain, for without measurement, analgesic medication remains problematic. If children have less sensitivity to pain as compared to adults then indeed they do require proportionately less medication. However, the assumption that children experience considerably less pain than adults must be held suspect until research is able to clarify the experience of pain in children. In chapter 4, we have recommended the development of quality assurance procedures to monitor and improve postoperative pain control in children. We feel that quality assurance may be the best way, at this time, of improving the standard of care.

2.3. Pain relief from injury or disease

A similar problem of poor pain control occurs when pain is the result of injury or disease. For example, Eland and Anderson (1977) reported that a child with second and third degree burns to 70% of the body received one dose of aspirin. Another child with similar burns to 70% of the body received one dose of acetaminophen.

The assumption that children do not experience pain or that they are likely to become addicted if they receive medication must be challenged. There is no evidence to confirm this assumption. Again, if we wrongly argue that children do feel pain, children come to little harm. However, if we wrongly assume that children do not have significant pain we cause considerable additional torment to children who are already suffering from an injury or disease. As we have repeatedly argued, the facile invoking of psychological cause for children's pain may be a way of ignoring significant pain that is difficult to treat.

We wish to emphasize in the strongest possible terms that there is, in our opinion, an ethical imperative to adequately treat pain in children.

3. Ethics in pediatric pain research

Ethical research on pain in children is constrained in two ways. First are the considerations of any pediatric research and second are the constraints that apply to pain research.

A number of codes of research ethics have been developed to help guide the behavior of researchers. We will first review and discuss concepts that are commonly invoked in these ethical codes and then suggest guidelines.

3.1. Research or clinical practice

It is important to define research in order to determine if the more rigorous restrictions, that are usually placed on research as compared to clinical practice, should apply. On the simplest level, for example, ethics committee approval and informed consent are usually required for research whereas no committee approval and less rigorous and more general consents are required for clinical practice. Research refers to a course of critical or scientific inquiry designed to discover scientific facts (Nicholson, 1986). The discrimination between research and clinical practice is quite simple when we examine some work but not when we examine others. For example, a randomized placebo-controlled trial (e.g., Feldman et al., 1987) of a therapeutic substance, drug or a pyschological intervention would be designated by almost everyone as research. Although involving a critical inquiry and hopefully contributing to scientific knowledge, few would say that a case description (e.g., Richlin et al., 1978) is research. But what about a case series (e.g., Miser et al., 1980) involving an innovative procedure or innovative use of a drug? Should a single case experiment (e.g., Varni et al., 1981) be considered research? The problem becomes particularly important for the clinician/researcher who is constantly moving from research to clinical practice and vice versa. We have no real answers to this question but would opt for a definition based on the intent of the clinician/researcher. If the primary purpose is to treat then it is treatment. If the primary purpose is scientific inquiry, the effort is research. We see no other reasonable way of making the distinction between clinical practice and research. However, care must be taken when one leaves responsibility to the individual investigator. The pressures on the clinician/ researcher is to avoid the bureaucratic hassles implicit in ethics review and get the work done. Recognizing this problem Nicholson (1986) recommended that the number of times an innovative therapy can be used before it is submitted as a formal research project be limited. Unfortunately Nicholson did not give an indication of how many times such procedures should be used or how the decision to determine when innovative therapy becomes research should be made.

3.2. Strategies of research

Research can consist of interventions and/or observations. Interventions refer to doing something whereas observations involve looking at something. Interventions can be invasive or non-invasive. Nicholson (1986) defined invasive interventions as any that involve entrance into the subject's body. For example, taking a sample of blood to determine serum levels of an analgesic would be invasive while asking a child if he had pain would be non-invasive. Although invasive procedures are generally more dangerous than non-invasive procedures, care should be taken not to confuse non-invasive with harmless. For example, questioning a teenage girl about her sexual practices in conjunction with a study of abdominal pain might involve considerable risk of psychological harm.

3.3. Therapeutic versus non-therapeutic research

Therapeutic research refers to research in which the subject may directly benefit whereas in non-therapeutic research there is no benefit to the participant but there may be benefit to others and to the advancement of knowledge. Conceptually, the distinction between therapeutic and non-therapeutic research is quite straightforward and, in some cases, is easily made. However, in practice, the distinction is sometimes very difficult. The

Canadian Medical Research Council has abandoned this dichotomy because of the difficulty of applying such distinctions (Medical Research Council, 1978). The major danger of maintaining the concepts of therapeutic versus non-therapeutic research is the tendency to assume, that simply because the research is therapeutic, it is somehow ethical. As Nicholson (1986) illustrated therapeutic research can be unethical. The reason for the dichotomy between therapeutic and non-therapeutic research is that a different set of rules should apply to the two. The risk that can ethically accompany therapeutic research is generally agreed to be greater than that can be associated with non-therapeutic research.

There is a problem of whether to consider controls in a therapeutic research project as participating in therapeutic research or non-therapeutic research. For example, children in the control group in a randomized controlled trial do not have the probability of direct benefit other than placebo effect, from the research. In some cases, children in the control group are offered the treatment on completion of the study if it has been shown to be effective. However, this is not possible in a long-term investigation.

3.4. Risk

Three levels of risk situations have usually been defined (National Commission, 1977; British Paediatric Association, 1980; Nicholson, 1986). The area is confusing because different groups have used different terms to refer to the same risk or the same term to refer to different levels of risk. For example, the British Paediatric Association (1980) used the terms: negligible, minimal and more than minimal. Negligible risk is defined as risk less than that run in everyday life. Minimal risk is risk questionably greater than minimal. More than minimal risk is used to refer to all other risks. The National Commission (1977) used the terms minimal, minor increase over minimal and greater than minor increase over minimal. These were adopted by the working group of the Institute for Medical Ethics (Nicholson, 1986) because they were more precise. As Nicholson (1986) pointed out, there are substantial risks of morbidity and mortality in everyday life. Nicholson (1986) argued for the quantification of risk and provided a thorough discussion of strategies for developing quantitative measures. They quantified minimal risk as carrying a risk of death of less than 1 per million, risk of major complication as less than 10 per million and risk of minor complication of less than 1 per thousand. Minor increase over minimal carries risk of death of up to 100 per million; risk of major complication of 10–1000 per million and risk of minor complications of 1–100 per thousand. Greater levels of risk are in the 'greater than minor increase over minimal'. An example of their argument is:

> It should be noted that although there are no precise risk figures available for collecting a sample of venous blood, the scarcity of anecdotes of harm arising from this procedure compared to the frequency with which such blood samples are collected suggests that it lies in the 'minimal' risk category *(Nicholson, 1986, p. 120)*.

Arterial punctures, lung and liver biopsy, cardiac catheterization would all be excluded from the minimal risk category.

In a study by Janofsky and Starfield (1981), pediatric department chairmen and pediatric clinical research directors rated various procedures for risk at different ages (0–1 year; 1–4 years; 5–6 years; 7–11 years; and 12–18 years). A majority (54–59%) rated bone scans as having no risk or minimal risk. Sixty-nine to 76% of respondents found i.m. placebo injections to have no or minimal risk. For children over 6 years of age, gastric/intestinal intubation was seen as carrying no or minimal risk by 52–59% of respondents. Questioning children aged 7–18 years about sexual practices and about illicit drug use were seen as minimal risk by a majority of respondents. Nicholson (1986, p. 105) notes that:

> It would appear that the chief conclusion to be drawn from this survey of the perceptions of paediatricians and paediatric researchers is that they are unrealistically optimistic about the risks of research.

3.5. Benefit

Benefit from research can occur to the subject, to other children, or to knowledge. As in risk, Nicholson (1986) noted that benefit can in some cases, be numerically described.

Benefit is also on occasion provided to the child in the form of compensation, usually monetary. Sternbach (1979) has argued that monetary compensation for subjects in non-therapeutic pain research is a requirement of ethical practice. However, most commentators are opposed to any compensation beyond expenses or a token of appreciation because of the danger of money being an inducement that would lead children or their parents to participate in research in a way that was not completely voluntary (Keith-Spiegel, 1976; Nicholson, 1986).

Some researchers believe that one of the benefits to the participant consenting to research is the social good in that the research may ultimately be of benefit to society even though it may have no direct benefit to the participant. McCormick (1976) is one of the most vehement supporters of this point of view:

To pursue the good that is human life means not only to choose and support this value in one's own case, but also in the case of others when the opportunity arises. In other words, the individual ought also to take into account, realize, make efforts in behalf of the lives of others also, for we are social beings and the goods that define our growth and invite to it are goods that reside also in others... If this is true of all of us up to a point and within limits, it is no less true of the infant *(quoted in Ackerman, 1980, p. 100)*.

McCormick (1976) argued that when risk, discomfort and pain are minimal, that there is a duty to consent to experimental research with children and infants on their behalf as social beings.

However, several investigators adamantly reject such a motive as sufficient for consenting to participation in research (Ramsey, 1976, 1978; Van de Veer, 1981).

3.6. Voluntary informed consent

Voluntary informed consent requires that the procedures, the risks and the benefits are known and appreciated by the person giving consent. The issue of being informed and the need for the subject to give voluntary consent can present difficulties.

3.6.1. Voluntary

Consent must be voluntary and it must not be accompanied by any perceived or actual coercion or inducement. As previously mentioned there is debate in some quarters about payment of subjects. Perhaps more important is the need for parents and children to feel free to decline research participation without jeopardizing future health care.

3.6.2. Informed

In some situations, providing information to the subject can be in conflict with the design of the study. Prior information is likely to influence the subject's responses during the study. Deception and concealment may be necessary to insure the reliability of the subject's response (Keith-Spiegel, 1976). Usually in research with adult subjects, debriefing at the conclusion of the study is used to insure that subjects were adequately informed. However, debriefing in pediatric research may only lead to further confusion rather than clarification (Brewster-Smith, 1967; Keith-Spiegel, 1976). In our opinion, the need for deception is rare. The onus is on the investigator to demonstrate that the research question requires deception. There is a further obligation to minimize any negative impact on the subject.

3.6.3 Consent

In pediatric research, there are two main issues. The first is who (child? parent? parent and child?) can give consent and the second is for what procedures can consent be given.

The issue of consent by children is a complex ethical and legal question that involves interaction among ethics, statutory law and common law. The legal issues in the U.K. are clearly described by Nicholson (1986) and the American legal issues are discussed in detail by Langer (1985).

The difficulty in pediatric research is determining when children are of sufficient age to give informed consent; whether parents can consent on behalf of their children; and whether experimental pediatric research, where there is little benefit to the research participant but benefit to society as a whole, can be consented to. We will discuss these problems in turn.

Informed consent must be carefully managed with children to ensure that the information regarding the study is presented to them in developmentally acceptable language. However, the question remains at what age can children sufficiently comprehend the nature of a research request without the tendency to comply to the request of an adult (Langer, 1985).

Parents have a right to consent to procedures on behalf of their children but this right is constrained. Some researchers have suggested that proxy consent by the parent or legal guardian on behalf of the child is sufficient to satisfy the ethical requirements of pediatric research (McCormick, 1976). Other investigators argue that parents are not always concerned with the child's best interests when giving consent and may be prompted by other motives (Wellman, 1983; Phillips and Dawson, 1985). Wellman (1983) considered proxy consent to be invalid because it assumes that the parent can act in the place of the child when it is acknowledged that the child is unable to act on its own behalf. Wellman (1983) supported the use of combined parental and child consent before a child is accepted as a research participant.

Whether experimental pediatric research, with children too young to provide informed consent, is permissible is a hotly debated topic. As was discussed earlier, McCormick (1976) believed that parents should consent to such research on behalf of their children when the research carried a minimal or non-existent risk. McCormick maintained that parents had a social obligation in this respect. However, Ramsey (1976, 1978) emphatically disagreed with this position and believed such research could not be ethically sanctioned. He wrote:

Only if one discovers some medical interest in treatment or research for a particular child, or some grounds in the moral nurture of the child or the capacity in the child to give supplementary consent ... can consent be given to experimental research with the child without doing violence to the deputyship of parents and guardians. It is not enough to ascribe an inherent 'sociability' to the child or 'reasonableness' measured by adult standards, or to base surrogate consent on the truth of the proposition that these attributes are inherent in children but not yet exercised. The deputyship of parenthood includes the duty to bring these out, but not to act as if such volitions toward beneficence were already actualized *(Ramsey, 1978, p. 67)*.

Despite these comments, Ramsey (1976) acknowledged that there were situations in which such experimental research, which did not directly benefit the child and had minimal or no risk, was necessary. However, he maintained that in conducting such research the investigator needed to be aware that a vital ethical principle was in violation:

Some sorts of human experimentation should ... be acknowledged to be 'borderline situations' in which moral agents are under the necessity of doing wrong for the sake of the public good. Either way they do wrong. It is immoral not to do the research. It is also immoral to use children who cannot themselves consent and who ought not to be presumed to consent to research unrelated to their treatment. On this supposition research medicine, like politics, is a realm in which men have to 'sin bravely' *(Ramsey, 1976, p. 21)*.

Other ethicists believe that it is permissible for parents to agree to the child participating in experimental research without direct benefit to the child as a means to teaching their child morally responsible behavior in the same way that parents may decide that their children should participate in other activities (Bartholome, 1978: Ackerman, 1980).

3.7. Ethical review

It is widely recognized that it is in the best interests of both children and investigators that a committee, that is not involved in the research, independently review the protocol to determine ethical acceptability of the research. Various specific suggestions have been made for the membership of the ethics committee. Most emphasize a broad base of investigators, clinicians and laypersons. Nicholson (1986) has detailed the functioning of ethics committees for pediatric research in the U.K. and has suggested detailed guidelines for the functioning of such committees.

4. Ethical guidelines

We present these suggestions based substantially on the recommendations of the Institute of Medical Ethics working group (Nicholson, 1986).

(1) Research that is not scientifically valid is not ethical. Research that is not scientifically valid cannot provide any scientific or therapeutic benefit and thus cannot be justified even if the work is essentially harmless.

(2) Research should not be done with children unless there is a specific need to do the research with children. Research that can be validly done with adults should not be done with children.

(3) Basic principles of ethical research must be followed. These principles have been outlined in the Helsinki Declaration (World Medical Association, 1964). These include: risks to subjects and number of subjects should be minimized; voluntary informed consent must be obtained from children or their parents before the research begins; there must be a free right to withdraw from the research and subjects must be withdrawn if they are being harmed; and, finally, privacy of subjects and confidentiality of data must be insured.

(4) The benefit of therapeutic research must exceed the risk. Therapeutic research must not only be of potential benefit to the child but the risks must be reasonable. For example if the risks are 'greater than a minor increase over minimal' the potential benefit to the child must be great. Nicholson (1986) outlines a number of examples of therapeutic research where the risk clearly was not worth the possible benefit. In the area of pain in childhood, for example, invasive or potentially harmful therapeutic research would not be justifiable for the benign self-limiting recurrent abdominal pain syndrome but might be justifiable in treatment of the serious and painful sickle cell disease.

(5) Non-therapeutic pain research with children can be ethical. Although the British Medical Research Council (1964) in its landmark position paper declared that children should not be subjected to non-therapeutic research, the American National Commission (1977) did foresee the ethics of non-therapeutic research as did the Institute of Medical Ethics working group (Nicholson, 1986). However, it is clear that the risk of non-therapeutic research must be minimal.

(6) Although expenses to subjects should be paid and nominal payment is permissible, strong financial inducements are not ethical.

5. *Future directions*

(1) The ethical acceptability of current clinical practice regarding pain from surgery, procedures and disease should be examined by the medical ethics committees of professional groups. Failure to address this issue by hiding behind facile and wrong assurances that infants do not feel pain, will result in unnecessary suffering by children, distrust by patients and parents, and lobbying by lay groups.

The realization that neonates are frequently not anesthetized is just beginning to dawn but is dawning with a vengeance. For example, in a recent editorial in Birth, on surgery on the paralyzed unanesthetized newborn, the editor concluded:

> It staggers the imagination that nursery and operating room personnel would participate in unanesthetized surgery, whether out of ignorance or fear of reprisal. Such were the excuses of those who stood by during similarly well-meaning, officially sanctioned activities of the Third Reich. No court in the world has accepted ignorance or coercion as excuses for torture *(Shearer, 1986, p. 79)*.

Similarly, in a recent editorial in Perinatal Press, titled Barbarism, Scanlon (1985) argued that surgery without anesthesia is barbarous.

(2) Research on the risks of research procedures needs to be undertaken. The perceived risk of various procedures needs to be examined.

(3) Research should examine the voluntariness of consent in clinical research.

(4) The prevalence of research that has not been ethically reviewed should be examined.

(5) The decision making of ethical review committees and of professionals and laypersons should be examined to determine the actual process of how people decide that a given project is ethical.

References

Abu-Saad, H. (1984) Assessing children's responses to pain. Pain 19, 163–171.

Ackerman, T.F. (1980) Moral duties of parents and nontherapeutic clinical research procedures involving children. Bioethics Q. 2, 94–111.

Anand, K.J.S. and Aynsley-Green, A. (1985) Metabolic and endocrine effects of surgical ligation of patent ductus arteriosus in the human preterm neonate: Are there implications for further improvements of postoperative outcome? Mod. Probl. Paediatr. 23, 143–157.

Anand, K.J.S., Sippell, W.G. and Aynsley-Green, A. (1987a) Randomized trial of fentanyl anaesthesia in preterm babies undergoing surgery: Effects on the stress response. Lancet i, 243–247.

Anand, K.J.S., Sippell, W.G. and Aynsley-Green, A. (1987b) Does the newborn infant require anaesthesia during surgery? Answers from a randomized trial of halothane anaesthesia. Vth World Congress on Pain, Hamburg. Pain suppl. 4, S451.

Bartholome, W.G. (1978) Central themes in the debate over involvement of infants and children in biomedical research: a critical examination. In: J. Van Eys (Ed.), Research on Children: Medical Imperatives, Ethical Quandries, and Legal Constraints (University Park Press, Baltimore, MD) pp. 69–76

Beyer, J., DeGood, D.E., Ashley, L.C. and Russell, G.A. (1983) Patterns of postoperative analgesic use with adults and children following cardiac surgery. Pain 17, 71–81.

Brewster-Smith, M. (1967) Conflicting values affecting behavioral research with children. Children 14, 53–58.

British Paediatric Association (1980) Guidelines to aid ethical committees considering research involving children. Arch. Dis. Child. 55, 75–77.

Downes, J.J. and Betts, E.K. (1977) Anesthesia for the critically ill infant. ASA Refresher Courses Anesthesiol. 5, 47–69.

Eland, J.M. and Anderson, J.E. (1977) The experience of pain in children. In: A.K. Jacox (Ed.), Pain: a source book for nurses and other health professionals (Little, Brown & Co., Boston, MA) pp. 453–473.

Feldman, W., Rosser, W. and McGrath, P.J. (1987) Primary Medical Care of Children and Adolescents. (Oxford University Press, New York).

Franck, L.S. (1986) A new method to qualitatively describe pain behavior in infants. Nurs. Res. 35, 28–31.

Grunau, R. and Craig, K. (1987) Pain expression in neonates: facial action and cry. Pain 28, 395–400.

Janofsky, J. and Starfield, B. (1981) Assessment of risk in research on children. J. Pediatr. 98, 842–846.

Keith-Spiegel, P. (1976) Children's rights as participants in research. In: G.P. Koocher (Ed.), Children's Rights and the Mental Health Professions (Wiley, New York) pp. 53–81.

Langer, D.H. (1985) Children's legal rights as research subjects. J. Am. Acad. Child Psychiatr. 24, 653–662.

Lawson, J.R. (1986) Letter to the editor. Birth 13, 124–125.

McCormick, R.A. (1976) Experimentation in children: sharing in sociality. Institute of Society, Ethics and Life Sciences, Hastings Center Report, pp. 41–46.

Mather, L. and Mackie, J. (1983) The incidence of postoperative pain in children. Pain 15, 271–282.

Medical Research Council (Canada) (1978) Ethical Considerations in Research Involving Human Subjects (MRC, Ottawa).

Medical Research Council (U.K.) (1964) Responsibility in investigations on human subjects. In: Report of the Medical Research Council for the year 1962–63 (HMSO, London) pp. 21–25.

Miser, A.W., Miser, J.S. and Clark, B.S. (1980) Continuous intravenous infusion of morphine sulphate for control of severe pain in children with terminal malignancy. J. Pediatr. 96, 930–932.

National Commission for the Protection of Human Subjects of Biomedical and Behavioral Research (1977) Research Involving Children (U.S. Department of Health Education and Welfare, Washington, DC).

Nicholson, R.H. (Ed.) (1986) Medical Research with Children: Ethics, Law and Practice (Oxford University Press, Oxford).

Owens, M.E. (1986) Assessment of infant pain in clinical settings. J. Pain Symptom Manage. 1, 29–31.

Owens, M.E. and Todt, E.H. (1984) Pain in infancy: Neonatal response to heel lance. Pain 20, 77–86.

Phillips, M. and Dawson, J. (1985) Doctors' Dilemmas: Medical Ethics and Contemporary Science (Methuen, New York) pp. 70–75.

Ramsey, P. (1976) The enforcement of morals: nontherapeutic research on children. Institute of Society, Ethics and Life Sciences, Hastings Center Report 6(4), 21–30.

Ramsey, P. (1978) Ethical dimensions of experimental research on children. In: J. Van Eys (Ed.), Research on Children: Medical Imperatives, Ethical Quandries and Legal Constraints (University Park Press, Baltimore, MD) pp. 57–86.

Richlin, D.M., Carron, H., Rowlingson, J.C., Sussman, M.D., Baugher, W.H. and Goldner, R.D. (1978) Reflex sympathetic dystrophy: Successful treatment by transcutaneous nerve stimulation. J. Pediatr. 93, 84–86.

Scanlon, J.W. (1985) Barbarism. Perinatal Press 9, 103–104.

Schechter, N.L., Allen, D.A. and Hanson, K. (1986) The status of pediatric pain control: A comparison of hospital analgesic usage in children and adults. Pediatrics 77, 11–15.

Shearer, M.H. (1986) Surgery on the paralysed, unanesthetized newborn. Birth 13, 79.

Sternbach, R.A. (1979) Ethical problems in human pain research. In: J.J. Bonica and V. Ventafridda (Eds.), Advances in Pain Research and Therapy, Raven, New York pp. 837–842.

Van de Veer, D. (1981) Experimentation on children and proxy consent. J. Med. Philosophy 6, 281–293.

Varni, J.W., Gilbert, A. and Deitrich, S.L. (1981) Behavioral medicine in pain and analgesia management for the hemophilic child with Factor VIII inhibitor. Pain 11, 121–126.

Ward, R.J., Crawford, E.W. and Stevenson, J.K. (1970) Anesthetic experiences for infants under 2500 grams weight. Anesth. Analg. 49, 767–772.

Waugh, R. and Johnson, G.G. (1984) Current considerations in neonatal anesthesia. Can. Anaesth. Soc. J. 31, 700–709.

Wellman, C. (1983) Consent to medical research on children. In: T.L. Beauchamp and T.P. Pineaud (Eds.), Ethics and Public Policy: An Introduction to Ethics (Prentice Hall, Englewood Cliffs, NJ) pp. 369–386.

Williamson, P.S. and Williamson, M.L. (1983) Physiologic stress reduction by a local anesthetic during newborn circumcision. Pediatrics 71, 36–40.

World Medical Association (1964) Declaration of Helsinki. Recommendations Guiding Physicians in Biomedical Research Involving Human Subjects (Adopted in Helsinki, 1964; amended in Tokyo, 1975; and in Venice, 1983).

CHAPTER 16

Service and research in pediatric pain

1. Introduction

The closing chapter of this book will examine general issues in service delivery and research in the field of pain in children and adolescents. There are a few issues that should be obvious. First of all, the field of pediatric pain, in terms of both clinical service delivery and research, is a multidisciplinary endeavour. Medicine and surgery (with their many subspecialities), nursing, psychology, social work, physiotherapy, pastoral care, occupational therapy, epidemiology, sociology and the lab sciences each have their contribution to make. That is not to say that every issue or problem in the area requires an interdisciplinary approach. Some clinical service and some research will be most efficiently undertaken by single disciplines. However, each of us, in our clinical practice and in our research, is in peril if we are not constantly cognizant of the multifaceted nature of pain. The premier professional body in the area of pain, the International Association for the Study of Pain is a good reflection of the need for cross-fertilization across disciplines. Founded under the leadership of John Bonica in 1973, the IASP is composed of members of all health disciplines and is dedicated to treatment and research of pain.

Pain in children, both in terms of clinical interest and research is expanding rapidly. Although it is difficult to measure the growth of interest in a topic such as pain in children, one indication is that scarcely any issue of journals devoted to pain is published without at least one article on pediatric pain.

Interest in pain in children has grown for a number of reasons: a realization that children may have been poorly treated by being undermedicated for postoperative pain relief; advances in pain measurement with children; and finally a realization that some of the keys to preventing the staggering human and financial costs of pain in adults might lie in a better understanding of its roots in childhood.

2. Service delivery

The advantages of pain clinics are considerable and yet there are few pediatric pain clinics. Is this simply because pediatric pain has lagged behind adult pain or are there specific reasons for the paucity of such clinics?

2.1. The pediatric pain clinic

In adult pain treatment, the pain clinic has become a major focus of clinical services. Some pain clinics are exclusively outpatient but many have both an inpatient and outpatient component. Some pain clinics are specialized and treat only one type of pain most commonly headache, back pain or orofacial pain but many take all types of pain problems. The growth of pain clinics, particularly in the United States has been phenomenal. The major advantages of the pain clinic (Rose, 1986) are the need for comprehensive multidisciplinary facilities, the development of clinical expertise, the relative ease of recruiting sufficient subjects for clinical research, the availability of specialized clinical teaching experiences and the administrative streamlining that is possible in a specialized clinic. In addition adult pain clinics can make good business sense. We will examine each of these in turn in the context of the pediatric pain clinic.

2.1.1. Comprehensive multidisciplinary facilities
Aronoff (1985) has emphasized that the multidisciplinary pain clinic and especially the inpatient clinic is the best strategy for treating the individual with debilitating chronic pain and the patient who has been unresponsive to conventional therapy and exhibits pain behavior, life disruption, depressive illness, drug-seeking behavior and entrenchment in the disability system. These individuals have particular difficulty obtaining the type of treatment they need in conventional health care delivery. In fact health care delivered by a single discipline with a narrow specialization may have made a major contribution to the patient's problem. These chronic intractable pain patients are intensive users of the health care system; they are difficult for professionals to deal with because they do not respond to traditional medical treatment.

2.1.2. Development of clinical expertise
Rose (1986) points out that the average practitioner will see relatively few patients of any given type and that it is unrealistic to expect every practitioner

to be competent in all areas. Specialization, which can be accomplished in pain clinics, has led to the development of expertise that would probably not be possible without them.

An important issue is whether or not the pain problems that children experience require special expertise that cannot be reasonably expected to be had by most practitioners.

2.1.3. Recruiting sufficient subjects for clinical research

Clinical research, in particular randomized trials, does require large numbers of subjects with similar diagnoses. Pain clinics do provide for the relatively easy aggregation of subjects who have sought tertiary care treatment. However, one of the disadvantages of research based exclusively in tertiary care settings is that referral biases may occur (Sackett et al., 1985). For example, children with abdominal pain who attend a pain clinic are likely to be different from children who visit their family doctor with pain.

2.1.4. Specialized clinical teaching

There are two elements to specialized clinical teaching. One is the expertise of the teacher; the second is the availability of clinical material. As we have been arguing the major pain problems in children are the common problems of recurrent pain and postoperative pain. Specialized clinics are not required to provide clinical teaching material. On the other hand, specialized clinics or units might encourage the development of the faculty expertise.

2.1.5. Administrative streamlining

A pediatric pain clinic could help facilitate cross-referral among professionals and consultation on cases. For example, in our own area referral to some specialists (e.g., pediatric psychologist) may take 6–8 months. Moreover, a pain clinic would allow for meetings which are always most difficult to coordinate with busy professionals.

2.1.6. Profit

The ability of a pediatric pain clinic to generate profit would depend on volume and cost of services. Generally pediatric medicine is not as well funded as adult medicine and a pediatric pain clinic would not have workmen's compensation or disability insurance payments. Since chronic intractable pain is relatively rare in children the volume of patients in a pediatric pain clinic might be low. Consequently, it is unclear if a pediatric pain clinic could be a viable business.

2.2. Generalist approach

An alternative model of service delivery is the generalist approach where all health practitioners are taught better management of pain in children. There are several strategies that are available: integration of pediatric pain issues into the undergraduate curriculum of nurses and doctors; development of in-service and extramural workshops on pediatric pain; publication of pediatric pain studies and reviews in the professional and scientific literature; public education about pediatric pain; development of educational material for professionals; consultation by specialists on a case-by-case basis; and inter-disciplinary research. Limited use of these strategies has been made because the recent emergence of the field has precluded their full development.

There are, in our opinion, three major advantages to a generalist approach rather than the pediatric pain clinic approach.

2.2.1. Pediatric pain cannot be taken out of clinics

The first advantage is that pediatric pain problems occur within medical clinics and cannot be isolated into a pain speciality clinic. For example, pain from cancer, postoperative pain, and pain from arthritis are best handled within their respective speciality clinic. The recurrent pains (headache, recurrent abdominal pain, and limb pain) are best handled within the pediatrician's or family practitioner's office. Pain clinics in adults deal mostly with chronic intractable pain. Fortunately, as we discussed in chapter 13, very few children and adolescents develop chronic intractable pain. Those who do, share many of the characteristics of adults with the syndrome and are very difficult to treat without intensive collaboration of different disciplines. It is unclear that there are sufficient cases to warrant a specialized clinic and perhaps the small number of cases should be handled on a case-by-case basis.

2.2.2. Onus on everyone to learn about pediatric pain

Pediatric pain is the responsibility of all health professionals. There is a danger that the creation of speciality clinics may relieve the rest of the health professionals of the obligation of dealing with pediatric pain problems. Pain is too important to be left to the specialist.

2.2.3. Opposition to pain clinics

In times of financial restraint, creation of new clinics in public institutions is difficult if not impossible. Since pain is not as glamorous as life-threatening diseases, pediatric pain clinics may have difficulty competing for scarce health dollars. In a fee for service milieu, a pediatric pain clinic that cannot draw on insurance funds for disabled workers may be at a financial disadvantage. Prejudice against considering children's pain seriously may further compromise attempts to form pediatric pain clinics. Consequently, in many situations the question of whether or not to have a pediatric pain clinic may be decided less on its merits and more on financial considerations. A generalist approach may be the only way to deliver service.

However, it is necessary to have a nucleus of individuals who have a commitment to clinical service, teaching and research in pediatric pain to exchange ideas. In our own hospital, a pain interest group (PIG) serves this purpose.

3. Overcoming prejudices

Whatever approach is used to delivery of services, one must be aware that there are major difficulties to overcome. Eland and Anderson (1977) suggested that the reasons that children were undermedicated may have been 'old nurses tales'. These clinical folktales, which are by no means limited to nurses, are hypothesized to interfere with adequate pain management. Such folktales include: (1) children do not feel pain with as much intensity as adults; (2) children do not remember pain; (3) pain in children cannot be accurately measured; (4) opioids are unsafe for children because of addiction and respiratory depression; (5) children 'need' to experience pain.

Little research has examined attitudes and behaviors in the administration of medication to children. Two papers have examined data on this issue. Burokas (1985) surveyed pediatric nurses requesting their responses to eight vignettes depicting children following surgery. No vignettes with adults were used. She found that close to 90% of the nurses would administer analgesics for the situations depicted. Demographic factors such as age, educational background and personal pain experience did not influence the decision to medicate. However, nurses who themselves had a child who had significant pain were more likely to opt for medication.

Schechter and Allen (1987) surveyed the pediatricians, family doctors and surgeons of an American city. One hundred and twelve physicians (57% of those contacted) responded to a one page survey asking questions about their attitudes and beliefs about children's pain. As can be seen from Table 1, there were some significant differences in the responses of the three groups of physicians with a tendency for more pediatricians to regard children as

TABLE 1

Attitudes and behaviors of pediatricians, family doctors and surgeons about pediatric pain. (Based on data from Schecter and Allen, 1987).

	Pediatricians (%)	Family physicians (%)	Surgeons (%)
Children experience adult-like pain by age 2 years	91[*]	75	59
Use opioid analgesics in 2-year-olds	80[*]	64	49
Use routine analgesics for postoperative medication in 2-year-olds	85	70	69
Use analgesia or anesthesia for lumbar puncture in 2-year-olds	52	59	61
Somewhat or significantly concerned about addiction in patients	33	50	42
Respiratory depression limits opioid usage	Approximately 63%		
Children experience less pain for same problem than do adults	6	0	25

[*]Statistically significant difference across groups.

suffering pain similarly to adults. More pediatricians were willing to use opioid analgesics than family doctors or surgeons. The differences for routine use of postoperative medication are similar but not significant. More surgeons would use analgesia or anesthesia for lumbar puncture in a 2-year-old but the differences were not significant. A surprisingly high percentage of the doctors were concerned about addiction in their pediatric patients. The fear of respiratory depression also was a major impediment to analgesic use.

It is difficult to compare the two studies (Burokas, 1985; Schechter and Allen, 1987) because of the differences between the two questionnaires and methodology. However, there is some indication that physicians especially surgeons may be somewhat more conservative in using analgesics than are nurses.

The underlying mechanism is not known. However, we have examined the belief of nurses about children's pain in general (McGrath et al., 1984). Using vignettes of pain situations, we asked nurses to rate their perception of the amount of pain experienced and the action that should be taken to alleviate the pain. Vignettes were of everyday experiences rather than medical events. We found no differences between the ratings given to child vignettes versus the same vignettes with an adult character. We concluded that differences in medication practices between adults and children could not be explained by an overall belief that children experience less pain than adults.

4. Research

Specific suggestions for research have been made in previous chapters. However in this chapter we would like to reiterate some general themes and to highlight some suggestions in applied research, administrative research and basic research that have not been previously mentioned.

4.1. Applied research

(1) Research is needed on the occurrence and severity of pain experienced by children and adolescents, in general, and in specific subgroups, such as children with cancer and children in the postoperative period.
(2) Validity and sensitivity of measures should be further researched.
(3) Research is needed on treatment safety and effectiveness in all pain problems.

4.2. Administrative research

(1) The effects of quality assurance and other administrative programs to improve patient care should be investigated in terms of the impact on pain control.
(2) Decision making in analgesic prescription and administration should be investigated.
(3) The costs of poor pain relief, in terms of longer hospital stay and increased morbidity should be examined.
(4) The effects on attitudes and behaviors of education in pediatric pain should be researched.

4.3. Basic research

(1) The role of learning in the development of pain responses should be elucidated in greater detail.

(2) Familial influences on pain deserve greater attention.
(3) Developmental changes in the biochemistry, anatomy and the physiology of pain should be mapped.

References

Aronoff, G.M. (1985) The role of the pain center in the treatment for intractable suffering and disability resulting from chronic pain. In: G.M. Aronoff (Ed.), Evaluation and Treatment of Chronic Pain (Urban and Schwarzenberg, Baltimore, MD) pp. 503–510.

Burokas, L. (1985) Factors affecting nurses' decisions to medicate pediatric patients after surgery. Heart Lung 14, 373–379.

Eland, J.M. and Anderson, J.E. (1977) The experience of pain in children. In: A. Jacox (Ed.), Pain: A Source Book for Nurses and Other Health Professionals (Little Brown, Boston, MA) pp. 453–473.

McGrath, P.J., Vair, C., McGrath, M.J., Unruh, E. and Schnurr, R. (1984) Pediatric nurses' perception of pain experienced by children and adults. Nurs. Papers 16, 34–40.

Rose, F.C. (1986) Headache clinics: Their role in health care systems and science. Headache 26, 112–116.

Sackett, D.L., Haynes, R.B. and Tugwell, P. (1985) Clinical Epidemiology: A Basic Science for Clinical Medicine (Little Brown, Boston, MA) pp. 162–163.

Schechter, N.L. and Allen, D. (1987) Physicians' attitudes toward pain in children. J. Dev. Behav. Pediatr. 7, 350–354.

Subject index